# Practical
# Radiation
# Protection and
# Applied
# Radiobiology

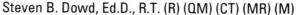

Steven B. Dowd, Ed.D., R.T. (R) (QM) (CT) (MR) (M)
Program Director
Associate Professor
Radiography Program
University of Alabama at Birmingham
Birmingham, Alabama

Elwin R. Tilson, Ed.D., R.T. (R) (QM) (M)
Professor and Clinical Coordinator
Radiologic Sciences
Armstrong Atlantic State University
Savannah, Georgia

# Practical Radiation Protection and Applied Radiobiology

## Second Edition

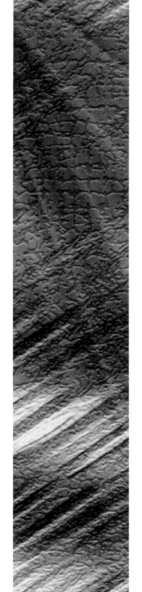

**W.B. SAUNDERS COMPANY**
*A Division of Harcourt Brace & Company*

Philadelphia   London   Toronto   Montreal   Sydney   Tokyo

**W.B. SAUNDERS COMPANY**

*A Division of Harcourt Brace & Company*

The Curtis Center
Independence Square West
Philadelphia, Pennsylvania 19106

**Library of Congress Cataloging-in-Publication Data**

Dowd, Steven B.
    Practical radiation protection and applied radiobiology / Steven
B. Dowd, Elwin R. Tilson – 2nd ed.
      p.  cm.
    Includes bibliographical references and index.
    ISBN 0-7216-7523-9
    1. Radiation—Safety measures.  2. Medical physics.
3. Radiobiology.  I. Tilson, Elwin R.  II. Title.
    [DNLM:  1. Radiation Protection—methods.  2. Radiation Effects.
3.  Radiation Injuries—prevention & control.  WN 650 D745p  1999]
RA569.D68  1999
616.9'897—dc21
DNLM/DLC                                98-43925

PRACTICAL RADIATION PROTECTION AND APPLIED RADIOBIOLOGY     ISBN 0-7216-7523-9

Printed in the United States of America.

Last digit is the print number:  9  8  7  6  5  4  3  2  1

*This book is dedicated to Lisa Dowd, my wife,
without whose support this text would not be possible.*

*This book is dedicated to
Charlene, Amber, and Autumn.
You are the reason.*

# Contributors

**Laurie Adams, Ed.D., R.T. (T)**
Department of Radiologic Sciences
Armstrong Atlantic State University
Savannah, Georgia
*Chapter 13: Applying Radiobiology and Protection to Radiation Therapy* (with Jan Carlisle)

**Jan Carlisle, M.A. Ed., R.T. (R) (T)**
School of Health Related Professions
Division of Medical Imaging and Therapy
University of Alabama at Birmingham
Birmingham, Alabama
*Chapter 13: Applying Radiobiology and Protection to Radiation Therapy* (with Laurie Adams)

**Siamak Shahabi, Ph.D**
Chief Technical Editor
Advanced Medical Publishing and Professional Radiation Resources
Madison, Wisconsin
*Chapter 9: Radiation Safety/Protection and Health Physics*

**Ann M. Steves, M.S., C.N.M.T.**
Associate Professor and Program Director
Nuclear Medicine Technology Program
University of Alabama at Birmingham
Birmingham, Alabama
*Chapter 1: The Basis for Radiation Protection* (with Steven B. Dowd)
*Chapter 12: Radiation Protection in Nuclear Medicine*

**Richard Terrass, M.Ed., R.T. (R)**
Massachusetts General Hospital
Department of Radiology
Boston, Massachusetts
*Appendix B: A Guide to Radiation Protection Resources on the Internet*

# Preface

The second edition of *Practical Radiation Protection and Applied Radiobiology* contains a number of exciting additions while retaining the clinical and pedagogical approach of the first edition. As the editor of the first edition, I (SD) made what I consider to be a very smart addition by asking Elwin Tilson to come in as my co-editor. This addition was helpful in that we share the view that we need to have textbooks that are educationally sound and foster the development of practical critical thinkers for the radiologic science profession.

A primary reason I added Elwin was his expertise as an instructional designer, which I think has led to some useful additions to the text. First, we now have three styles of text boxes that call out important information. The two additional types are designed to bring out what we consider "advanced" topics. "More Information" boxes call out short, important advanced topics in the text as they appear. "Advanced Information" boxes appear at the back of some chapters and are designed to provide advanced information that may be important, especially in undergraduate programs in the radiologic sciences.

We have always been critical of second editions that just rehash the first edition, maybe with different-colored diagrams, but provide no real new information. With that in mind, we have added something to each chapter and have added a new chapter. Ann Steves, who wrote Chapter 12 on nuclear medicine for this edition as well as for the first edition, helped in Chapter 1 to refine some of our ideas as to why radiation protection is important. Elwin used his physics and science background to refine Chapters 2, 3, and 4. We paid special attention in Chapters 5–8 on radiobiology to retain the clinical focus but also to rewrite the material in a way that would heighten the critical thinking of students by stressing research findings and the "why?" of radiobiology. Chapter 9 was revised by Siamak Shahabi, and we feel his expertise will be very helpful, especially to those technologists who have to perform RSO duties in a managed-care environment—just another form of "cross-training."

Chapters 10 and 11 also reflect more critical thinking and include explanatory material that we hope will encourage students to think about the best ways to provide effective radiation protection to their patients as well as to protect themselves. Ann again revised her chapter with the newest regulations and recommendations in nuclear medicine. Two excellent radiation therapy educators from our own institutions, Jan Carlisle and Laurie Adams, improved Chapter 13 on radiation therapy, and also provided us with input on how we could make the radiobiology chapters attractive to therapy instructors without sacrificing the main intent of the book, the effective instruction of all radiologic science students.

We are particularly proud of the new chapter, Chapter 14, although we also offer it with a bit of trepidation. We believe that radiation protection has a significant patient education role, and we express our views in that chapter. We cannot help but think that the need for effective patient education will increase in the future, and we offer this chapter with that in mind.

One completely new aspect of this text is the use of the Internet as a resource for technologists in practice. Appendix B, new to this edition, lists some of the most important (at the time of this writing) Internet sites that deal with radiation protection and radiobiology. One exciting aspect of this Internet listing is that an Internet Web page now exists that constantly updates the links to the sites listed in Appendix B plus any new sites that we find to be useful to technologists. The Web site list includes addresses for advisory bodies, comprehensive sites, dosimetry sites, general safety information sites, health effects of radiation sites, fluoroscopy safety sites (an area that has become very important recently), low-level exposure research sites, radiation history sites, human radiation experiment sites, population registries/data base sites, professional organi-

zation sites, publication sites, radiation safety training guide sites, governmental regulation sites, and e-mail discussion (listserves) sites. The address of the comprehensive Web page linking to all the sites listed in Appendix B is http://www.radscice.com/dowd.html. Another Internet-related addition to this text is "Tales from the Listserve," where actual conversations about various aspects of radiation protection have been taken from Internet listserves and reprinted here.

As always, we are looking for input on how even an excellent text can be improved. We used many of the ideas of educators in revising this edition, and look forward to more constructive criticism of this edition.

Steven B. Dowd, Ed.D., R.T. (R) (QM) (CT) (MR) (M)

Elwin R. Tilson, Ed.D., R.T. (R) (QM) (M)

# Contents

# The Basis for Radiation Protection

Steven B. Dowd • Ann M. Steves

## Chapter Objectives

At the end of this chapter, the student should be able to:

1. Define radiation protection.

2. Give basic risk–benefit comparisons.

3. List the three common goals of radiologic technologists (radiologic science professionals).

4. Describe the professional attitude toward radiation protection.

5. List some radiation protection practices to be emulated and some to be avoided.

6. Describe the role of motivation and attitude in radiation protection.

7. Define ethics as it relates to radiation protection.

8. State the legal issues related to radiation safety and protection.

| Important Terms | law |
|---|---|
| | licensure |
| ALARA | negligence |
| beneficence | plaintiff |
| benefit | positive beam limitation |
| certification | radiation protection |
| diagnostic efficacy | radiologic science professional |
| ethics | radiologic technologist |
| genetically significant dose | risk |
| health physicist | therapeutic efficacy |

## WHAT IS RADIATION PROTECTION?

Radiation protection (also called radiation safety) is applied radiation physics and radiobiology. The goal of this text is to provide the student with both the knowledge and the attitude necessary to provide radiation protection. Each year my goal as an educator teaching radiobiology and radiation protection is to ensure that students receive the knowledge they need to protect the patient, themselves, and others from the potentially harmful effects of radiation. This includes motivating them to want to provide radiation protection. That is also the goal of this book.

Radiation protection includes the private and public promotion of those practices that limit exposure to ionizing radiation to the smallest amount. When the principles of radiation physics and radiobiology are intelligently applied in the clinical setting, the dose to the patient is limited to the lowest amount possible.

ALARA is an acronym standing for *as low as reasonably achievable*. It is based on an assumption that radiation can cause harm, and any exposure to radiation should be kept as low as possible, within limits. This philosophy of keeping the potential benefit of an examination high, and the risk low, will be stressed throughout the book.

Often we practice radiation protection more based on what we do not know rather than on what we know. We can view radiation protection in the same light as the patient care principle of Universal Precautions, which views each patient as potentially infectious. Similarly, we view each radiation exposure as having some potential for harm. Thus, even though we may not know the potential effect, we act to provide radiation protection since a harmful effect *may* occur.

## BASIC CONCEPTS OF RISK VERSUS BENEFIT

Radiation protection could be practiced mechanically without an understanding of the risks and benefits of radiation. It can be practiced well only by an individual who understands the risks and benefits of radiation. This understanding encourages a professional technologist to seek creative means to limit exposure while maximizing the diagnostic and therapeutic efficacy of an examination.

Humans have been exposed to a certain amount of natural background radiation since the beginning of human existence. Since the discoveries of x-ray and radionuclides, they have also been exposed to man-made radiation. Use Figure 1–1 to determine your own yearly exposure to all types of radiation. On the average, the medical doses of ionizing radiation are not greater than natural background radiation.

Some authorities have stated that this proves that medical doses of radiation must be safe since they do not exceed normal background levels of radiation. Develop a critique of this statement while reading through the chapter. This will help you understand risk considerations in greater detail. The answer can be found at the end of the chapter.

# PERSONAL RADIATION DOSE

We live in a radioactive world—always have. Radiation is all around us as a part of our natural environment. It is measured in terms of millirems (mrems). The annual average dose per person from all sources is about 360 mrems, but it is not uncommon for any of us to receive far more than that in a given year (largely due to medical procedures we may have done). As an example, international standards allow up to 5,000 mrems a year exposure for those who work with and around radioactive material.

| | Common Sources of Radiation | Your Average Annual Dose (mrems)* |
|---|---|---|
| **Where you live** | Cosmic radiation at sea level (from outer space)........................................................ | 26 |
| | For your <u>elevation</u> (in feet) - add this number of millirems: ........................... | ............ |
| | up to 1000 ft.= 2   2-3000 ft.= 9   4-5000 ft.= 21   6-7000 ft.= 40   8-9000 ft.= 70<br>1-2000 ft.= 5   3-4000 ft.= 15   5-6000 ft.= 29   7-8000 ft.= 53 | |
| | Elevation of some U.S. cities (in feet): Atlanta 1050; Chicago 595; Dallas 435; Denver 5280; Las Vegas 2000; Minneapolis 815; Pittsburgh 1200; St. Louis 455; Salt Lake City 4400, Spokane 1890. | |
| | Terrestrial (from the <u>ground</u>):<br>  If you live in states that border the Gulf or Atlantic Coasts (from Texas east, and then north) add 23 | ............ |
| | If you live in the Colorado Plateau Area (around Denver)........................add 90............. | ............ |
| | If you live in Middle America (rest of the U.S.)...................................add 46............. | ............ |
| | House construction:<br>  If you live in a stone, brick or concrete building.....................................add 7............. | ............ |
| **What you eat and drink** | Internal radiation (in your body):<br>  From food and water - U.S. average<br>  From air (radon) - U.S. average | 40<br>200 |
| **How you live** | Weapons test fallout (less than 1)** | 1 |
| | Jet plane travel:<br>  For each 1000 miles you travel.................................................add 1 | ............ |
| | **If you have porcelain crowns or false teeth***.............................add 0.07 | |
| | If you use gas lantern mantles when camping.................................add 0.003 | |
| | **If you wear a luminous wristwatch (LCD)..................................add 0.06** | |
| | **If you use luggage inspection at airport (using typical X-ray machines)....................add 0.002** | |
| | **If you watch TV (value is less than 1)....................................add 1**** | |
| | **If you use a video display terminal (less than 0.1).......................add 1**** | |
| | **If you have a smoke detector................................................add 0.008** | |
| | **If you wear a plutonium-powered cardiac pacemaker........................add 100** | |
| | If you have had medical exposures:***<br>  **Diagnostic X-rays (e.g., upper and lower gastrointestinal, chest X-rays) - U.S. average....add 40** | ............ |
| | **If you have had nuclear medical procedures (e.g., thyroid scans) - U.S.average.............add 14** | ............ |
| | **If you live within 50 miles of a nuclear power plant (pressurized water reactor) - U.S. average add 0.009** | |
| | **If you live within 50 miles of a coal-fired electrical utility plant................................add 0.03** | |
| Copyright © 1990 by the American Nuclear Society | | **My total annual mrems dose** |

*Some of the radiation sources listed in this chart result in an exposure to only part of the body. For example, false teeth result in a radiation dose to the mouth. The annual dose numbers given here represent the "effective dose" to the whole body.

**The value is less than 1, but adding a value of 1 would be conservative.

***These are yearly <u>average</u> doses. If you have had many such procedures, your dose would be much greater.

Primary sources for this information are National Council on Radiation Protection and Measurements Reports: #92 Public Radiation Exposure from Nuclear Power Generation in the United States (1987); #93 Ionizing Radiation Exposure of the Population of the United States (1987); #94 Exposure of the Population in the United States and Canada from Natural Background Radiation (1987); #95 Radiation Exposure of the U.S. Population from Consumer Products and Miscellaneous Sources (1987); and #100 Exposure of the U.S. Population from Diagnostic Medical Radiation (1989).

**Note:** Boldface items are man-made radiation; others are naturally occurring.

**Figure 1–1** Personal radiation dose. (Courtesy of the American Nuclear Society, La Grange Park, IL; © 1990 American Nuclear Society.)

## Means of Expressing Risk

Comparing risk and benefit is based on human nature. We are willing to take on a risk so long as the potential benefit is greater. These kinds of comparisons are difficult to make, so we usually assign numbers to the risks. It would be better, of course, if we had one standard unit such as the roentgen to compare risk. This is the idea behind the BERT, described later. However, this is only weakly possible.

We can say, for example, that the risk of 1 rad of radiation is equivalent to driving 220 miles on a freeway. That means that an equal number of people are thought to die from cancer due to radiation as those driving 220 miles on a freeway. Yet there are so many confounding variables. These include the health status of the individual and the type of automobile driven. This weakens the validity of the comparison. When we compare radiation exposures, we must also be careful of confounding variables such as the type of radiation used. With no other way to quantify or assign numbers to risk, we are forced to use imperfect measures.

This chapter defines risk as any potential threat to the well-being of a human being. Benefit is defined as improvement of the quality of life of a human being. There are a variety of ways of expressing risk and benefit, and of comparing the two. These are described in the following section.

## Perceived Risk and Risk Comparisons

Two common means of expressing risk are perceived risk and risk comparisons. Perceived risk asks individuals or groups of individuals to express their perception of risk. Perceived risk is an excellent awareness tool. For example, asking the individuals to first rank a list of five items for potential risk allows them to express their opinion. The instructor or group facilitator then provides the group with information that presents the actual risk of the item. This provides a basis for group discussion, disagreement, and critical thinking about items that did not agree with expert opinion.

In these and other cases, perceived risk is often used with risk comparisons. Risk comparisons make comparisons between two or more activities. For example, getting a chest x-ray can be compared with smoking a cigarette in terms of life span shortening. Table 1–1 lists the loss of life expectancy associated with certain risks.

One authority, Dr. John Cameron, has recommended the use of an actual unit called the BERT, which stands for Background Equivalent Radiation Time. This would compare a chest x-ray, for example, with natural background radiation. A patient might be told that the x-radiation received was worth 10 days of natural background radiation. This idea is somewhat sound but falls short in that too many comparisons are made. First, as Cameron himself notes, "The values vary greatly from one medical center to another." Also, a chest x-ray uses a dif-

**Table 1–1**  Loss of Life Expectancy Associated with Risk

| Familiar Risks | Life Expectancy Lost |
| --- | --- |
| Smoking a cigarette | 10 minutes |
| Construction employment from age 20 years | 94 days |
| Home accidents | 95 days |
| Coal mining from age 20 years | 155 days |
| Overweight by 20% | 2.7 years |
| **Ionizing Radiation Risks** | |
| 1 mrad of radiation | 1.5 minutes |
| 1 rem occupational exposure | 1 day |
| Medical x-rays (U.S. average) | 6 days |
| Radiation work at 500 mrem/year from age 20 years | 7 days |
| Radiation work at 5 rem/year from age 20 years | 68 days |

rem = roentgen equivalents (equivalent of 1 rad × relative biological effectiveness); mrem = millirem (0.001 rem); mrad = millirad (0.001 rad). (Reprinted with permission from Dowd SB, Steves AS: Patient Education: Communicating Radiation Risk. Albuquerque, NM, ASRT, 1996.)

## Table 1–2  Comparisons of Radiation Levels*

| | |
|---|---|
| Natural background | 50 chest x-rays per year* |
| Nuclear imaging | 100 chest x-rays |
| Beginning of acute radiation syndromes | 30,000 chest x-rays per day |
| Lethal dose to half the population | 300,000 chest x-rays per day |

*The assumption for comparisons is that whole-body dose is being compared. These doses also vary based on a variety of factors; for example, different technical factors used for chest x-rays in different facilities.

ferent type of radiation, for the most part, than is seen in natural background radiation (see Table 1–2 for some comparisons of relative radiation levels).

A League of Women Voters group rated nuclear power as the number one risk on a list of 30 potential risks (such as smoking, surgery, mountain climbing, pesticides), with diagnostic x-radiation 23rd. College students ranked nuclear power first also, placing x-radiation 18th. Business and professional club members ranked nuclear power 9th and x-radiation 24th. For actual number of deaths, x-radiation is ranked 9th as a risk and nuclear power 20th. Each group overrated the potential danger of nuclear power and underrated the potential risk of diagnostic x-radiation (Figure 1–2).

### The Risk–Benefit Continuum

Radiation protection guidelines usually assume that there is no threshold or level below which no effects will be seen. If no threshold is assumed, any dose of radiation could have a potential effect. The lack of a threshold has led to risk versus benefit considerations for both patients and radiologic technologists. If a threshold is not assumed, every use of radiation involves a potential small risk. However, use of radiation in the healing arts results in such numerous benefits that, if well used, the benefits of radiation can greatly exceed the very small risk to the individual.

Without ionizing radiation, the health of the population would decline because we would lack

the ability to diagnose disease and to pinpoint trauma. This can be graphically represented by a bell-shaped curve (Figure 1–3) in which the health of the population is seen as compromised with nonuse of ionizing radiation. The health of the population improves when radiation is well used; it declines when radiation is overused.

A similar concept applied to the individual is the risk–benefit continuum (Figure 1–4). Obviously, there is no need for an examination if it carries only a risk, and the patient should refuse it. When the risk is small and the potential benefit great, the patient should have the examination. Most radiologic examinations carry a very small risk in relation to the potential benefit. The risk–benefit continuum is a useful tool for personal and classroom learning of risk versus benefit. For example, what personal, numeric value would the radiographer assign to a career in radiation work? Which is greater—the risk of radiation or the potential benefits?

The goal of the risk–benefit continuum is not to show, exactly, the relationship between risk and benefit. That is not possible. The relationship between risk and benefit is a value decision that is only poorly put into numbers. Thus, the numbers do not have meaning except to show how strong or weak the end value of radiation is.

For example, a patient who will die without the use of radiation can be assigned a +3 in terms of risk. That is, if the patient does not have the examination, he or she will die. Thus, any potential long-term effects such as cancer induction (5 to 20 years in the future) poses little threat to an individual who will die tomorrow if the examination is not undertaken. If the examination will, with an almost 100% degree of probability, find a curable cause of the disease, that examination is assigned a +3 in terms of benefit. That total of +6 indicates that the examination should be done. However, even if the examination has only a weak chance of finding the cause (e.g. a +0.5; total of 3.5) the benefits still outweigh the risk.

As the numbers approach 0, the question of why an examination is performed must be asked. A classic example is the 98-year-old patient referred for a barium enema. Although the problem may be diagnosed, if no intercession is possible (i.e. no surgery or other means will cure the problem), why subject the patient

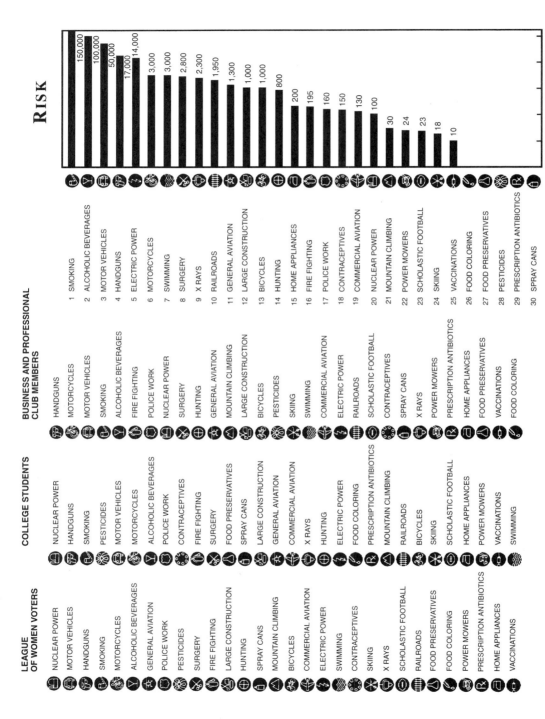

**Figure 1–2** Perception of risks. (Reprinted from Whalen JP, Balter S: Radiation Risks in Medical Imaging. Chicago, Year Book Medical Publishing, 1984, p 20–21.)

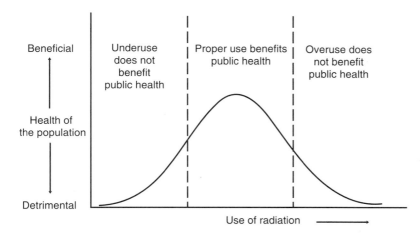

Figure 1–3 Bell-shaped curve showing relation between radiation exposure and public health. (Redrawn from Thompson MA, Hall J, Hattaway P, Dowd S: Principles of Imaging Science and Protection. Philadelphia, WB Saunders, 1994.)

to the examination? This question is not easily answerable, and certainly each physician has specific reasons for ordering a diagnostic examination that may not be known to us.

Pelvimetry (an x-ray examination of the pelvic proportions to determine whether a fetus can be delivered by the normal route) is an examination that few students encounter in their clinical experience. The risks are not great, but other examinations provide the same information without ionizing radiation. For example, let's assume that through a class discussion we had established the facts given in Examples No. 1 and No. 2:

**EXAMPLE NO. 1**

Risk of procedure      −1 (risk to both mother and fetus)

Benefit of procedure   −1

This is an overall risk–benefit ratio of −2. Ultrasound can provide the same information with little or no risk to the mother and the fetus.

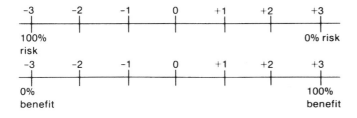

**Total**
−6   Patient should not undergo examination
−3   Patient and physician may decide that patient should not undergo examination because of high risk-benefit ratio
0   Difficult decision for patient and physician; risk and benefit equal
+3   Good risk-benefit ratio; patient probably should undergo examination
+6   Patient should undergo examination

Figure 1–4 Risk–benefit continuum. (Reprinted with permission from Dowd SB: A continuum for evaluating risks and benefits of ionizing radiation. Appl Radiol 13:81, 1984.)

**EXAMPLE NO. 2**

Most students will have heard by now or will hear about "defensive medicine"— ordering of imaging tests not because they are needed but because the physician wants to be sure that a lawsuit is out of the question. Let's assume that a physician orders an entire extremity examination (whole arm from hand to shoulder) in a case in which the patient fell and is in pain, but otherwise is asymptomatic.

What risk do you assign to the procedure?
What is the potential benefit?
What is the overall risk–benefit ratio?

## THE PROFESSIONAL ROLE OF THE RADIOLOGIC TECHNOLOGIST

Another definition to be used in this book is that of the radiologic technologist, also called the radiologic science professional. This text assumes three common goals to the three radiologic science professions that use ionizing radiation—radiographers, nuclear medicine technologists, and radiation therapists. The three common goals are:

1. To promote diagnostic/therapeutic efficacy of examinations. This means that imaging professionals (radiographers and nuclear medicine technologists) strive to perform examinations that provide the most information possible. Radiation therapists strive to use radiation in a manner that destroys malignant tissue.
2. To provide radiation protection. This is achieved in balance with goal number 1. Thus, imaging examinations are performed to provide a maximum of information at the lowest possible dose of radiation to the patient, and therapeutic examinations must strive to spare normal tissue while destroying malignant tissue.
3. To provide the highest level of patient care possible. This includes the above technical aspects of patient care as well as

providing a safe, nurturing environment to patients while they are in the professional's care.

Radiologic technologists must balance a technical knowledge of equipment and physics with empathy and concern for the well-being of others. This combination of science and art translates into effective radiation protection practices.

Radiologic technologists, along with radiologic physicists and physicians (primarily radiologists and radiation oncologists), are the individuals who are responsible for providing radiation protection to the patient and others who may be exposed to radiation. A 1980 position statement by the American College of Radiology (ACR), a group of radiologists, supports the professional role of the radiologic technologist. This document noted that "the application of proper radiologic techniques and radiation protection measures involves both initiative and independent professional judgment by the radiologic technologist." One of the underlying assumptions of this text is that radiologic technologists are in many cases the patient's front-line defense against excessive ionizing radiation exposure.

The purpose of this text is not to comment on the competence of physicians. It cannot be assumed, however, that every physician is an expert in the use of radiation. In most cases (with the exception of radiologists and radiation oncologists), the radiologic technologist receives a much greater education in the safe use of ionizing radiation than does a physician. Consider the results of a survey of fourth-year medical students by Janssen and Wellen:

- 53% thought objects in an x-ray room emitted a small amount of radiation following an x-ray examination.
- 43% thought that angiographic contrast media were radioactive.
- 49% thought that gamma rays were more hazardous than x-rays.
- 10% thought that radionuclides used in medicine were potentially explosive.
- 21% would have ordered a magnetic resonance (MR) scan on a patient with a metallic respirator.

● 45% thought that radiologists had shorter life spans than other physicians.

In addition to radiologists, radiation oncologists, and radiologic physicists, radiologic technologists must recognize that they possess the greatest knowledge on the health care team regarding the safe uses of ionizing radiation.

## Why Provide Radiation Protection?

### The Professional Attitude

One of the battles that technologists face today is a battle for professional recognition. You will have little doubt, after completing your professional studies, that technologists are professionals. However, some outside groups do not recognize technologists as professionals. There are many aspects to this fight. For the practicing technologist, image and professional knowledge are of most importance. Technologists who do not show their professionalism by limiting patient exposure are a burden on the profession.

Such technologists do not realize that they hold an important responsibility. They are the individuals *best* able to limit the dose of the public to ionizing radiation. Radiologic and health physicists calibrate equipment and design new means of protection. Without the technologist to practice these techniques or use the new equipment effectively, however, their efforts would be limited. The public's first line of defense against excess radiation is the radiologic technologist. This role should never be taken lightly.

Despite laws to protect patients, and developments such as better equipment and rare earth screens, both of which minimize patient exposure, the genetically significant dose (GSD) has been steadily rising. The GSD is a measure of the genetic exposure to the population from diagnostic and other forms of ionizing radiation. It indicates the genetic load on the population.

This measure of radiation exposure is rising, despite measures to minimize it, as ever-increasing numbers of individuals are undergoing diagnostic procedures. In addition to defensive med-

icine, there are a variety of valid reasons for the increase in diagnostic exposures. These include the aging of the population and the better diagnostic and therapeutic efficacy of examinations.

### Public and Patient Attitudes

The public remains interested in stories about the effects of x-radiation and other forms of radiation. This heightened interest is well founded. All of us want what is best for us and our relatives. The radiologic technologist must protect the public from excessive radiation exposure. Giving up that obligation limits our professional status. Some studies, for example, have focused on the best ways to educate the consumer (patient) to make the operator of diagnostic x-ray equipment provide gonadal shielding. The fact that such studies have been conducted indicates that there are technologists who shirk their responsibility.

Unfortunately, people cannot always distinguish that the medical uses of radiation are only distantly related to other uses of radiation such as nuclear power plants. Also, many media and other reports on radiation often contain more nonsense than good sense. Figure 1–5 contains a radiologic health survey. There are "correct" answers based on the opinions of a majority of health physicists. Take this quiz to see if your views match those of scientists who work with radiation. The answers can be found at the end of the chapter.

People often fear that which they do not understand. It is the obligation of the technologist to alleviate patient fears. Securing a diagnostic film is just one positive outcome of an imaging examination. Shrinking a tumor is just one part of radiation oncology. The patient rarely sees the film produced. Patients assume that technologists are competent in the administration of radiation. What the patient sees is what the technologist does. This includes, for total patient care, alleviating patient fears about radiation exposure, no matter how silly they are.

In many cases, the best information for radiographic studies that can be given patients is the entrance skin exposure (ESE) when they ask about their radiation exposure. For radiographic

Indicate on the dotted line whether you agree, are undecided about, or disagree with each of the 10 statements below.

| | Agree | Undecided | Disagree |
|---|---|---|---|
| 1. Making a full set of dental radiographs on a yearly basis is not a health risk. | _____ | _____ | _____ |
| 2. Too many chest radiographs can lead to sterility. | _____ | _____ | _____ |
| 3. Airport x-ray baggage detectors yield harmful levels of radiation. | _____ | _____ | _____ |
| 4. Microwave ovens leak harmful levels of radiation. | _____ | _____ | _____ |
| 5. Exposure to sunlamps is unsafe. | _____ | _____ | _____ |
| 6. Radar installations are sources of harmful levels of radiation. | _____ | _____ | _____ |
| 7. Color TV sets leak harmful levels of radiation. | _____ | _____ | _____ |
| 8. Amounts of radioactive fallout from nuclear weapons testing have reached safe levels. | _____ | _____ | _____ |
| 9. Nuclear power plants are unsafe. | _____ | _____ | _____ |
| 10. The level of radioactivity in a person's body varies with diet. | _____ | _____ | _____ |

**Figure 1–5** Radiation health survey. (From Weinstein RD: Radiological health attitudes of college students. Radiol Technol 30(3): 1978. Reprinted with permission of Radiologic Technology, the official journal of the American Society of Radiologic Technologists, © 1978.)

studies, the Center for Devices and Radiological Health (CDRH) of the U.S. Food and Drug Administration has developed an IBM computer program to calculate tissue doses such as bone marrow and gonadal dose from the ESE. This is provided free of charge to interested institutions, who may make copies as they see fit.

The CDRH has also gone on record as advocating the use of personal radiation record cards. It provides the physician and patient with a record of exposures. Also, repeat examinations are limited by making physicians aware of comparison films.

A technologist cannot diagnose. This is seen in principle 6 of the ASRT Code of Ethics discussed later in this chapter. However, the technologist has a professional responsibility to advocate examinations and treatments that are medically necessary. This means that the patient must be provided with sufficient information to understand and grant consent for procedures. This balance is delicate, is practiced differently in different institutions, and is best learned through experience.

## Developing a Respect for Radiation

Technologists learn about radiation in all its aspects, including the physical aspects of radiation and its potential for biologic damage. Why, then, new students often ask, are some technologists apathetic about radiation? Why would they not provide gonadal shielding to all patients, for example? The answer may lie in the old saying, "Familiarity breeds contempt." Ionizing radiation in almost all cases today does not produce immediate effects. Thus, it is easy to adopt an attitude that radiation causes no real harm. Some technologists shun lead aprons and scoff at giving a gonadal shield to an 80-year-old woman. This woman may not know much about radiation, but her fears should certainly not be taken lightly. Some use fluoroscopy to localize structures and limit their own repeat rates for films. This exposes the patient to more radiation than a normal repeat examination.

Students must be careful to respect radiation rather than fear it or scoff at its potential for harm. Radiation exposure poses a risk. It is a smaller risk than many other risks, but we must be careful not to compound it. These risks were discussed in general earlier in this chapter and are specifically handled throughout the book.

## The Role of Motivation

In 1982, in the professional journal *Radiologic Technology,* Franz indicated that there were two modes of practicing radiation protection. One was the apathetic attitude in which technologists avoided unnecessary radiation only as much as they were compelled to do so. These individuals practiced radiation protection only by mandate of law or departmental rules.

Franz's contention was that apathetic technologists hurt the profession of radiologic technology more than the patient. While the patient is guaranteed some amount of radiation protection by law, apathetic technologists

do not strive to reduce radiation exposure to the patient. They bring about a declining professional role for the technologist that can never be recovered.

If technologists provide radiation protection only because they are forced to do so, they cannot be considered professionals. This is reflected in the earlier statement by the ACR, which assumed "initiative and independent judgment" in radiation protection by the professional radiologic technologist. A variety of laws regulate the manufacture of equipment that promotes radiation safety, such as positive beam limitation (PBL; automatic collimation). A technologist whose only motivation to provide radiation safety is based on a requirement of law is practicing an occupation, not a profession.

Luckily, apathetic technologists are in the minority. Franz's other category was the actively involved technologist. This individual recognizes professional responsibility by practicing radiation protection. Radiographers and nuclear medicine technologists ensure that diagnostic images are obtained with a minimum of exposure to the patient and other individuals. Radiation therapists ensure that the radiation given to the patient is as therapeutic as possible, while sparing normal tissue.

Franz's actively involved technologist takes the professional responsibility of radiation protection very seriously. An actively involved radiographer limits the size of the beam, if possible, to an area *smaller* than is possible with PBL (automatic collimation). This individual will go out of his or her way to find a lead apron for anyone who needs one.

The actively involved technologist also is a contributing member of professional societies and engages *willingly* in continuing education. The individual who waits for a mandate to keep current in medical imaging or therapy is lacking one of the most important professional attributes—engaging in a positive activity willingly rather than being forced. Professionals know why something must be done. Nonprofessionals wait to be forced to do something.

Your instructors in radiologic technology recognize this dilemma. One of the most important (possibly *the most* important) aspects of learning is motivation. Each instructor strives to ensure that his or her students join the actively involved majority of technologists. Unfortunately, some students are swayed to be apathetic, adopting a "What's in it for me?" attitude. Ideally, an instructor hopes that each year all students decide to be active practitioners of radiation protection.

## The Radiologic Technologist as Educator

This text carries Franz's model of motivation one step further by including some of the views of motivation held by adult educators. Chapter 14 contains a full description of the role of the technologist as an educator, more specifically as related to educating patients. Radiologic technologists must realize that one of their roles is education. Radiologic technologists provide education to patients, other health care workers, the general public, and radiologic technology students. The *Essentials and Guidelines of an Accredited Program for the Radiographer,* for example, states that the radiographer is able to "provide patient/public education related to radiologic procedures and radiation protection/safety."

One of the greatest problems noted by health physics societies is the lack of education of the lay public regarding radiation. This includes risks but also the potential of radiation to provide great benefit for humankind. There are simply not enough health physicists to provide large-scale education about radiation. This may be a role radiologic technologists want to assume for their own professional standing.

Cyrile Houle, an adult educator, has developed a list of six orientations to learning. The first is the *oblivious* person. An example might be the "average" patient, who willingly undergoes radiation procedures without questioning or complaining. This person is not ready, or willing, to learn about radiation. The second type is the uninvolved person. This person is definitely not willing to learn and does not want to be bothered with the information.

These two orientations might be acceptable for patients. However, the technologist will encounter situations in which patients do not want to undergo certain examinations, which, assuming they are adults of sound mind, is always their right. However, the technologist must try, *gently,* to persuade patients of the low risk and high benefit associated with diagnostic and therapeutic uses of radiation. This requires a sound knowledge of radiation and considerable professional tact.

The oblivious and uninvolved orientations are definitely not acceptable for technologists. A technologist who is oblivious or unwilling to learn must be persuaded that radiation protection is the one of the three basic obligations of the radiologic technologist. These are, again, to promote diagnostic and therapeutic efficacy of examinations, to provide radiation protection, and to provide the highest level of patient care possible.

Houle gives specific reasons why individuals fall into his third category of the *resistant* person. This category, along with the first two, is similar to Franz's apathetic technologist. However, this individual is almost "anti–radiation protection."

One reason for being resistant is that these individuals believe that factors in life are beyond their control. A technologist might lament, "Well, *everything* causes cancer," and thus feel that radiation protection is hardly worthwhile. Another is the person who always says, "Someday." This person plans to be more effective in radiation protection at some future date. This date rarely comes.

Another reason may be bad previous experiences. Perhaps this individual has been chastised for an excessive repeat rate for films. Rather than learn the right way to do things, this person has learned how to cheat. This may involve using fluoroscopy as a localizer or hiding repeat films. A similar, final reason is fear of the process. Some people see learning as painful and find it easier to resist learning than to fulfill professional duty.

The category of the *focused* person is similar to Franz's actively involved technologist. This person is interested in radiation protection because he or she knows that this learning enhances his or her effectiveness as a professional. Some people also enjoy the process of learning as its own reward.

Others have specific goals. A technologist may want to be promoted and recognizes that administration sees the technologist who learns about, promotes, and practices radiation protection as one who is deserving of pro-

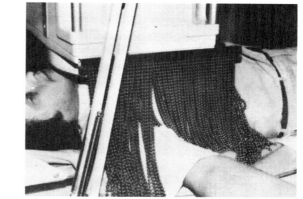

**Figure 1–6** Winkler protective curtain. (Courtesy of AliMed Inc., Dedham, MA.)

motion. Many aspects of quality assurance, for example, relate to radiation protection. It is doubtful that administration would promote a technologist in the radiology department to quality assurance technologist if that individual was sloppy in radiation protection. On the contrary, the combination of providing protection, taking advantage of local seminars related to the profession, and being a member of societies that promote professional practice shows professionalism.

The final category is the *comprehensive* person. This can be seen as an extension of Franz's actively involved technologist, perhaps a "super-actively involved" technologist. This person wants to know everything possible about radiation protection. This individual wants to know about radiation protection for personal benefit, for the benefit of the patient and others who may be exposed, and simply out of curiosity.

### The Radiologic Technologist as Leader

Radiologic technologists must also realize that they can and should serve as leaders within their profession. This includes developing new means of radiation protection as well as practicing radiation protection and educating others about radiation.

One example of a radiologic technologist's serving as a leader is the development of the Winkler protective curtain (Figure 1–6) by Norlin Winkler, RT(R), a Fellow of the American Society of Radiologic Technologists (FASRT).

This means of radiation protection was developed based on Winkler's education, knowledge, and clinical experience, combined with his desire to come to a solution for more effective protection of the operator of a fluoroscope. This is the mark of a professional leader. Winkler also wrote what is still one of the best presentations of the radiographer's role in promoting radiation protection in volume 41 (1969) of *Radiologic Technology*, the professional journal for radiologic technologists.

### Ethical Issues and Radiation Protection

An important distinction must be made between law and ethics. Laws are rules of behavior that must be followed. Law may be based on ethics, particularly the ethics of society. However, ethics and law cannot be seen as the same thing. When the courts have reviewed ethical issues, guidelines may exist. However, professionals must follow ethical standards that call for a higher level of care than the law requires.

### What Is Ethics?

Ethics are *not* rules of behavior. They involve general guidelines that translate into practice. Ethics are not simple will or will not scenarios such as "Never call a patient by his or her first name." They are *not* good manners, nor are they legal mandates. In situations in which one individual has power over another, ethics are of importance. One issue in ethics is how that power is used. The technologist has power over the patient and can choose, within limits, to provide or not to provide radiation protection.

There are personal and professional codes of ethics. For example, the ethical principle called beneficence is usually viewed in terms of a "good" patient outcome. The term means doing good. To the physician, a diagnostic film might be the "good" outcome. Thus, a physician might want to continue an examination regardless of patient refusal. Legally, the technologist might escape conviction because the physician might be seen as ultimately responsible. However, that would not be an ethical consideration but a legal one.

A technologist has an ethical obligation to act in the best interest of the patient. The questions from the ethical standpoint are, "What is the best interest of the patient? When does the need for a film outweigh the patient's right to choose? Does it ever?"

Another example of beneficence is the use of fluoroscopy as a localizer, as previously mentioned. It is possible to use the fluoroscope to localize an organ. This reduces the chances of needing a repeat film to almost zero. The technologist uses the fluoroscope, makes a mental note of the position of the organ, and then takes the regular films required. There is a definite "good" outcome in that the films generated are of good quality and no repeats were required. Yet, the dose from fluoroscopy—often as high as 5 rad/min—is much greater than what a set of repeat films would have required. Thus, this technologist is not thinking about the negative aspects of excess exposure, seeing only the final film as the good outcome.

Ethics involves some issues that are very clear and others that are not so clear. As well as "book learning," it takes experience in the clinical setting for the student to understand ethics.

## Codes of Ethics

The technologist professional societies concerned with promoting the best use of ionizing radiation possible to increase the diagnostic and therapeutic efficacy of examinations and radiation protection are the American Society of Radiologic Technologists (ASRT) and the Technologist Section/Society of Nuclear Medicine (TS/SNM). These organizations have each developed a Code of Ethics to guide professional practice (Figures 1–7, 1–8). Technologists registered by the American Registry of Radiologic Technologists (ARRT) agree to conduct themselves in a manner consistent with the ASRT Code of Ethics.

A code of ethics is a *guideline* for practice; it does not set specific behaviors for practice. The underlying expectation is that a professional is able to take general guidelines and translate them into personal behavior. A more specific code would not be valuable; professionals encounter few situations on a daily basis that lend themselves to a specific code.

Principle 7 of the ASRT Code of Ethics specifically addresses the obligation of the technologist to protect the patient, self, and others from unnecessary or excessive radiation exposure. All of the other principles address radiation protection indirectly except for principles 3 and 8. This befits the status of radiation protection as one of the main roles of a radiologic technologist.

The TS/SNM Code of Ethics deals with radiation protection indirectly. Principles 3 and 4, complying with laws and regulations and performing clinical duties competently, certainly include the use of radiation protection practices.

## Legal Issues and Radiation Protection

In addition to more general aspects of health care law that students learn in courses or sections of courses, they must learn laws related to radiation protection. Some of these topics, such as pregnancy, the law, and radiation exposure, are discussed in greater detail in later chapters. Equipment laws in terms of state and federal regulations for equipment are also discussed in greater detail in subsequent chapters.

With an increased recognition of radiographers as health care professionals goes an increased responsibility. Today's patients are customers, and they expect high levels of service.

## Equipment Laws

In addition to laws mandating the provision of certain radiation protection equipment, laws

# ASRT code of ethics

1. The Radiologic Technologist conducts himself/ herself in a professional manner, responds to patient needs and supports colleagues and associates in providing quality patient care.

2. The Radiologic Technologist acts to advance the principal objective of the profession to provide services to humanity with full respect for the dignity of mankind.

3. The Radiologic Technologist delivers patient care and service unrestricted by concerns of personal attributes or the nature of the disease or illness, and without discrimination, regardless of sex, race, creed, religion or socioeconomic status.

4. The Radiologic Technologist practices technology founded upon theorectical knowledge and concepts, utilizes equipment and accessories consistent with the purpose for which they have been designed, and employs procedures and techniques appropriately.

5. The Radiologic Technologist assesses situations, exercises care, discretion and judgement, assumes responsibility for professional decisions, and acts in the best interest of the patient.

6. The Radiologic Technologist acts as an agent through observation and communication to obtain pertinent information for the physician to aid in the diagnosis and treatment management of the patient, and recognizes that interpretation and diagnosis are outside the scope of practice for the profession.

7. The Radiologic Technologist utilizes equipment and accessories, employs techniques and procedures, performs services in accordance with an accepted standard of practice, and demonstrates expertise in limiting the radiation exposure to the patient, self and other members of the health care team.

8. The Radiologic Technologist practices ethical conduct appropriate to the profession, and protects the patient's rights to quality radiologic technology care.

9. The Radiologic Technologist respects confidences entrusted in the course of professional practice, protects the patient's right to privacy, and reveals confidential information only as required by law or to protect the welfare of the individual or the community.

10. The Radiologic Technologist continually strives to improve knowledge and skills by participating in educational and professional activities, sharing knowledge with colleagues and investigating new and innovative aspects of professional practice. One means available to improve knowledge and skills is through professional continuing education.

*Adopted by: The American Society of Radiologic Technologists, The American Registry of Radiologic Technologists*

**Figure 1–7** ASRT Code of Ethics. (Courtesy of the American Society of Radiologic Technologists, Albuquerque, NM; © 1989.)

---

**TS/SNM Code of Ethics**

Nuclear medicine technologists, as members of the health care profession, must strive as individuals and as a group to maintain the highest ethical standards.

The principles listed below were adopted by the Technologist Section and Society of Nuclear Medicine at the 1985 Winter Meeting. They are not laws, but standards of conduct to be used as a quick guide by nuclear medicine technologists.

**Principle 1–** The nuclear medicine technologist should provide service with compassion and respect the rights of patients.

**Principle 2–** The nuclear medicine technologist should hold in strict confidence all privileged information concerning the patient.

**Principle 3–** The nuclear medicine technologist should comply with the laws and regulations governing the practice of nuclear medicine.

**Principle 4–** The nuclear medicine technologist should be responsible for competent performance of assigned duties.

**Principle 5–** The nuclear medicine technologist should strive continuously to improve knowledge and skills.

**Principle 6–** The nuclear medicine technologist should not engage in fraud or deception.

**Principle 7–** The nuclear medicine technologist should be willing to assume responsibility to participate in activities that promote community and national response to health needs.

---

**Figure 1–8** TS/SNM Code of Ethics. (Reprinted by permission of the Society of Nuclear Medicine from Society of Nuclear Medicine-Technologist Section. Code of ethics. Journal of Nuclear Medicine Technology, 1985; 13:60.)

exist at the federal level in which technologists are required to report problems with medical devices. This obligation is usually fulfilled by reporting the problem to the employer. In 1991, the Safe Medical Devices Act went into effect, which authorized civil penalties to technologists and other health care workers who do not report defects and failures in medical devices. A technologist should recognize an obligation to report defects from a safety and radiation protection standpoint.

## Certification and Licensure Laws

Licensure is the process by which some competent authority grants permission to a qualified individual or entity to perform certain specified activities. In the state of Illinois, the Illinois Department of Nuclear Safety grants qualified individuals the right to apply ionizing radiation to human beings in the areas of radiography, nuclear medicine, radiation therapy, and chiropractic radiography. The goal of such licensure is to *protect the public* from excessive ionizing radiation, not to raise professional standing of practitioners. Licensure carries more obligations than it does privileges; this is in accordance with protecting the patient from harm.

Most state licensure laws are an outgrowth of the Consumer–Patient Radiation Health and Safety Act of 1981 (Title IX of Public Law 97-35), which was signed into law in August 1981 by President Ronald Reagan. This law provides standards for accreditation of programs for educating individuals responsible for administering radiation to patients and licensing standards for radiologic technologists. Recently the ASRT has began an initiative to secure national licensure, that is, licensure in all 50 states.

Students may be asked to support or lobby for licensure or the maintenance of licensure standards in their state. In late 1997, 13 states still did not have licensure of radiologic technologists. This is an improvement of 8 states over the last edition of this book. Remember that the goal of licensure is patient protection, and all individuals involved in licensure legislation should bear this in mind. Once you become involved in licensure fights for any reason other than to improve patient care, you will rapidly become burnt-out. You will not see a financial gain. Most likely you will end up paying an extra fee for licensure. The reason to lobby for licensure is to ensure that operators without training become trained and meet the same standards that you do. This is another aspect of being a leader in the field.

## Lawsuits and Other Legal Actions

In the early days of radiology, before radiation protection standards were developed and the effects of radiation exposure known, lawsuits were filed against the users of diagnostic and therapeutic equipment. This 19th-century lawsuit brought by a 37-year-old man that received x-rays of the ankle serves as an example:

> On September 19, 1896, x-ray photographs were made, each sitting occupying from 35 to 40 minutes, the tube being placed 5 or 6 inches from the ankle. While under the exposure, the patient complained of sharp, tingling pains, . . . . An intensely painful ulcer formed, for which condition amputation of the foot was performed.

This man won $10,000, not a small sum in 19th-century America.

The most likely charge that could be brought for "radiation injury" from low levels of radiation today would be cancer induction, or in the case of a pregnant patient, a defect to the fetus. Negligence law would most probably form the basis for the suit. To prove negligence, four items must be satisfied:

1. It must be shown that a *duty* on the part of the professional exists.
2. If a duty is shown, a *breach* of duty must be shown.
3. The *cause* must be due to an action on the part of the professional.
4. If cause is proven, an *injury* must be proven.

The plaintiff (the person bringing the suit) faces an uphill battle in proving cause. To show direct causation, the plaintiff must isolate the harm-causing agent, trace the pathway from the agent to the victim, and prove medically that the agent caused the disease. As we will see later, radiation causes no unique (radiounique) effects that are not seen in nature. A variety of other agents can cause the same effects as radiation.

In the case of a fetal defect, there is a certain normal incidence of fetal defects. Thus, proof must exist that shows that radiation caused the defect. This is almost impossible.

Another problem is that the effects of low doses of radiation take many years to show themselves. In the case of cancer induction, there is a latent period of many years. The statute of limitations limits the period in which a suit can be brought. Thus, a patient with a radiation injury that lies dormant for 30 years may not be able to bring a lawsuit.

The fact that a lawsuit against a technologist is close to impossible may limit the legal liability of the technologist in the case of radiation injury. However, it *increases* this individual's *moral* liability. Because the public has little recourse in cases of poor radiation protection practices, they must put an added trust in the radiologic technologist. This is one of the hallmarks of professionalism.

## The Student's Role in Radiation Protection

Schools and programs are accredited so that students may take the national certification examinations. The *Essentials and Guidelines* developed for these programs speaks both to developing student competence and radiation protection of the patient throughout. However, mandates for radiation protection are seen most strongly in the clinical education section.

For example, in radiography and nuclear medicine technology programs, documentation must exist that the student has received basic instruction in radiation protection and the sponsor must support the ALARA concept.

All radiologic technology programs must be competency based, which ensures that students do not attempt procedures until they are competent to do so. This limits patient doses and increases the diagnostic efficacy of examinations.

Students must also realize that they have obligations in such a system. They must not attempt examinations until they are ready to do so. Sometimes technologists are eager to let students try new procedures to help them learn. These individuals are not always familiar with the policies of the program or the student's competency level. Students need to *do* procedures to learn *how to do* procedures. However, they must document ability before they attempt a procedure. This is often achieved through laboratory practice or simulation.

## SUMMARY

Radiation protection includes the private and public promotion of those practices that limit exposure to ionizing radiation to the smallest amount. When the principles of radiation physics and radiobiology are intelligently applied in the clinical setting, the dose to the patient is limited to the lowest amount possible.

The goal of radiation protection is to maximize the benefit of an examination or procedure while limiting the risk to as low as reasonably achievable. This concept is often referred to as ALARA. There are a variety of means of expressing risk, including perceived risk, risk comparisons, and the risk–benefit continuum.

The radiologic technologist is the professional—in conjunction with other professionals on the health care team such as radiologists and radiologic physicists—who is responsible for radiation protection of patients, self, and others. The practice of radiation protection requires, along with knowledge, a professional attitude that includes motivation, a willingness to educate others, and leadership.

One of the ethical duties of the radiologic technologist is to practice sound principles of radiation protection. The ASRT Code of Ethics includes both specific and general guidelines for the practice of radiation protection. The TS/SNM Code of Ethics contains more general guidelines that allude to radiation protection.

Laws related to radiation protection include equipment laws, licensure law, and potential lawsuits based on malpractice law. Laws are designed to protect the public, but the radiologic technologist should recognize a higher professional obligation based on professional ethics and professional trust by patients.

Students must also realize that, as beginning professionals, they too are obligated to practice radiation protection. This means participating in the competency-based educational system offered by their program and not engaging in examinations until they are ready to do so.

*Answer to Question:* This statement does not recognize the possible compounding of risk. You cannot state with certainty that driving 220 miles twice, for example, is the same or different than driving 440 miles once. The most logical assumption would be, however, that as driving distance increases, the risk increases by some amount. Similarly, it might be assumed that, even though one dose of 50 mrad is safe, two doses of 50 mrad would increase the risk by some amount. Also, if there is no threshold, every dose of radiation involves some risk, even if the risk is very small.

## Answers to Radiation Health Survey (Fig. 1–5)

| | *Expert Opinion* |
|---|---|
| 1. Making a full set of dental radiographs on a yearly basis is not a health risk. | Disagree |
| 2. Too many chest radiographs can lead to sterility. | Disagree |
| 3. Airport x-ray baggage detectors yield harmful levels of radiation. | Disagree |
| 4. Microwave ovens leak harmful levels of radiation. | Disagree |
| 5. Exposure to sunlamps is unsafe. | Disagree |
| 6. Radar installations are sources of harmful levels of radiation. | Agree |

7. Color TV sets leak harmful levels of radiation.  Disagree

8. Amounts of radioactive fallout from nuclear weapons testing have reached safe levels.  Agree

9. Nuclear power plants are unsafe.  Disagree

10. The level of radioactivity in a person's body varies with diet.  Agree

## Questions

1. The genetically significant dose is increasing as a result of:

    I. laws designed to limit patient exposure.
    II. defensive medicine.
    III. increased diagnostic efficacy.

    a. I and II only
    b. I and III only
    c. II and III only
    d. I, II, and III

2. Which of the following are the technologist organizations responsible for promoting professionalism among technologists?

    I. ARRT
    II. ASRT
    III. TS/SNM

    a. I and II only
    b. I and III only
    c. II and III only
    d. I, II, and III

3. If it is assumed that there is no threshold dose of radiation, this means that:

    a. there is no risk from radiation below a certain amount.
    b. the risk associated with radiation outweighs its benefit.
    c. even small amounts of radiation are potentially harmful.
    d. the ALARA concept is not applicable to clinical practice.

4. Which of the following is a visible outcome, to the patient, of a diagnostic procedure?

    a. radiographic image
    b. technologist's actions
    c. hospital facilities
    d. department facilities

5. Which individual or group of individuals does the apathetic technologist hurt the most?

    a. hospital administration
    b. patients
    c. general public
    d. other technologists

6. Which of the following describes the relationship between law and ethics?

    a. Ethics is based on law.
    b. Law is based on ethics.
    c. Ethics and law are the same thing.
    d. Ethics is not related to law.

7. What is the primary purpose of licensure?

    a. to increase technologists' salaries
    b. to improve professional status of technologists
    c. to improve patient care
    d. to meet hospital accreditation standards

## Exercises

1. What is radiation protection?

2. What groups do radiologic technologists educate?

3. What are the three common goals of all radiologic technologists?

4. What is involved in the professional attitude toward radiation protection?

5. Why might a technologist or student become apathetic about radiation protection?

6. Why do patients fear radiation?

7. What type of technologist has the best chance of promotion?

8. What factor reduces the chances of lawsuits from radiation damage?

9. How is risk minimized and benefit maximized?

10. How do ethics translate into practice?

## Answers

Questions

| | |
|---|---|
| 1. c | 5. d |
| 2. c | 6. b |
| 3. c | 7. c |
| 4. b | |

Exercises

1. Radiation protection includes the private and public promotion of those practices that limit exposure to ionizing radiation to the smallest amount. The intelligent application of the principles of radiation physics and radiobiology in the clinical setting limits the dose to the patient to the lowest amount possible.

2. Technologists provide education to patients, other health care workers, the general public, and radiologic technology students. This teaching role includes radiation protection and the benefits of intelligent uses of radiation.

3. The three common goals of all radiologic technologists, to be sought in unison, are:
   a. to promote diagnostic and therapeutic efficacy of examinations.
   b. to provide radiation protection.
   c. to provide the highest level of patient care possible.

4. Technologists hold an important responsibility—they are the individuals *best* able to limit the dose of ionizing radiation to the public. Technologists who do not show their professionalism by limiting patient exposure are a burden on the profession.

5. One possibility among many is the fact that once individuals do not see an immediate effect from radiation exposure, they may scoff at the potential of radiation to do harm. Although radiation should not be feared, it should always be respected.

6. Patients may fear radiation because they do not understand it. It is difficult for some patients to separate the nonsense from the sense in media reports of radiation.

7. A technologist who is goal oriented recognizes that practicing radiation protection will be noticed by administration. Showing positive motivation is an important aspect of gaining promotions in health care.

8. The fact that there are no radiounique effects limits the number of successful lawsuits, as well as the fact that a good deal of assurance (proof) must exist that radiation caused the effect.

9. Risk is best minimized and benefit is best maximized by realizing that any dose of radiation might have an effect, but that with the proper uses of radiation, benefit will outweigh the risks.

10. Ethics are guidelines for practice. Professionals use these guidelines to direct their clinical practice. Ethics that consist of very specific mandates would not be useful to the professional, who encounters a variety of situations each workday.

## Further Discussion Questions

1. Make up a list of ten items that carry a risk on a piece of paper, and rank these risks from greatest to least risk. Ask two people to do the same. Do your rankings agree?

2. Develop a set of risks and benefits for one of the items on the list in question #1. Analyze these using the risk–benefit continuum.

3. Discuss how other ethical principles (except for ASRT principle 7) of the ASRT and TS/SNM Code of Ethics address radiation protection. Under which principle would the fluoroscopy example mentioned in this chapter fall?

4. How can students serve as leaders in radiation protection?

5. What is your personal orientation to radiation protection? What are your radiation protection learning goals?

6. How can you determine other's people attitude toward radiation protection.

7. In what ways can radiologic technologists show the public their role as one of the main professionals responsible for radiation protection to the public.

8. Use the radiologic health survey with a group of your friends, relatives, or technologists. How well did their answers match expert opinion?

9. On example 2 for the risk–benefit continuum, is it appropriate for the technologist to tell the physician that the examination does not seem necessary? What should the technologist say to the patient, if anything?

## CHAPTER 2

# The Production of X-Radiation

## Steven B. Dowd • Elwin R. Tilson

## Chapter Outline

## Chapter Objectives

At the end of this chapter, the student should be able to:

1. Define x-ray.

2. List the physical properties of x-rays.

3. Describe medical and nonmedical uses of x-rays.

4. List the components of an x-ray tube.

5. Describe the process of x-ray production.

6. Relate x-ray tube design to patient dose.

7. Discuss the use of fluoroscopic equipment.

8. Relate fluoroscopic design to patient dose.

## Important Terms

anode
alternating current
bremsstrahlung
C-arm
cathode
computed tomography
characteristic radiation
differential absorption
digital radiography
diode
direct current
electromagnetic
energy
falling load
filtration
fluoroscopy
half-value layer (HVL)

| | |
|---|---|
| heterogeneous | remnant radiation |
| image intensifier | root mean square value |
| input phosphor (screen) | rotor |
| isotropic | scattered radiation |
| kilovoltage peak (kVp) | secondary radiation |
| leakage radiation | single phase |
| mammography | thermionic emission |
| milliampere-seconds (mAs) | three phase |
| output screen | tomography |
| plain-film radiography | tungsten |
| polyenergetic | useful beam |
| potential difference | waveform |
| radiography | x-ray |
| rectification | |

## INTRODUCTION

The purpose of Chapters 2, 3, and 4 is to give the student an overview of radiation production and equipment, ionizing radiation, and radiation interactions. These chapters are *not* designed to replace information found in physics texts and courses, but rather to serve as a review for the student who has had physics or as a brief introduction for the student who will be taking a later course in physics.

In this chapter, basic radiation production, x-ray tubes and generators used in diagnostic radiology, and image intensification units are discussed. In the informational text boxes of the chapter, a number of additional areas such as the effect of generation types on patient dose, mammography units, filtration, and linear accelerators are covered for the advanced student and the specialists. The equipment and production overview will also be helpful to students later studying for certification examinations who need an overview of the topic before studying the material in depth.

## THE PRODUCTION OF X-RAYS

This chapter will define x-rays, give the physical properties of x-rays, and describe how x-rays are used in medical imaging and other settings. Some of this material will be discussed again in Chapter 3, when x-radiation and gamma radiation are presented together.

### Definition

X-rays are a form of *electromagnetic radiation*. They are similar to visible light but are of shorter wavelength. X-rays have no mass or charge but behave as both waves and particles depending on how they are viewed. When we talk about x-rays, we either talk about the wavelength and energy, which are aspects of waves, or we talk about photons, which are particle-like packets of energy.

### Physical Properties

The following are the physical properties of x-rays:

- They are the most penetrating *electromagnetic* waves. This is one of the aspects of x-ray first noted by Roentgen, its ability to pass through matter. This is the reason x-rays are useful for seeing "inside" the body.
- They are *heterogeneous* (many different wavelengths) and *polyenergetic* (many different energies). Along with varying thicknesses of parts and atomic number of tissue, this is the basis for differential absorption of

x-rays, as some x-rays will be absorbed and others will not.

- Any given x-ray photon travels in a straight line at the speed of light. X-rays diverge from the source and are emitted *isotropically* (in all directions) in the same way light usually travels in a straight line and diverges in all directions from the bulb. The fact that x-rays are emitted in all directions necessitates lead shielding around the tube except for the window. Early operators of x-ray equipment did not shield their tubes, which exposed them to large amounts of leakage radiation and caused radiation injuries.

- Although x-rays are in many ways similar to visible light, they cannot be focused by a lens nor do they reflect off surfaces. This characteristic necessitates the use of various other means to control the x-ray beam, including collimation and filtration.

- They are electrically neutral. X-rays differ from some other forms of ionizing radiation, such as alpha and beta radiation, in two important ways. First, an x-ray is electromagnetic in nature, which means that it is pure energy and therefore does not have any mass or particle associated with it. Second, because it is not made up of particles, an x-ray also has no electrical charge.

- They produce secondary and scattered radiation when interacting with matter. Secondary radiation is radiation produced inside an object by an interaction between an x-ray which is completely absorbed and the atoms inside the object. Scattered radiation is produced when x-rays interact with matter and have their direction and/or energy level changed. Scattered radiation and especially secondary radiation are the sources of most of the exposure to operators of diagnostic x-ray equipment.

- They cause certain crystals to fluoresce or give off light (also called luminescence). This is the basis of operation for intensifying and fluoroscopic screens.

- They affect photographic film. This is the basis of medical imaging and the basis of operation for film badges.

- They ionize (knock off electrons) all matter including gases. This is the basis of opera-

tion of ionization chambers used to detect radiation. Some automatic exposure controls (phototimers) also use this principle.

- They cause biologic changes. These potential changes must be understood by the radiologic technologist to effectively practice radiation protection both for themselves and the patient.

## Uses

The basic medical diagnostic use of x-rays is to direct them toward an object (the patient or some part of the patient). Some of the x-rays will pass through and some will be absorbed (*differential absorption*). This differential absorption will be recorded on a film (a radiograph) or some other recording medium such as a television screen in the form of an image. This simple concept has formed the basis for a variety of types of imaging, including:

*Plain-film radiography* refers to most forms of radiography. The production of a typical radiograph and the devices used to produce that radiograph are shown in Figure 2–1.

*Fluoroscopy* is dynamic radiography, or radiography of motion.

*Tomography,* also called body-section radiography, uses motion of tube and film to blur out structures above and below a structure of interest so that only the areas of interest are clearly visible on the radiograph.

*Mammography* is radiography of the breast. Typically, this is performed on the female breast, but a growing number of mammograms are being performed on males as their value is proved.

*Computed radiography* (CR) refers to all forms of radiography (but not CT) that use a computer to process the image in lieu of capturing the image on a sheet of film.

*Computed tomography* (CT or CAT) scans involve the production of a thin slice, transverse image of an area of the patient's body using sophisticated mathematical modeling and high-speed computers.

Radiography has also been used in a variety of nonmedical situations. Among other uses in industry, radiography has been used to deter-

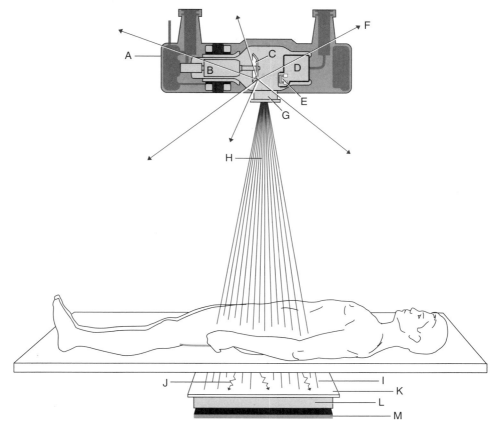

**Figure 2–1** Production of a radiograph. A, tube housing; B, anode; C, target; D, cathode; E, filaments; F, leakage radiation; G, collimator; H, primary beam; I, remnant beam; J, secondary and scatter produced with the patient; K, grid; L, ionization chamber-type automatic exposure control; M, film.

mine the integrity of pipes used in nuclear power facilities and airplane wings. X-rays of very low energy (called Grenz rays) have been used to authenticate paintings. In scientific laboratories, x-rays are used to determine the structures of crystals (x-ray crystallography).

## RADIOGRAPHIC EQUIPMENT

### X-Ray Tube

#### Components

The x-ray tube (Figure 2–2) is the device that generates x-rays. It is a specially designed vac-

uum tube with two electrodes (a *diode*). The three basic components of an x-ray tube are:

- an evacuated glass envelope to maintain a vacuum.
- a cathode, which is negatively charged.
- an anode, which is positively charged.

X-ray tubes are contained within a lead-lined protective housing to prevent leakage radiation from exposing the patient and other personnel. The housing also supports the tube and is insulated against electric hazards.

The glass envelope contains two electrodes (the cathode and anode) and is usually made of glass that is structurally strong and resistant

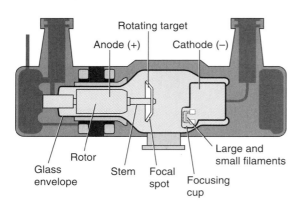

**Figure 2–2** X-ray tube.

to both heat and chemicals, such as Pyrex glass. The window is a thin area of the glass envelope designed to let x-ray photons pass through with a minimum of absorption.

The cathode is the negatively charged electrode in the tube. It is the source of electrons used to produce x-rays and consists of three main components: a large filament, a small filament (both made of tungsten wire), and a negatively charged focusing cup.

The anode is the positive electrode in the tube. Most anodes used in radiology are rotating to help dissipate heat in the tube. The three main portions of a rotating anode are the target, the stem, and the rotor. The rotor is an induction motor and rotates the target. The stem attaches the rotor to the target. The target is made of a tungsten alloy and is struck by the high-speed electrons to produce x-rays.

## Function

The basic method of operation of the x-ray tube is as follows. First, the filament of the cathode is heated by a low-voltage, high-amperage electrical current. This current heats up a filament (similar to those found in incandescent light bulbs) and "boils off" a stationary cloud of electrons. This is called *thermionic emission,* or the release of electrons by heat.

The unit of *milliampere-seconds* (mAs) is used in measuring the number of electrons moving from the cathode to the anode of the x-ray tube. Adjustments in the mAs settings actually control the heat of the filament by varying the voltage and/or the amount of current flowing through the filament (mA) and the length of

time the electrons are allowed to flow to the anode (s). The amount of filament heat controls the number of electrons produced, which in turn controls the amount of radiation produced at the target. There is a direct relationship between the mAs setting and radiation production: doubling the mAs doubles the amount of radiation produced.

Recall, electrons have a negative electrical charge and are attracted to a positive charge. To attract the electrons to the target of the anode, a high *potential difference* (voltage) is applied across the tube, significantly increasing the negativity of the cathode and making the anode highly positive. In an x-ray tube, that voltage is measured at its maximum level in units of thousands of volts, or *kilovoltage peak* (kVp). The electrons are so forcefully attracted to the anode that they are traveling at very high speed by the time they strike the target. The speed depends on the kVp applied but can be over half the speed of light. At the target, the kinetic (motion) energy of the electrons is changed, mostly to heat (99% or greater) but some to x-ray (1% or less).

The kVp determines the maximum energy of the x-rays produced and the penetrating ability of the radiation produced. The penetrating ability influences the scale of contrast on the radiograph: higher kVp radiographs show a longer scale of (less) contrast because the radiation is able to penetrate more objects and fewer areas of the image remain "white." The kVp also influences the quantity (amount) of radiation produced, as a high kVp will pull more electrons from the cathode to the anode and therefore produce more radiation. A high kVp is preferred from a radiation protection standpoint but must be balanced with the scale of contrast needed for a diagnostic radiograph.

X-rays are generated by two processes when the high-speed electrons are stopped by the target. The first involves an interaction of the electrons with the nucleus of the atoms of tungsten in which the electron slows down to change direction. This is called *bremsstrahlung,* German for "braking radiation." Bremsstrahlung radiation is emitted at all energies from just above 0 to the maximum set energy (the kVp). The second process is a collision of the high-speed (incident) electrons and an electron in one of the inner shells of the tungsten atom which knocks the electron out of the atom. This is called *characteristic radiation,* in reference to the fact that the energy produced is related to the binding energy of the atom and is always the same for (characteristic of) a specific target atom.

The radiation produced in the tube is called *primary radiation.* The radiation that passes through the window of the tube is called the *useful* or *primary beam.* X-rays exiting other than through the window are called *leakage radiation.* Portions of the primary beam that pass through the patient without interacting are called *remnant radiation.* The American Registry of Radiologic Technologists (ARRT) prefers the terms *exit radiation* or *image-forming radiation* to *remnant radiation.* Radiation that has interacted with the patient and is particularly absorbed is called *scatter radiation.* Scatter radiation usually has a different direction and always has a lower energy than the original radiation. Radiation generated in the patient's

## The Effect of Filtration and HVL on Patient Dose

Filtration and the half-value layer have a significant impact on the energy of the radiation reaching the patient and consequently also have a significant impact on the radiation dose received by the patient.

In general diagnostic radiography, filtration is used to remove the low-energy, long-wavelength x-ray photons from the beam. Because these photons are of such low keV (thousands of electron volts), they rarely have enough penetration power to pass through the body part and reach the film or detector. Thus, they only add dose to the patient and do not improve the radiographic image. Aluminum has such a low atomic number that it tends to absorb only low-energy photons, which is exactly the type of interaction that reduces patient dose.

In mammography, the filters are significantly different. They are made up of molybdenum and/or rhodium. Because these metals have a higher atomic number, they will absorb both high- and low-energy photons. The low-energy photons are absorbed due to the relationship of energy to penetration, in which low-energy photons tend to be absorbed and higher-energy photons tend to penetrate. Molybdenum/rhodium filter also absorb higher-energy (20–25 keV) photons due to photoelectric interactions. In these interactions, the energy of the photon matches the binding energy of one of the inner shell electrons and is totally absorbed by that electron and removed from the beam. These types of filters remove both low- and high-energy photons. (See the text box "Mammography Equipment" for more information about mammography equipment.)

A half-value layer (HVL) is a measure of the quality of a radiographic beam, in other words, the ratio of the percentage of low-energy photons to the percentage of high-energy photons in a beam. What an HVL actually measures is the amount of (usually) aluminum necessary to remove half of the photons from the beam. When a beam has a large percentage of high-energy photons (compared to low-energy photons), it requires more aluminum to remove half of them. With any HVL measurement, the higher the amount of aluminum, the "harder" the beam and the lower the patient dose. See the text box "Mammographic Units, Tubes, and Filtration" for related information.

body is called *secondary radiation* and, like radiation inside the tube, moves in all directions.

## Generators

An electrical current is used in the production of x-ray radiation in an x-ray tube. The nature or *waveform* of the electrical current has a major impact on the type and amount of radiation produced inside the tube and ultimately on the amount of radiation absorbed by the patient. In normal commercial or household current, the electrons in a current move in one direction and then reverse their direction over and over again. The waveform of the electricity moves from a positive polarity (if one were only looking at a single wire in the pair) to neutral to a the negative polarity and back again to neutral (see Figure 2–3A). This type of electrical current is referred to as *alternating current* (AC) because the electrons alternate directions. Unfortunately, if this type of electrical current were used in an x-ray tube, it would damage the tube itself. In order to prevent this damage, the current is modified through a process called *rectification.*

Rectification is the process of converting the negative electrical pulses into positive pulses, which changes the alternating current into pulsating *direct current* (DC). With this type of current, the electrons only move in a single direction. The waveform of this DC current may be changed in a number of ways depending on the type of rectification. Three common types of rectification are single-phase rectification, three-phase rectification, and high-frequency rectification.

### Single Phase

In single-phase rectification (Figure 2–3B), the negative pulses are inverted into positive pulses. In the United States, electrical power has 60 cycles per second. So, instead of sixty negative and sixty positive pulses per second (one each per cycle), the waveform ends up with 120 positive pulses per second (two positive pulses per cycle). This prevents damage to the tube but is a very inefficient way to produce x-rays. The problem with single-phase rectification is that voltage or potential difference across the tube (which is measured in keV) is not constant at all. The voltage varies

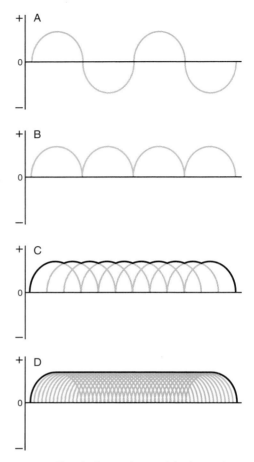

**Figure 2–3** Electrical Waveforms. (*A*) Alternating Current: In alternating current, the electrical current (such as the electrical current used in hospitals) pulses go from no voltage (zero) to a maximum positive voltage to no voltage to maximum negative voltage and back to zero. (*B*) Single-Phase Rectified Current: In an x-ray machine the current is rectified so that the negative electrical pulses are transformed to positive pulses, which go from no voltage (zero) to maximum positive to no voltage then back to maximum positive voltage. (*C*) Three-Phase Rectified Current: With three-phase power, three sets of positive pulses are used at the same time. The voltage goes from zero to maximum positive, drops a little, and then moves back to maximum positive. (D) High-Frequency Current: Inside the x-ray unit itself, either single- or three-phase current is converted to a current with several hundred sets pf pulses which are superimposed. The voltage goes from zero to maximum positive and stays within a couple percentages of the maximum.

from zero to the peak kV (the kVp) and then back to zero. At times when the voltage is a zero, no x-rays are produced, and at times when the voltage is less than the peak, the quality of the radiation produced is less. The *root mean square value* (a measure of the average *energy* in the beam) being only 70.7% that of the peak voltage. Thus, an 80-kVp setting would generate root mean square (RMS) voltage of about 57 keV (.707 × 80 = 57).

## Three Phase

A three-phase generator uses the most common form of rectification. It is more efficient than a single-phase generator, combining three waveforms of current slightly out of step with each other (Figure 2–3C). There are two main advantages to this type of waveform. First, the voltage never goes all the way to zero except at the start and stop of the current flow. In this type of rectification, the electrical company supplies a power line to the facility that has three different electrical currents on it at the same time. The net effect is that the voltage goes from zero to maximum, drops a small amount until the next rising pulse moves it back up to the maximum, starts to drop again, and so on. With this waveform, the voltage stays near the maximum at all times, with the average voltage generated by a three-phase generator being as high as 97% of the peak voltage. With this type of generator, an 80-kVp setting would generate a root mean square voltage of 78 keV. Although a three-phase generator is more efficient, it is not necessarily superior from a radiation protection standpoint to a single-phase generator because of technical factor selection. See the text box "The Effect of Generation Type and Waveform on Patient Dose" later in this chapter for more information.

The second advantage of the type of generator is that the three-phase power can be used as it comes off the feed line and gives 6 pulses per cycle (three-phase, 6-pulse power) or the three-phase power can be altered to give not three waveforms but six waveforms, ending up with 12 pulses per cycle. The root mean square value for 12-pulse power is near 97% and is higher than for 6-pulse power, which can be as low as 92%.

## High Frequency

The newest type of radiation generation is high-frequency generation. In this process, power converters inside the actual x-ray unit are used to change the incoming electricity from 60 Hz (cycles per second) to as much as 6000 Hz (Figure 2–3D). In high-frequency generation, the average voltage is similar to that of three-phase generation but the maximum is achieved in far less time. High-frequency generators are becoming popular, as they are less expensive to manufacture than traditional three-phase equipment and can be used with either three-phase or single-phase waveforms. In either case, the root mean square value of the system is in the 97%–98% range.

## Falling Load

The number of electrons moving through an x-ray tube is measured in milliamperage (mA). In most x-ray units, the mA for any given exposure is fixed (e.g. 300 mA, 500 mA, etc.). In falling-load generators, the mA is not constant but is allowed to fall during the exposure. With these types of units, the mA at the beginning of the exposure is as high as possible. During the exposure, the number of electrons (mA) moving through the tube is constantly reduced. The main purpose of this type of unit is to reduce the exposure time and permit a better use of the tube limits, especially in allowing shorter times in heavy-load situations. These units are also simpler to operate. However, the radiographer can set only the mAs but not the mA or time independently. This removes control of these factors from the operator but has no impact on radiation safety, as the amount of radiation received by the patient is the same with fixed- and falling-load units. These generators are becoming common in high-end units but are not widely used at this time in low-end units.

## Other Types

Other types of generators include capacitor-discharged generators and battery-powered generators, both of which are used for mobile equipment. The major advantage of the capacitor-discharged generator is its size. Unfortunately, it is very hard or impossible to maintain the set mA or kVp with such units. A battery-powered unit is superior for providing consistent mA and kVp and does not have to be charged immediately before each use. Consistent mA and kVp are important for radiation protection as well as image quality, especially on larger patients and parts such as abdomens. The size and weight of the units are the main disadvantages of battery-powered units.

## The Effect of Generation Type and Waveform on Patient Dose

Based only of the physics of x-ray generation, there should be an appreciable difference in the patient dose when using single-phase equipment versus three-phase or high-frequency equipment. This difference has to do with the distribution of photons in the beam. With a single-phase unit, the voltage ranges from zero to the peak (kVp) and the root mean square value of the beam is only 70.7% of the peak. With three-phase and high-frequency units, the RMS is 92% to 97% of the peak. What this means is that there are many more high-energy photons in the beam of a three-phase unit than there are in a single-phase unit at the same kVp. The impact of this higher-level distribution in three-phase and high-frequency generation is that there is less patient absorption and less contrast. A rule of thumb is that a three-phase unit produces an image with contrast similar to that of a single-phase unit with a peak 7 kV higher peak. Based solely on this, three-phase and high-frequency equipment should reduce patient dose.

Unfortunately, many technologists have been taught or ordered by radiologists to lower the kVp with three-phase units in order to keep the contrast of the image at the same level as they had with a single-phase unit. The net effect of lowering the kVp is to lower the average energy of the entire beam, which increases patient dose and increases contrast. The best approach to reducing patient dose in factor selection is the use of optimum kVp factors. The reader is referred to Chapter 11 for more information on this approach.

## FLUOROSCOPIC EQUIPMENT

### Definition

*Fluoroscopic imaging* is dynamic imaging or the imaging of motion. Fluoroscopy is used in a variety of settings to show motion, such as in upper gastrointestinal examinations, barium enemas, angiography, and cardiac catheterization, to name a few examples. The term *fluoroscopy* also implies the use of a fluorescent screen (a material that emits light when struck by x-rays). The basic fluoroscopic equipment is an x-ray tube designed to give off continuous radiation exposure, an image receptor such as an intensification screen, and a patient. On all modern fluoroscopic units, the intensification screen is part of an image intensification unit, a device which improves the brightness of the image. The image from the image intensifier is thentransmitted to a TV monitor for viewing. The x-ray tube and image receptor are mounted on a *C-arm,* which maintains the alignment of tube and film and reduces radiation exposure to the patient and others in the room (Figure 2–4).

Fluoroscopy uses lower mA settings than those found in conventional radiography—1 to 3 mA—and kVp settings of 90 to 120. However, the exposure times in fluoroscopy are measured in minutes as opposed to milliseconds. The role of a radiographer in fluoroscopy is typically to function as a physician's assistant, although in some states, it is now legal for "advanced" radiographers to perform fluoroscopy without direct physician supervision. Duties of a technologist during fluoroscopy typically include positioning

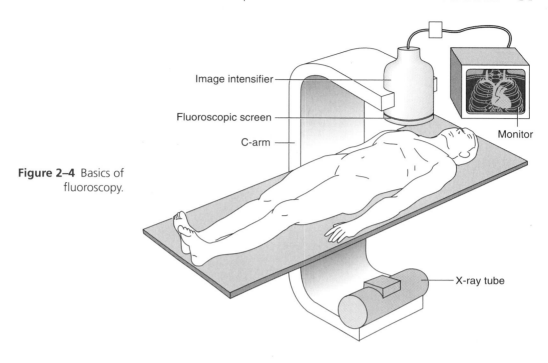

**Figure 2–4** Basics of fluoroscopy.

and communicating with the patient, along with other patient care duties such as barium administration, loading and unloading spot films, setting and resetting the 5-minute timer, monitoring and recording fluoroscopy time, and adjusting image quality on the television screen.

The weakest link in the fluoroscopic imaging process is the TV monitor used to display the images. The amount of resolution of an image is measured by determining how many objects can be seen in the space of 1 mm, which is about the thickness of a U.S. dime. Because there must be a space between each object, the objects are referred to as *line pairs.* The TV monitor displays a resolution of about 1 to 2 line pairs per millimeter (lp/mm). Radiographic film and screens can display about 5–9 lp/mm. Contrast, sharpness, and noise all impact the fluoroscopic image and are also related the radiation dose. For example, solving the problem of quantum mottle (a form of noise resulting from the use of intensifying screens) by increasing the milliampere-seconds setting increases patient dose. More information about the relationship between the use of fluoroscopy and radiation dose is given in Chapter 11.

## Image Intensifier

Modern fluoroscopic equipment uses an image intensification tube to amplify the brightness of the image. The total brightness gain is a product of the gain due to making the image smaller (the minification gain) times the flux gain (brightness increase due to speeding up the electrons inside the intensifier). The minification gain is calculated by the ratio of the area of the *input phosphor (screen)* to the *output screen* squared. Thus, with an input screen of 7 inches and an output screen of 1 inch, the minification gain would be 49. The flux gain is a constant based on the potential difference across the tube. A tube with an input screen of 7 inches, an output screen of 1 inch, and a flux gain of 100 would have a total brightness gain of 4900. The image is 4900 times brighter. The brightness gain of image intensifiers tends to range from 5000 to 20,000.

The process of image intensification is as follows (Figure 2–5):

1. The remnant beam (after the patient) passes through the glass front of the image intensifier, striking the input phosphor.

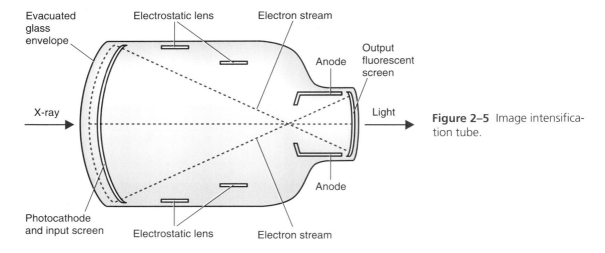

**Figure 2–5** Image intensification tube.

The crystals of cesium iodide produce light proportionally to the intensity of the beam.

2. The light photons strike the photocathode. It emits electrons proportionally to the intensity of the emitted light.
3. The electrostatic lens focuses, accelerates, and inverts the stream of electrons.
4. The anode further attracts the electrons.
5. The output screen converts the electrons into light photons.

Although the original goals of image intensification were to improve image quality and to reduce radiation dose to the patient from fluoroscopy, image intensification has served primarily to improve image quality. Since this leads to an increase in diagnostic efficacy, it is a positive outcome. Increasing the benefit of examinations while maintaining a low level of risk can be seen as practicing sound radiation protection.

## SUMMARY

*X-rays* are a form of *electromagnetic radiation* produced in the x-ray tube; they have a variety of physical properties; they are highly penetrating, heterogeneous, polyenergetic rays that travel at the speed of light and diverge isotropically from the source; they cannot be focused by a lens; they are electrically neutral; they produce secondary and scatter radiation; they cause some crystals to luminesce; they affect photographic film; they ionize gases; and they cause biologic changes.

To produce x-rays, the filament is heated with a low-voltage, high-amperage current controlled by the mA. This produces a cloud of electrons, which are available to produce radiation. A high-voltage current (kVp) is applied across the tube, increasing the negativity of the filament and making the anode (target) highly positive for a predetermined length of time. This causes the electrons to move at high speed to the target. The target stops the electrons and converts the kinetic energy of the electrons to heat (99%) and x-ray (1%).

Fluoroscopy is dynamic radiography, or radiography of motion. The basics of fluoroscopy are an x-ray tube and an image receptor mounted on a C-arm. Modern image receptors use an image intensifier to increase the brightness of the image. The total brightness gain of an image intensifier is the ratio of the input phosphor to that of the output phosphor squared times the flux gain.

## Questions

1. Which of the following would be a typical mA setting for a fluoroscopic unit?

   a. 2               b. 20
   c. 200             d. 2000

2. The positive electrode in the x-ray tube is the:

   a. cathode.        b. focusing cup.
   c. anode.          d. filament.

3. The ionization of gases is the basis of operation of:

    I. ionization chambers.
   II. automatic exposure controls.
  III. fluoroscopic screens.

    a. I and II only      b. I and III only
    c. II and III only     d. I, II, and III

4. The high-voltage current applied across a diagnostic x-ray tube is:

    a. mAs.                b. kVp.
    c. thermions.       d. flux gain.

5. A single-phase generator would generate what average energy with a setting of 90 kVp?

    a. 45 keV           b. 63 keV
    c. 87 keV           d. 90 keV

6. On which type of generator is the radiographer unable to set amperage or time?

    a. thermionic       b. single phase
    c. three phase      d. falling load

7. Which of the following are part of the anode?

    I. filament
   II. target
  III. rotor

    a. I and II only      b. I and III only
    c. II and III only     d. I, II, and III

8. The penetration of the beam in diagnostic x-ray is controlled by the:

    a. grid.                 b. filament.
    c. mAs.                d. kVp.

9. The brightness gain of image intensifiers tends to range from:

    a. 100 to 1000.      b. 1000 to 5000.
    c. 5000 to 20,000.   d. 10,000 to 100,000.

## Exercises

1. Outline the basic process of x-ray production.
2. Outline the basic process of image intensification.
3. Describe each of the types of generators.
4. Which of the properties of x-ray are especially important from a radiation protection standpoint?

## Answers

Questions

    1. a                6. d
    2. c                7. c
    3. a                8. d
    4. b                9. c
    5. b

Exercises

1. The filament is heated with a low-voltage current (mA). This produces a cloud of electrons. A high-voltage current (kVp) is applied across the tube for a set time (a), increasing the negativity of the filament and making the anode (target) more positive. This causes the electrons to move at high speed to the target. The target stops the electrons and converts the kinetic (motion) energy of the electrons to heat (99%) and x-ray (1%).

2. The remnant beam strikes the input phosphor. Light is produced proportional to the intensity of the beam. The light photons strike the photocathode, which emits electrons proportional to the intensity of the emitted light. The electrostatic lens focuses, accelerates, and inverts the stream of electrons. The anode further attracts the electrons. The output screen converts the electrons into light photons.

3. A single-phase generator allows the voltage to drop to zero and has an a root mean square value of 70.7% of the maximum (kVp). A three-phase generator uses three waveforms, each slightly out of step, and can provide root mean square values of up to 97% of maximum (kVp). A high-frequency generator has a root mean square value similar to that of three-phase generation. A falling-load generator has the potential to be the most efficient but does not allow the technologist to set mA or time, which limits its effectiveness.

4. Although all the properties of x-rays can be considered important from a radiation protection standpoint, the following two are probably of greatest importance: x-rays

## Advanced Information:
## An Overview of Linear Accelerators

Although cobalt-60 units are still used in some instances for radiation therapy, most facilities now use linear accelerators (linacs). Other devices, such as Van de Graaff generators or betatrons, have not shown the clinical utility of linear accelerators or cobalt-60. A linear accelerator is a device used to accelerate subatomic particles for radiation therapy, radionuclide production, and physics research. Linear accelerators used in radiation therapy accelerate electrons by stationary or traveling electromagnetic waves of microwave frequency.

### Components

Although linear accelerators consist of many components (Figure 2–6), four are basic to their operation: the modulator, the electron gun, the radiofrequency (RF) power source, and the accelerator guide. Understanding the function of these four components assists in understanding the operation of a linear accelerator. These four components will be described sequentially according to location.

The modulator amplifies the local power supply to 30 to 50 keV prior to rectifying the AC current to DC. The modulator is located in the gantry, in the support stand for the gantry, or in a separate cabinet.

The modulator also pulses the electron gun. The electron gun injects pulses of electrons of 15 to 40 keV into the accelerator guide. Electron guns are typically diodes (two electrodes) or triodes (three electrodes, including an electronic grid to obtain finer control of the ejected electrons).

The RF power used to generate electromagnetic waves for a linear accelerator is generated through one of two means. Magnetrons are usually used in low-energy linacs of 10 megavolts or less. They generate a high-

frequency power. Higher-energy machines use a klystron, which amplifies the high-frequency waves by using a radiofrequency driver.

The accelerator guide consists of a number of specially shaped, microwave-resonant, copper cavities brazed together to form one structure. Its function is to accelerate the electrons to the required energy. The electrons injected interact with the electromagnetic field of the microwaves and gain energy through the sinusoidal electric field in a process similar to that of a surfer riding ocean waves.

A heavy metal target of tungsten at the end stops the electrons, producing megavoltage x-rays through bremsstrahlung. The generated beam emerges in a forward-directed lobe, and the intensity distribution must be flattened through the use of a flattening filter.

### X-Ray Beams

Whereas diagnostic units provide a range of about 10 to 1200 mA, with times of 0.001 to about 10 seconds and a kVp of 20 to 150, therapeutic units operate below 20 mA, with times of 1 to 60 minutes and energies of 4 to 40 MV. According to Khan, since the x-ray beam is heterogeneous in nature, the designation MV is preferred; for the relatively monoenergetic electron beam, MeV is used.

### Electron Beams

If the target is removed and an electron-scattering foil of thin lead is used, an electron beam rather than an x-ray beam is produced (Figure 2–7). Some x-rays are still produced through bremsstrahlung; however, this is minimal. Electron beams are typically used to treat superficial tumors overlying cartilage and bone. They are particularly useful in the treatment of head and neck tumors.

## An Overview of Linear Accelerators *(Continued)*

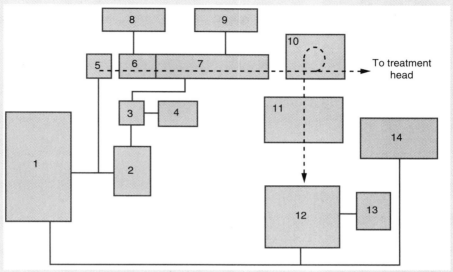

**Figure 2–6** Block diagram of linear accelerator. 1, modulator; 2, klystron or magnetron; 3, circulator; 4, water load; 5, electron gun; 6, buncher section of accelerator guide; 7, accelerator section of accelerator guide; 8, vacuum system; 9, cooling system; 10, bending magnet; 11, treatment head; 12, treatment couch; 13, pendant; 14, control console.

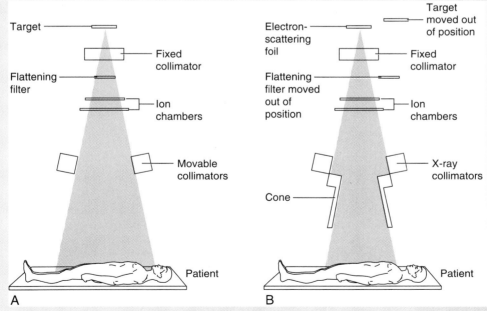

**Figure 2–7** (*A*) A basic set-up for x-ray beams. (*B*) The set-up for electron beams. The target and flattening filter are moved out of position, and a cone is added.

produce secondary and scattered radiation when interacting with matter, and they cause biologic changes. The first necessitates protection of the operators of equipment, as well as patients, and the second is important to both patients and personnel. A radiologic technologist must understand the biologic effects of radiation to be best able to practice radiation protection.

## Advanced Information:
## Mammography Units, Tubes, and Filtration

Mammography equipment differs from conventional radiographic equipment in a number of ways. Whereas conventional equipment uses a variety of types of generators, today dedicated mammographic units use single phase high-frequency generators that allow extremely precise control of factors such as mA, time, and kVp. The major differences between a conventional x-ray unit and a mammographic unit are:

| Mammographic | Conventional | Rationale |
|---|---|---|
| kVp of 25–28 | kVp of 40–150 | As breast tissue is a very low-density soft tissue, high kVps would give too little contrast for diagnosis. |
| One AEC detector | Three AEC detectors | Automatic exposure control need not average exposures to breasts. |
| Focal spot of 0.1 mm or 0.3 mm. | Focal spot of 0.6 to 1.0 mm. | Focal spot size strongly influences the resolution, and good resolution is needed as breast masses are often quite small. |
| SIDs of 60–65 cm | SID of 100 cm to 180 cm | Long SIDs are needed to offset the effects of object–film distance, which is minimal in mammography. |
| HVL of only 0.3 mm Al. | HVL of 2.8 mm Al. | The half-value layer (HVL) is a measure of the ratio of high- to low-energy photons. As mammographic images are done at low kVp, the HVL is also lower. |
| Anode made of molybdenum or rhodium. | Anode made of tungsten alloy. | The x-ray photons produced by the conventional tubes have too high an energy for mammography. |
| Molybdenum or rhodium filters. | Aluminum filter. | See below. |
| Beryllium port. | Glass or aluminum port. | Beryllium does not filter out the photons needed for mammography as does glass or aluminum. |

These differences make radiation exposure and imaging concerns a bit different from conventional radiography. Unlike the filtration in conventional radiography machines, for example, which exist to eliminate primarily low-energy photons, mammography filtration seeks to eliminate both the low-energy photons, which would be absorbed in the breast and thereby increase dose without adding to the image, and the high-energy photons of 20 to 30 keV that would degrade image contrast.

Mammographers need to be careful *not* to transfer one technique they learned in conventional radiography—increasing the density compensation circuit when the backup time is reached and a repeat radiograph is needed. In mammography, a higher kVp

## Mammography Units, Tubes, and Filtration *(Continued)*

is needed, as the problem is with the inability of the photons to penetrate the breast; thus, increasing mAs through the density setting will have no effect. Increasing the density compensation circuit will only cause the back-up time to be reached again.

The largest concern for radiation exposure to the patient is during magnification views taken to enhance microcalcifications or to show very small structures. Radiation exposure can be two to three times that of normal views. Long exposure times are used due to a reduction in mA, which can increase the possibility of patient motion, and thus repeats.

## CHAPTER 3

# Ionizing Radiation

### Steven B. Dowd • Elwin R. Tilson

## Chapter Outline

Introduction

## Chapter Objectives

At the end of this chapter, the student should be able to:

1. Define radiation and ionizing radiation.

2. Differentiate between types of ionizing radiation.

3. Define particulate and electromagnetic radiation.

4. List radiation units.

5. Give the use of each type of radiation unit.

6. Convert between traditional and SI units.

7. Define types of instruments for detecting radiation.

8. Determine the type of personnel monitoring system best suited for specific situations.

## Important Terms

absorbed dose
alpha radiation
atomic (Z) number
atomic mass unit (amu)
back scatter

| | |
|---|---|
| becquerel (Bq) | ionized |
| beta radiation | kerma |
| biologic effects | neutron |
| brachytherapy | nuclear disintegration |
| coulombs per kilogram (C/kg) | nucleus |
| curie (Ci) | particulate radiation |
| dosimeter | personnel monitors |
| dosimetrist | photomultiplier |
| dosimetry | pocket ionization chamber |
| electromagnetic radiation | proton |
| electron | quality factor (QF) |
| exposure | rad |
| f-factor | radiation |
| field survey instrument | radiation safety officer |
| film badge | radioactive |
| gamma radiation | radioactive decay |
| Geiger-Mueller (GM) counter | rem |
| gray (Gy) | roentgen® |
| half-life | scintillation counter |
| ionization chamber | self-reading dosimeter |
| ionizing radiation | sievert (Sv) |
| isotopes | thermoluminescent dosimeter |

## INTRODUCTION

The purpose of this chapter is to give an overview of the types of radiation commonly used in radiology, discuss the units used to measure radiation, and outline the various types of field survey instruments and personal dosimeters. Again, the discussion of radiation types is not intended to replace a physics text but to give students without a background in physics enough information to understand the nature of the radiations used. For the student who has had physics, the first part of the chapter can serve both as a review of the physics course material and for the national boards.

The information text boxes in the chapter cover the following additional topics: confusion in radiation units, badges, film badge construction, common mistakes in the use of film, basic rules of using field survey instruments, and other types of radiation.

## DEFINITIONS

### Radiation

*Radiation* is a general term used to describe the process of emitting radiant energy in the form of waves or particles. Simply, radiation can be defined as energy in transit. When no modifier (a term, such as *microwave,* placed in front of a word) is used, the term *radiation* usually refers to ionizing radiation.

### Ionizing Radiation

In 1895, Roentgen found that certain types of electronic tubes could emit radiant (radiation) energy. He named this radiant energy *x-radiation,* using the letter *x* to stand for an unknown quantity. In 1896, Becquerel discovered that certain naturally occurring substances emitted radiation. He discovered three different types

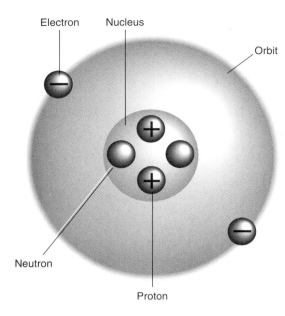

**Figure 3–1** Atom.

of radiation. Each had different physical properties. Ernest Rutherford, an English physicist, later named them alpha, beta, and gamma, the first three letters of the Greek alphabet.

*Ionizing radiation* produces positively and negatively charged particles as it passes through matter. Sources of ionizing radiation can be man-made—for example, x-ray, nuclear power, and nuclear waste—or natural background such as cosmic rays from the sun or the radioactive material in the earth's crust. It can be in the form of particles (*particulate radiation*) such as alpha and beta radiation or pure energy having neither mass or charge (*electromagnetic radiation*) such as x- and gamma rays.

An understanding of ionizing radiation necessitates a basic understanding of the atom (Figure 3–1). This is important both in understanding how radiation is produced and in discussing the interactions of radiation with matter, which we do in the next chapter. In essence, the atom consists of three types of particles:

> *Electron,* Very light particles with a charge of −1.
> *Proton,* Particles with a mass about 2000 times that of the electron; they possess a charge of +1.

> *Neutron,* Particles with about the same mass as a proton; they are electrically neutral.

Atoms are electrically neutral, having the same number of electrons as protons. Protons and neutrons are concentrated in a dense central core called the *nucleus;* electrons revolve around the nucleus in orbits.

The number of protons in the nucleus is known as the *Z* or *atomic number.* This determines the identity of the element (e.g. oxygen) as well as its chemical properties. Different forms of the same element may exist in what are called *isotopes.* These elements have the same number of protons, maintaining chemical identity, but different numbers of neutrons. Changing the number of neutrons in the nucleus of the atom often makes it *radioactive* (or go through *nuclear decay*). It would then emit particulate (alpha or beta) or electromagnetic (gamma) ionizing radiation.

## Alpha Radiation

*Alpha radiation* (symbolized by the Greek letter α) is made up of four particles and does not penetrate matter as easily as other types of radiation. As particulate radiation goes, alpha is huge. In fact, it is the Mack truck of the radiation world. It is very large and slow moving, and it carries a lot of energy. As alpha radiation is made up of two protons and two neutrons, it has a mass of 4 amu (*atomic mass units* are each equivalent to the matter or mass of one proton), a charge of +2, and is best described as a helium atom nucleus. It is produced by *nuclear disintegration,* primarily of heavy atoms such as plutonium. Alpha particles have a range in air of about 1 cm for each million electron volts (MeV) of energy, and most naturally occurring alpha particles travel 4 to 8 cm. Alpha particles are so large and have such a strong electrical charge that they interact with matter very quickly and normally are unable to penetrate even a sheet of paper. Because of their low penetrating ability, there are no medical uses for alpha particles, and they are dangerous if taken inside the body. Personnel monitoring devices are not normally sensitive to alpha radiation.

It has been shown, by irradiating a gas-filled vessel for some time, that alpha particles are helium nuclei. Helium gas builds up in the vessel, whereas there was no helium before irradiation. Having a charge of +2 causes the particle to capture two negatively charged electrons to become a neutral helium atom.

## Beta Radiation

*Beta radiation* (symbolized by the Greek letter β) is produced only in or near the nucleus of the atom and essentially consists of high-speed electrons. Each beta particle has a mass of 0.00055 amu and a charge of −1 or +1. A negatron (negative electron) is produced by nuclear disintegration. A positron (positive electron) is produced by nuclear disintegration or x-ray/matter interaction called *pair production.* Beta particles are similar to a speeding bullet in that they are small and fast moving. Because they have less mass and a smaller electrical charge, they are more penetrating than alpha particles. Beta particles can travel approximately 3 meters/MeV of energy in air and up to several millimeters in tissue. One medical function of beta radiation is the use of radioactive phosphorus (P-32) to reduce fluid accumulation in the serosal (pericardial or peritoneal) cavities resulting from metastatic carcinoma. Iodine-131 ($^{131}$I) also emits beta and gamma radiation, and is used to treat thyroid carcinoma. Positrons are used in

nuclear medicine in positron emission tomography (PET) studies.

Beta particles can be shown to be electrons by observing the behavior of beta rays in the presence of a magnetic field. When beta rays travel through a magnetic field, their course is deflected or changed, suggesting that they consist of streams of charged particles. The direction and amount of deflection is used to determine the charge (+1 or −1) and mass (0.000555 amu) of the particles.

## X-Radiation and Gamma Radiation

*X-rays* and *gamma rays* (radiation)—along with visible light, radio waves, and microwaves—are electromagnetic waves that form part of the electromagnetic spectrum. However, of these, only x-rays and gamma rays are both ionizing radiation and electromagnetic waves.

Electromagnetic waves have properties similar to other types of waves, such as ripples in a body of water. As do other waves, they have characteristic frequencies (number of waves per second), wavelengths (distance between waves), and amplitudes (height of waves). Electromagnetic waves differ from other wave phenomena in that they do not require a physical medium for travel: they can travel through empty space. Electromagnetic waves can be visualized as electric and magnetic fields moving through space (Figure 3–2).

Figure 3–3 illustrates the electromagnetic spectrum in terms of frequency. All electromagnetic waves travel with the same velocity: $c = 10 \times 10^8$ meters per second. As velocity (speed) is constant, what varies are the frequency and wavelength of the radiation. This is related to the amount of energy in the wave. The higher the energy, the shorter the wavelength and the higher the frequency. X-rays and gamma rays have the highest energy of all electromagnetic waves; thus, they have the shortest wavelength and the highest frequency.

X-rays are produced outside the nucleus by accelerating electrons in a vacuum using a high voltage and having them strike a metal target, preferably of a high atomic number such as tungsten (Figure 3–4). The voltages typically range from 20,000 to 200,000 volts (20 to 200 keV). The high-speed electrons are slowed down or stopped in the target by interacting with

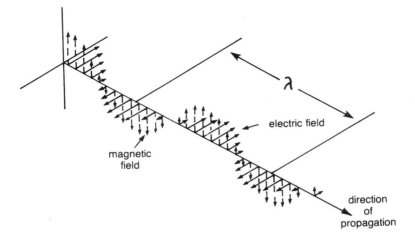

**Figure 3–2** Visualization of electromagnetic radiation. (Reprinted with permission from Nave CR, Nave BC: Physics for the Health Sciences, 3rd ed. Philadelphia, WB Saunders, 1985, p 325.)

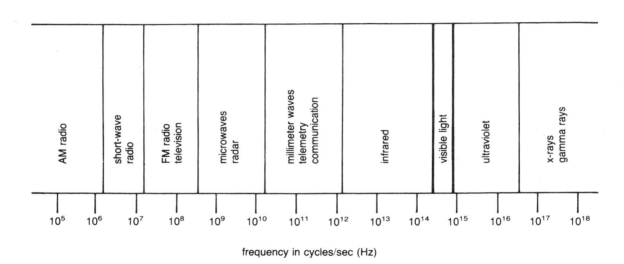

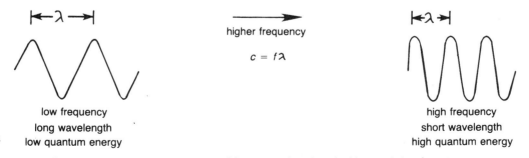

**Figure 3–3** Electromagnetic spectrum in terms of frequency. (Reprinted with permission from Nave CR, Nave BC: Physics for the Health Sciences, 3rd ed. Philadelphia, WB Saunders, 1985, p 326.)

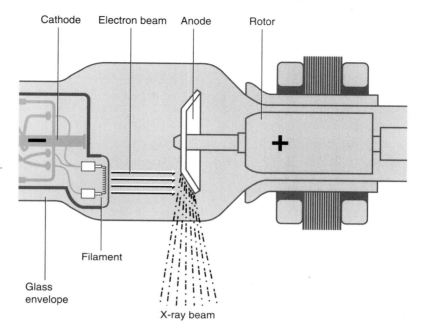

**Figure 3-4** X-ray production.

atomic nuclei or the electrons in orbit around the nuclei. This kinetic (motion) energy is given off as heat (99% or more) and x-rays (1%). A wide range of energies are produced at the target, because different electrons are decelerated at different rates. For this reason, x-ray beams are often called *heterogenous* or *polyenergetic* since they possess energies ranging from 0 to the maximum kilovoltage peak (kVp) applied to the tube.

Gamma rays are electromagnetic radiation produced in the nucleus and are identical to x-rays in energy, wavelength, and frequency. As with x-rays, they have no mass or charge. What makes gamma rays different from x-rays is their origin. Gamma rays originate from within the nucleus; x-rays originate from outside the nucleus. Most radioactive materials used in medicine emit gamma rays—for example, I-131 (radioactive iodine), Cs-137 (cesium used for brachytherapy), and Co-60 (cobalt used for teletherapy). Brachytherapy (*brachy* means "short," implying a short distance) is the irradiation of cancer close to the surface of the body (interstitial) or within the body (intracavitary) using sealed radioactive sources. Brachytherapy takes advantage of the inverse square law by placing the source of radiation close to the tumor, sparing normal tissue. Teletherapy (tele = distant) is irradiation of cancerous lesions with the source of radiation distant from the body.

Table 3–1 compares types of ionizing radiation.

## RADIATION UNITS

Four units are used to express an amount of radiation (Table 3–2). They are described next. There are two types of units: traditional and SI (Système International). In the United States, it is still customary to use the traditional units. Some texts also call these units *customary units.* In most other countries, SI units are used.

### Exposure in Air

The *roentgen* (R; traditional unit) or *coulombs per kilogram* (C/kg; SI unit) is a measure of the ionization of air produced by x-radiation and gamma radiation below 3 million electron volts (3 MeV). These units are considered units of *exposure* in air. Simply put, the roentgen is a measure of the amount of ionization (number

Table 3–1  Types of Ionizing Radiation

| Type | Mass (amu) | Charge | Description | Production Source |
|------|-----------|--------|-------------|-------------------|
| Alpha particle | 4 | +2 | Doubly ionized helium atom | Radioactive decay, mostly heavy atoms |
| Beta particle (negation) | 0.00055 | −1 | Negative electron | Radioactive decay |
| Beta particle (positron) | 0.00055 | +1 | Positive electron | Radioactive decay; pair production |
| Protons | 1 | +1 | Hydrogen nuclei | Van de Graaff generators; cyclotrons |
| Negative pi-mesons | 0.15 | −1 | Negative particle | Accelerators |
| Heavy nuclei | Varies | Varies | Atom stripped of one or more electrons | Accelerators |
| Neutrons | 1 | 0 | Neutron of atom | Atomic reactor; cyclotrons |
| Gamma rays | 0 | 0 | Electromagnetic radiation | Radioactive decay radiation |
| X-ray | 0 | 0 | Electromagnetic radiation | X-ray tube; rearrangement of orbital electrons |

---

### *More Information:*
### Other Types of Radiation

Linear accelerators are very large and expensive devices used to accelerate charged particles such as electrons and protons to very high speed using a series of electromagnetic fields. (See "An Overview of Linear Accelerators" in Chapter 2.) Accelerators produce a number of particles beyond the electron, proton, and neutron. Negative *pi-mesons* (pions) have a mass of 0.15 amu and a charge of −1. These negatively charged particles have a mass 273 times that of an electron and are produced by linear accelerators. Some facilities are experimenting with the use of pions in radiation therapy.

Heavy nuclei are also produced by an accelerator and have a range of masses and charges. Any atom stripped of one or more electrons and accelerated becomes an ionizing particle. Examples of ionizing particles include deuterons, which are nuclei of "heavy hydrogen" (1 proton and 1 neutron as opposed to just 1 proton in the nucleus).

---

of electrons knocked off atoms) produced by x-radiation or gamma radiation in air. The definition of the roentgen is somewhat complicated and very exact. It is defined as the quantity of x-radiation or gamma radiation such that the associated corpuscular emission per 0.001293 g of dry air (1 cm$^3$ at 0°C and 760 mm Hg) produces in air ions carrying 1 electrostatic unit of electrical charge of either a positive or negative sign.

The coulomb is the SI unit of electric charge.

Table 3–2  Radiation Units

| Quantity | Traditional Unit | SI Unit |
|----------|-----------------|---------|
| Exposure (measured in air) | roentgen (R) | coulombs per kilogram (C/kg) |
| Absorbed dose | rad | gray (Gy) |
| Dose equivalent (occupational) | rem | sievert (Sv) |
| Radioactivity | curie (Ci) | becquerel (Bq) |

It is defined as the charge (number of electrons) moving through a conductor by a steady current of 1 ampere in 1 second. Simply put, it represents a given number of electrons. The kilogram measures the quantity of air. Thus, this unit also measures an electric charge (electrons) in a quantity of air.

### Absorbed Dose

The *rad* (an acronym for *r*adiation *a*bsorbed *d*ose; traditional unit) and *gray* (Gy; SI unit) are used to express the *absorbed dose*. They are also refereed to as units of *kerma,* which stands for *k*inetic *e*nergy *r*eleased in *ma*tter. When radiation interacts with any matter, energy is transferred from the photons to the electrons of the atoms, moving them into a higher energy shell. That energy is the kerma. A subset of this concept, air kerma, has implications in radiation protection. Air kerma is the transfer of radiation energy to atoms of air. When talking about diagnostic levels of x-rays, the energy transferred to air by 1 rad is approximately equal to an exposure of 1 R. See "Confusion in Radiation Units" for more information on practice implication of this concept.

The rad is defined as an energy transfer of 100 ergs (a small unit of energy) per gram of any absorbing material. One rad equals 1/100 gray. The amount of radiation absorbed depends on the energy or penetrating ability of the radiation and the composition of the absorbing material. The higher the energy, the less likely that photon will interact and transfer energy, but the more dense the material (like lead), the more likely it is that the photon will interact and transfer energy. The ratio between the number of roentgens (exposure) and the number of rads (energy transfer) is called the *f-factor.*

The rad and gray can be used for any type of ionizing radiation, and patient dose is often expressed in these units. The drawback in the two units lies in the fact that the biologic effect of 1 rad or 1 Gy varies with the type of radiation. For example, 1 rad of x-ray will do less biological damage than 1 rad of beta radiation, so discussing radiation in terms of rads—or for that matter, roentgens—is not as useful for protection as using units of rems or seiverts.

### Occupational Exposure (Dose Equivalent)

The *rem* (acronym for *r*adiation *e*quivalent *m*an; traditional unit) and the *sievert* (Sv; SI unit) are units of *biological effect*. Rems are determined by multiplying the absorbed dose (rad) times a *quality factor* (in essence, a measure of the biologic impact or damage of a particular type of radiation) and are expressed as dose equivalence. The most common use of rems is for personnel radiation monitoring. The rem can also be informally defined as the quantity of any ionizing radiation that has the same biologic effectiveness of 1 rad of x-ray. It was formerly believed that the quality factor used for converting rad to rem was the same as the relative biologic effectiveness (RBE; see Chapter 5). It is now recognized that these are similar but not identical units.

The sievert is equivalent to 100 rem. It is the SI unit that produces the same biologic effect as 1 Gy of x-ray.

### Radioactivity

The *curie* (Ci; traditional unit) and becquerel (Bq; SI unit) are not strictly measures of radiation intensity like the roentgen. Instead, they measure rate of nuclear disintegration (decay) of a material. Specifically, with any radioactive material, a certain *percentage* of all the atoms in any sample will break apart (disintegrate) per second. The curie is defined as $3.7 \times 10^{10}$ disintegrations per second of any radioactive substance. The becquerel is defined as one decay per second of any radioactive substance; thus, the curie is a very much larger unit than the becquerel.

The activity of a radiation source does not remain constant but tends to decrease with time. This is known as *radioactive decay*. The characteristic time of radioactive decay is known as the *half-life*, the time it takes a radioactive material to decay to 50% of original activity. For example, if there were 1,000,000 atoms of a radioactive material and it took 6.4 hours for 500,000 of them to decay, the half-life of that element would be 6.4 hours.

The relation among roentgens, rads, rems, and curies is illustrated in Figure 3–5.

## Confusion in Radiation Units

It is not uncommon in practice to hear technologists and physicians talking about radiation using the terms *rad, rem,* and *R* almost as though they were interchangeable. This habit on the part of some people causes a lot of confusion on the part of others because using those terms indiscriminately does not convey if we are talking about exposure in air, the energy transferred by the radiation (dose), or how much biologic damage was done. It is essential for the practitioner to have a good understanding of these units and to use them correctly. Roentgens measure exposure and are used for measuring the "intensity" of the radiation. Rads are used to measure absorbed energy and are used to talk about "dose" from radiation. Rems are used in dosimetry and measure biologic effects.

The confusion of these units comes about from how they were defined. As noted in the text, the amount of energy transferred to air atoms by 1 R of exposure is approximately the same as the amount of energy transferred by 1 rad of dose. Also, the unit rem is defined relative to the biological impact of 1 rad of dose from 250-keV x-rays to human tissue. Consequently, one R of exposure gives about one rad of dose and about one rem of impact. The problem with this relationship is that it holds true if, and only if, (1) we are talking about human exposure, (2) the radiation is x-ray, and (3) the x-rays are in the diagnostic range. Unless all three of these conditions are met, the comparisons do not hold true. Therefore, it is important that practitioners be precise in their use of these terms.

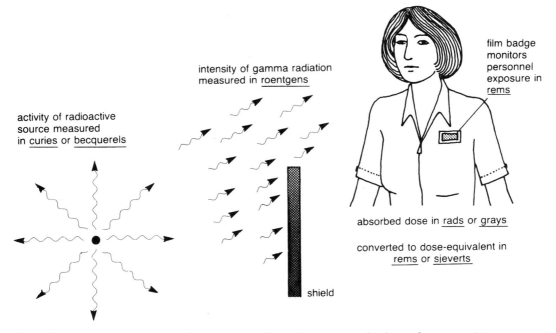

activity of radioactive source measured in curies or becquerels

intensity of gamma radiation measured in roentgens

shield

film badge monitors personnel exposure in rems

absorbed dose in rads or grays

converted to dose-equivalent in rems or sieverts

**Figure 3–5** Relationship between the four units of radiation intensity. (Redrawn from Nave CR, Nave BC: Physics for the Health Sciences, 3rd ed. Philadelphia, WB Saunders, 1985, p 373.)

**Table 3–3** Common Conversion Terms for Powers of Ten

| Power of Ten | Multiplication Factor | Symbol | Prefix | Example |
|---|---|---|---|---|
| $10^6$ | 1,000,000 | M | mega | megavolt |
| $10^3$ | 1,000 | k | kilo | kilogram |
| $10^{-3}$ | 0.001 | m | milli | milliroentgen |
| $10^{-6}$ | 0.000001 | μ | micro | microgram |
| $10^{-9}$ | 0.000000001 | n | nano | nanometer |

## Conventions for the Use of Units

### Practice

Since the traditional units of radiation intensity represent such large amounts of radiation, the prefix *milli* is often added to signify one thousandth of the unit. Thus, the milliroentgen (mR) is 1/1000 roentgen; the millirad (mrad) is 1/1000 rad; and the millirem (mrem) is 1/1000 rem. In the case of curies, the millicurie (mCi) and the microcurie (μCi) are preferred units. The mCi is 1/1000 curie; the μCi is one millionth of a curie. For a more complete listing of common power of ten conversions, see Table 3–3.

Few individuals in the United States use SI units, although they are the units of choice in almost the entire rest of the world. There is a movement to convert to SI units, but it is hard to change accepted practice. Some scientific organizations and publications use SI units, but it is more difficult to make changes at the practitioner level, that is, among radiologists, radiologic technologists, and radiologic physicists employed in clinics.

In some cases, one sees the SI units used in a way that is perhaps more palatable to the American reader. For example, some texts now use the centigray (cGy) as the unit of absorbed dose. This is 1/100 gray and equivalent to the rad.

### Conversions

To convert from roentgens to milliroentgens, rads to millirads, and rems to millirems, multi-ply the larger (first) unit by 1000. To convert from the smaller unit to the larger unit, perform the reverse: divide by 1000. Alternatively, multiply by 0.001.

---

**EXAMPLE 1**

5 R is how many milliroentgens?

$5 \times 1000 = 5000$ mR

---

**EXAMPLE 2**

50 mrad is how many rads?

$50/1000 = 0.05$ rad

$50 \times 0.001 = 0.05$ rad

---

The radiologic technologist must have an awareness of SI units that includes knowing how to convert from traditional units to SI units and from SI units to traditional units. To convert from traditional to SI, perform the following multiplications:

| | | | |
|---|---|---|---|
| 1 R | $\times$ | $(2.58 \times 10^{-4}) =$ | coulombs per kilogram (C/kg) |
| 1 rad | $\times$ | $0.01 \quad =$ | grays (Gy) |
| 1 rem | $\times$ | $0.01 \quad =$ | sieverts (Sv) |
| 1 Ci | $\times$ | $(3.7 \times 10^{10}) =$ | becquerels (Bq) |

The shaded (middle) area is the conversion factor between units. Converting from SI units to conventional units requires division by the appropriate conversion factor. Since the conversion factors are the same (0.01) between absorbed dose (rad to grays) and dose equivalent (rem to sieverts), they are usually the easiest to remember.

---

**EXAMPLE 1**

10 rad is equivalent to _____ grays.

$10 \times 0.01 = 0.1$ Gy

---

**EXAMPLE 2**

100 rem is equivalent to _____ sieverts.

$100 \times 0.01 = 1$ sievert

---

**EXAMPLE 3**

1 gray is equivalent to _____ rads.

$1 \times 0.01 = 100$ rad

---

When converting from milliroentgens, millirads, and millirems to the whole units of coulombs per kilogram, grays, and sieverts, these units must first be converted to their whole unit by dividing the unit by 1000. Alternately, milliroentgens can be multiplied by $2.58 \times 10^{-7}$ to convert to coulombs per kilogram; millirads can be multiplied by 0.00001 to convert to grays; and millirems can be multiplied by 0.00001 to convert to sieverts. These and other conversions are covered in greater detail in Appendix A.

## DETECTION INSTRUMENTS

Radiation is not detectable by ordinary means; that is, we cannot see, hear, taste, or feel it. The detection of radiation requires instruments specifically designed to detect ionizing radiation. This is done indirectly by measuring the effect radiation has on a medium such as air (ionization) or film (density).

*Dosimetry* is the determination by scientific methods of the amount, rate, and distribution of radiation emitted from a source of ionizing radiation. A *dosimeter* is a device used to detect and measure exposure to radiation. In radiation therapy, a *dosimetrist* is an individual who plans an optimal radiation treatment dosage pattern or who establishes a radiation distribution pattern for radiation therapy.

Two general classes of instruments are used to detect ionizing radiation. *Field survey instruments,* such as ionization chambers and *Geiger-Mueller counters,* record the amount of ionizing radiation in air. *Personnel monitors* are used by the radiographer to monitor personal exposure to radiation on a regular basis. Usually, these are film badges or TLDs (see below). They also are used when guests such as nurses visit the department to assist with patients and procedures. Refer to Chapter 10 for the regulations on personnel monitoring.

### Field Survey Instruments

There are three basic types of field survey instruments: the ionization chamber, the Geiger-Mueller detector, and the portable scintillation detector. Each has its own best use, and these devices are not equally sensitive in the detection of radiation.

### Ionization Chamber

The *ionization chamber* (Figure 3–6) determines the amount of radiation by collecting ions in a chamber filled with gas (usually helium or argon). The chamber has a central electrode (usually positively charged) running down the middle of the chamber and another electrode (usually negatively charged) along the edges. When radiation ionizes the gas, the freed electron moves to the positively charged electrode and can be measured. As there is a direct relationship between the amount of radiation striking the chamber and the number of electrons liberated, the radiation amount can be closely estimated by measuring the number of electrons. Ionization chambers are most widely used in measuring either the dose (total amount of radiation) in milliroentgens or the

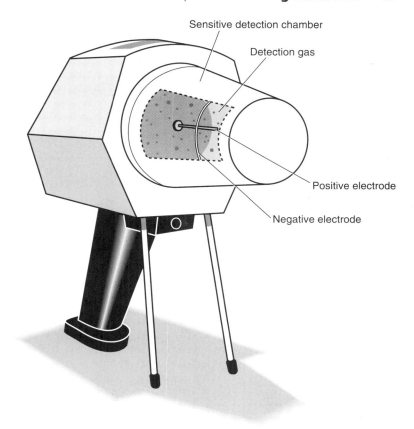

Sensitive detection chamber

Detection gas

Positive electrode

Negative electrode

**Figure 3–6** Ionization chamber. (Redrawn from Thompson MA: Principles of Radiation Protection for Nurses and Other Medical Facility Personnel. Birmingham, AL, University of Alabama at Birmingham, 1986.)

exposure rate in milliroentgens per hour. They are widely used as they are accurate, are sensitive to a wide range of radiation energies (from about 10 mR to several hundred R), and are portable. Examples would include the determination of acceptable time limits that staff and visitors could spend in the room with a patient with a radioactive implant or measuring the amount radiation in a given exposure. Ionization chambers are good at detecting x-rays, gamma rays, and high-energy beta radiation. They are not well suited to detecting alpha radiation or low levels of radiation such as a very small radioactive contamination.

## Geiger-Mueller Counter

Geiger-Mueller (GM) counters (Figure 3–7) also determine the amount of radiation by collecting ions in a gas. This gas (usually helium, argon, or neon) is housed in the detector probe. This probe has a very thin window that allows for the detection of alpha, beta, and gamma radiation. It is not sensitive to very low-energy alpha, beta, and gamma radiation, however.

GM counters are most useful in the detection (rather than measurement) of radiation sources and low-level radioactive contamination. They should not be used for exposure or rate measurements. An example of a common use of a GM counter is in a nuclear medicine lab where radioactive materials are stored. A meter is placed in a central location to give an audio alert if there is any contamination from the radioactive isotopes.

## Scintillation Counter

The *scintillation counter* (Figure 3–8) uses a sodium iodide or cesium iodide crystal that produces small flashes of light (called scintillations) upon exposure to radiation. The light is

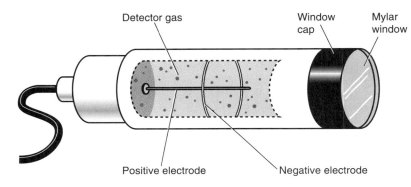

**Figure 3–7** Geiger-Mueller counter probe. (Redrawn from Thompson MA: Principles of Radiation Protection for Nurses and Other Medical Facility Personnel. Birmingham, AL, University of Alabama at Birmingham, 1986.)

detectable by a *photomultiplier* tube. This tube converts the flashes of light into electric impulses, which can be measured. As in the ionization chamber, the electrons measured can be related to a specific radiation dose. Radiography students who have completed a course in radiologic physics or equipment will recognize that this is a method of operation similar to the automatic exposure control found in the x-ray unit.

The scintillation counter is the most sensitive detector of x-radiation and gamma radiation. It is also useful in the detection and subsequent location of lost radiation sources.

### Personnel Monitoring

There are three basic types of personnel monitors: film badges, thermoluminescent dosime-

ters, and pocket ionization chambers. The desirable characteristics of personnel monitoring devices are (1) portability, (2) ruggedness (ability to withstand stress), (3) sensitivity, (4) reliability, and (5) low cost. Each of these criteria must be evaluated when deciding which personnel monitoring system is to be used in specific situations. In general, monitoring is performed in any situation in which an individual is expected to receive 10% of the effective dose equivalent (formerly called the MPD, or maximum permissible dose).

### Film Badges

*Film badges* (Figure 3–9) have been in use since the 1940s. They are the most common type of personnel monitor and are most often used

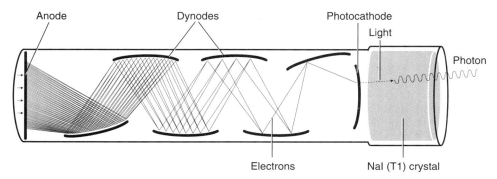

**Figure 3–8** Scintillation counter. (Redrawn from Thompson MA: Principles of Radiation Protection for Nurses and Other Medical Facility Personnel. Birmingham, AL, University of Alabama at Birmingham, 1986.)

*More Information:*
**Basic Rules of Using Field Survey Instruments**

Nuclear medicine technologists are most likely to routinely handle field survey instruments. Other radiologic technologists handle these instruments on a more infrequent basis. Some radiologic technology programs use these devices for performing experiments in the energized laboratory.

The following rules should be followed when using field survey instruments:

1. Always read the instructions before the use first.

2. Check batteries before use. If infrequently used, batteries should be removed prior to storage.

3. Handle any instrument carefully.

4. Ensure that the instrument has been recently calibrated by qualified personnel.

5. The instrument should be stored securely, but it should also be accessible for quick use.

to measure whole-body irradiation. The film badge is a plastic holder with a clip on the back to attach to clothing, a film holder and a series of filters and unfiltered areas in the middle, and the open front portion of the film badge, called the *window.* A small piece of film is placed inside a badge containing a variety of metal filters that allow estimation of the radiation dosage and energy because the energy level of the radiation interacts differently with each filter. Because of the series of filters, this design also allows determination of exposure to radiation that entered from the posterior of the person as well as *back scatter,* which is secondary radiation created inside the body of the wearer and then exits at the site of the film badge. A characteristic curve similar to one used in determining film speed and contrast is constructed after the film is processed by plotting the amount of exposure for each type of filtration (Figure 3–10). As the amount of exposure changes and/or the energy level changes, the graph also changes.

The traditional length of time before changing the film in a badge is 1 month, since they can fog easily as a result of temperature and humidity changes. Recently, dosimetry services have been giving institutions the option of changing film badges every 3 months. However, this is rarely done in educational institutions, as most persons acting as the *radiation*

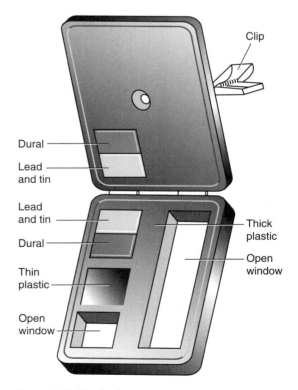

**Figure 3–9** Film badge.

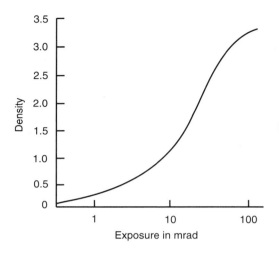

**Figure 3–10** Characteristic curve for film badge.

*safety officer* (RSO) feel that students need to be monitored more often than every 3 months.

Film badges are sensitive down to about 10 mrem (0.1 mSv), with the upper limit on sensitivity having been reported as anywhere from 700 to 2000 rem. Badges are most sensitive to an energy of 50 keV, which is not a problem since the film badge is designed primarily to detect low-energy scatter radiation. The range of stated accuracies of film badges has been cited as anywhere from ±25% to ±50%. However, since most practitioners receive relative low doses, this also is not a problem. For example, with a reading of 20 mrem, an accuracy rate of ±50% would mean that the practitioner received anywhere from 10 to 30 mrem—well within acceptable limits.

The advantages and disadvantages of film badges are these:

*Advantages*

- In use for many years
- Inexpensive
- Easy to handle
- Easy to process
- Permanent record of exposure
- Wide range of sensitivity

*Disadvantages*

- Must wait for reading
- Accurate only at 10 mrem and higher
- Limited accuracy, especially when compared to TLDs

- Fogging due to humidity, temperature, moisture, and light leaks.

**Guidelines for Use.** Different states have different requirements for the use of film badges, although all states at least adhere to minimum federal requirements. Also, institutions practice radiation protection in terms of how they interpret the concept of ALARA (*as low as reasonably achievable*), which is discussed in depth in Chapter 9. For example, since students ordinarily work far fewer clinical hours in a year than full-time employees and are not experienced in the safe use of radiation, radiologic technology programs often have more restrictive requirements. An example is given on page 60.

Recommendations for the location of the dosimeter differ from one source to another. National regulatory recommendations are that the dosimeter be worn at the level of the waist on the anterior side. In Canada, the recommendation is to wear the dosimeter under the lead apron, whereas in the United States, no specific recommendation is made. Most state regulatory agencies recommend that the dosimeter be worn at the level of the sternum and outside the apron when used, so unless otherwise directed by the radiation safety officer, the dosimeter should be worn at the level of the sternum. The collar of the lab coat is a common site (Figure 3–11). Also, unless directed otherwise, the film badge should be

## More Information:
## Film Badge Construction

As noted in the text, film badges are made up of a film holder that has a number of filters over the film in order to estimate the amount and types of radiation making the exposure. In most film badges, the holder is made of plastic. The filters used in the holder vary from manufacturer to manufacturer. One common filter set is the one shown in Figure 3–9, using two plastic filters, a lead/tin filter, a lead/cadmium filter, a Dural filter made up mostly of aluminum with copper and magnesium added, and an open window. Another common filter set uses a copper filter, an aluminum filter, a lead filter, and an open window. Note that these two filter sets are similar in that they use aluminum, copper, lead, and an open window.

The physical interaction that radiation has with specific atoms is well known. That has to do with one of the ways radiation interacts with matter. If the energy level of the radiation is almost the same as the binding energy that holds the electron in orbit around the nucleus, a photoelectric interaction is likely to occur and the radiation photon will be totally absorbed (see Chapter 4 for more detail). This is most likely to occur with electrons in the K-shell (nearest to the

nucleus) or the L-shell (the next shell out). The binding energy of the electrons of all common elements is well known. The following are the K-shell binding energies of materials used in filters:

| | |
|---|---|
| Carbon (plastic) | 0.28 keV |
| Magnesium | 1.3 keV |
| Aluminum | 1.5 keV |
| Copper | 8.9 keV |
| Cadmium | 26.7 keV |
| Tin | 29.2 keV |
| Lead | 88.0 keV |

As can be seen by the binding energies, in the materials from carbon (used in the plastic) to tin, the K-shell energy are in the same range as scatter radiation. The lead K-shell energy is in the range of the diagnostic primary beam and/or scatter from high-energy radiation such as cobalt. With the knowledge of these relationships and measurements of the relative densities of the film behind each of these filters, both the energy level and amount of exposure can be calculated.

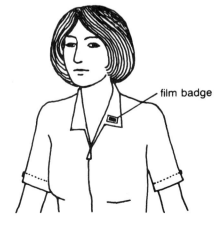

**Figure 3–11** Proper site of film badge.

## Common Mistakes in the Use of Film Badges

In one medical center, the radiation safety officer (RSO) received a report that showed one of the staff technologists had received an amount of very high-energy radiation exposure. The RSO was quite concerned about this, as the technologist should have had no access to very high-radiation sources. After extensively questioning the technologists about where she had worked, what she had done, and where besides the department she had taken the badge, the RSO still could not determine where or if the exposure reported had occurred. Several days later, the RSO happen to run into the technologist in the hallway and, on the spur of the moment, asked to see her film badge. When he opened it, it turned out that the film was improperly inserted into the badge so no part of the film was covered by a filter. That explained why the badge showed very high-energy exposure—only very high-energy radiation would give the appearance of almost no filtration.

In another facility, the RSO had a dosimetry report that showed that one staff technologist had received almost the legal limit of exposure for a year in just 1 month. What was really worrisome about this was that the technologist had been on vacation for most of the time reported. Neither the technologist nor the RSO could determine why the exposure was so high until the RSO noticed that the technologist clipped the dosimeter to the outside of the lead apron itself. When asked, the technologist stated that she was the only one who wore the apron when she was there so she always left it on the apron. It turned out that during the vacation time, the apron had traveled almost as widely as the technologist had. The apron, with the film badge still attached, had been used almost nonstop in fluoroscopy, as a patient shield in the department, and for portables, or it was left hanging on the portable unit during a multitude of patient exposures.

In one radiography program in Florida, the dosimetry report showed the readings for one student to be invalid due to heat exposure of the film badge. The program director had been very clear in explaining to the students that leaving a film badge on the dash of a car would have this exact effect. When the student was asked if she had left the film badge in the car, she denied it. The next month, the same thing happened again. This time the program director specifically asked where the student kept the film badge when she was not wearing it. The student replied that, as she should not keep it in the car, she kept it in the trunk of the car. Obviously, the heat and humidity in the trunk of the car had damaged the film.

A QC technologist was giving an inservice session on radiation safety during portable examination for nurses who worked in the recovery room. This was deemed essential because of the large number of examination done in the recovery room. During the talk, one of the nurses stood up and stated, "This is all well and good, but we all wear film badges, so why do we need to be concerned about the rest of this stuff when the badges absorbed all the radiation?"

worn outside the lead apron, as recommended by the ASRT. The rationale for this is that the highest dose received is to the approximate level of the sternum and outside of the apron. A badge at the collar will receive about 10 to 20 times the exposure of the protected trunk in fluoroscopy. Some authorities feel that this overestimates actual exposure and recommend wearing two badges, one over and one under the apron, for a better estimation of exposure.

Common mistakes in wearing film badges include:

1. Leaving the film badge on the lab coat and washing the lab coat. This renders the readings invalid.

2. Leaving the film badge on the lead apron and hanging the apron back on a rack in the room. This exposes the badge to radiation in the room while overhead films or later films are taken.
3. Removing the film badge and leaving it sitting on the dash of a car. This exposes the film badge to cosmic radiation and heat from the sun.
4. Not always wearing the film badge.
5. Not correctly inserting the film packet in the plastic badge holder.

**Film Badge Reports.** A sample film badge report is shown in Figure 3–12. This is more accurately called a radiation dosimetry report since it can report doses from both film badges and thermoluminescent dosimeters (TLDs). Note the existence of a control badge or badges. These are kept in an area away from radiation. If fogging of this badge happens, there may have been fogging of the whole set of badges sent to that department. Any reading above M (which stands for minimal or possibly no exposure) is subtracted from all readings in that batch of badges by the dosimetry service.

A film badge report is usually sent to the individual within the institution considered to be the radiation safety officer (RSO). The report usually arrives 4 to 6 weeks after the badges have been returned to the vendor. The RSO reviews the report first to ensure that doses are within normal limits and will usually want to meet with individuals who have exceeded institutional or regulatory guidelines. In educational institutions, the institutional limits are often lower than the regulatory guidelines. The primary rationale for this is to minimize students' exposure according to the ALARA concept. The other rationale is that students rarely work 5 full days a week in a radiation area and regulatory guidelines are based on that assumption.

In a typical dosimetry report as presented in Figure 3–12, the individual is assigned a participant identification number such as a badge number, with the name and social security number also listed for identification purposes. Special notes indicating potential problems with the reading are listed next, after which the type of dosimeter is listed. In this report, G1 signifies a film badge and U3 a ring badge. Reports are given for deep and shallow radiation for the exposure period (usually 1 month), calendar quarter, year to date, and permanent (the total dosage). *Deep* refers primarily to penetrating radiation such as x-radiation and gamma radiation, *shallow* to nonpenetrating radiation such as beta and very low-energy x-radiation and gamma radiation. These readings are usually given in the form of millirems.

It is important that student radiologic technologists make a habit of reviewing the film badge report. On graduation, or when changing jobs, information from the report (especially the vendor used) may be needed so that the new employer can issue a film badge. Personnel dosimetry records are considered legal documents; they usually require your signature before exposure records can be released to other individuals, such as new employers. These records must be maintained for a number of years based on regulatory requirements for the area in which they received the exposure.

In states in which student radiologic technologists may also hold jobs in radiology departments administering radiation to patients, a different monitor should be worn for the job than is worn as a student technologist. Some radiology departments/imaging centers may ask the student to wear a second monitor that they issue so that they have their own record of radiation exposure to students. Technologists who hold more than one job also often wear a separate badge for each site.

### Thermoluminescent Dosimeters

*Thermoluminescent dosimeters* (TLDs; Figure 3–13) use lithium fluoride (LiF), which stores radiation energy by alterations in its crystalline structure. This energy is released when the crystal is heated to several hundred degrees. This stored energy is emitted as light and is measured. The dose to the TLD can be calculated, as there is a direct correlation between the amount of radiation exposure and the amount of light released. TLDs can be worn for up to 3 months, can be reused, and are more sensitive than film badges (to about 5 mrem or 0.05 mSv). The accuracy of TLDs has been reported to be ±7%. One advantage of TLDs is that, unlike film, they absorb radiation approximately the same way human tissue does. Another advantage is that low amounts of heat have very little effect on TLDs

UNIV OF ALA/BIRMINGHAM
OCCUP HEALTH & SAFETY
933 SOUTH 19TH STREET
SUITE 445
BIRMINGHAM    AL 35294

# RADIATION DOSIMETRY REPORT

| ACCOUNT NO. | SERIES CODE |
|---|---|
| 35133 | RS |

| PROCESS NO. | REPORT DATE | DOSIMETER RECEIVED | REPORTING TIME IN WORK DAYS | PAGE NO. |
|---|---|---|---|---|
| 5335 8A | 5/27/93 | 5/19/93 | 6 | 1 |

*Landauer*
Landauer, Inc.  2 Science Road  Glenwood, Illinois 60425-1586
Telephone: (708) 755-7000  Facsimile: (708) 755-7016

Accredited by the
National Institute of Standards and Technology
through NVLap
DUPLICATE COPY

| QUALITY CONTROL RELEASE |
|---|
| RAM |

2S - PR 5161 - 71825

Figure 3–12 Sample film badge report.

*(Tabular radiation dosimetry report with columns for Participant ID Number, Name, Social Security Number, Dosimeter Type/Use, Radiation Quality, Exposure to Badge, Cumulative Totals (Calendar Quarter, Year to Date, Permanent), Adjustments, Sex, Birth Date, Number Badge Reports, Inception Date of Permanent Total.)*

Selected entries:

FOR EXPOSURE PERIOD 09/01/92 — THIRD 1992
03775 FURR EMILY  458287814 — SHALLOW 50 (NO CONTROL DOSIMETER OR AN INVALID CONTROL DOSIMETER WAS RETURNED WITH THE FOLLOWING PERSONNEL DOSIMETERS.)

FOR EXPOSURE PERIOD 03/01/93 — 03/31/93 — FIRST 1993
0000RS CONTROL
0000RS TLD CONTROL
03775 FURR EMILY  458287814
04113 GISH ADIE  212812914
04113 GISH ADIE  212812914
04251 RATTLES HYMIE  207832714
04251 RATTLES HYMIE  207832714
04428 PEKE SANDY  031772814
04428 PEKE SANDY  031772814
04680 PAYNE ETHELBERT  073485033
04680 PAYNE ETHELBERT  073485033

FOR EXPOSURE PERIOD 04/01/93 — 04/30/93 — SECOND 1993
0000RS CONTROL
0000RS TLD CONTROL
00423 SHAKESPEARE Z.  018904714
00423 SHAKESPEARE Z.  018904714
02721 THATCHER TRUDY  219527914
02721 THATCHER TRUDY  219527914
03697 HARVEY AMBROSE  648289614
03697 HARVEY AMBROSE  648289614

USE CODE (COLUMN 6)
1-WHOLE BODY      3-RIGHT FINGER   5-RIGHT WRIST   7-OTHER EXTREMITY
2-LENS OF EYE     4-LEFT FINGER    4-LEFT WRIST    8-OTHER WHOLE BODY
                                                   9-MONITOR

AN "H" HIGH ENERGY DESIGNATION, WHEN ONLY LOW ENERGY
EXPOSURE IS POSSIBLE, MAY INDICATE THAT THE FILM PACKET
WAS EXPOSED OUT OF THE FILTERED HOLDER.

IMPORTANT: SEE REVERSE SIDE FOR ADDITIONAL EXPLANATIONS

as opposed to film badges. Very high amounts of heat can cause the device to register lower radiation exposure than was actually received, as the heat will cause the crystalline structure to revert to the unexposed condition. This is different from the film badge, which fogs (shows increased exposure) when exposed to heat.

The biggest disadvantage of TLDs is that they do not provide a permanent record (other than the report generated by the measuring device), unlike film badges, which are superior legal documents (although film does fade with age). The initial cost of the TLD is higher, although this should not be a factor over time since the TLD can be reused. Also, the processing fees for TLDs are higher than those for film badges, but that is often offset by using TLDs for 3 months at a time. TLDs are sometimes called *film badges* in error.

The previous section mentioned ring badges on the dosimetry report. These are TLDs worn on the hand that could potentially receive the greatest radiation exposure. This would normally be the dominant hand—that is, the right hand of a right-handed individual. Radiographers rarely wear ring badges; most often, these are worn by nuclear medicine technologists because of the exposure to their hands from handling radioisotopes.

Another use of TLDs is the personal monitoring program developed by Personal Monitoring Technologies of Rochester, New York. Individuals interested in knowing their dosage from diagnostic x-ray exposures can enroll in a program that provides them with TLDs contained on a credit card–type card. One TLD is a control; another is given to the radiographer to tape in the field during exposures. Results from the control and the examination are sent to the individual. As consumers become increasingly interested in their exposure, it can be expected that usage of these kinds of programs will increase.

The advantages and disadvantages of TLDs follow:

*Advantages*

- Are tissue equivalent
- Can be worn for 3 months
- Can be reused
- Are highly accurate (sensitive)
- Do not fog

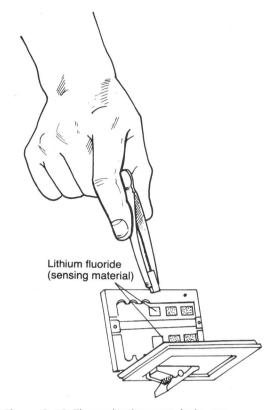

**Figure 3–13** Thermoluminescent dosimeter.

*Disadvantages*

- Are expensive
- Provide no permanent record
- Potentially higher cost

## Pocket Ionization Chambers

*Pocket ionization chambers* (Figure 3–14) have the advantage of providing immediate readings but are not in wide use because they must be recalibrated daily and must be read immediately, as the electrical charge inside the dosimeter bleeds off and shows less than actual exposure with time. Also, if the exposure exceeds the range of the dosimeter, the additional amount of exposure cannot be determined. In addition, they are easily affected by mechanical trauma such as being dropped or bumped and can measure only x-radiation and gamma radiation. Ionization chambers are usually used in short-term situations,

*(In the figure)* Lithium fluoride (sensing material)

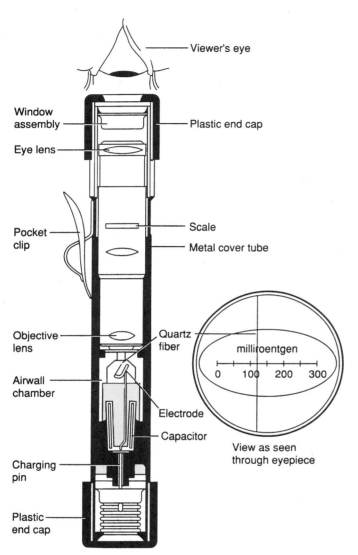

Viewer's eye

Window assembly

Plastic end cap

Eye lens

Pocket clip

Scale

Metal cover tube

Objective lens

Quartz fiber

Airwall chamber

Electrode

Capacitor

Charging pin

Plastic end cap

millidoentgen

0    100    200    300

View as seen through eyepiece

**Figure 3–14** Schematic drawing of a pocket dosimeter. (Redrawn from Thompson MA, Hattaway M, Hall J, Dowd S: Imaging Science and Protection: Philadelphia, WB Saunders, 1994.)

such as when a nurse or other health care worker accompanies a patient to the department. In California, regulations state that *everyone* who is in a room where radiation is being used must have a dosimeter. In many states, regulations state that a health care worker in a room with radiation must have a dosimeter, or all aspects of the exposure must be recorded permanently. In both of these situations, a pocket ionization chamber would be a viable choice. Technologists are also sometimes in situations in which two readings, one short-term and the other permanent, are required. In such cases, a pocket dosimeter can supplement the film badge or TLD.

A pocket dosimeter is similar to other ion chambers and consists of two electrodes in an air-filled chamber. The electrodes are charged positively prior to operation, which causes them to repel each other. One electrode is stationary; the other, a thin quartz wire called a *hair* or *fiber*, is movable. When totally charged, the fiber aligns with the zero point on the reading scale.

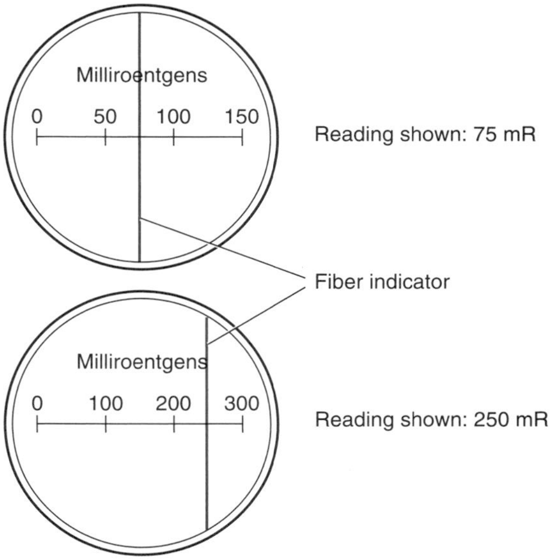

**Figure 3–15** Schematic drawing of a docket dosimeter reading scale. (Redrawn from Thompson MA: Principles of Radiation Protection for Nurses and Other Medical Facility Personnel. Birmingham, AL, University of Alabama at Birmingham, 1986.)

As air in the chamber is *ionized* (electrons are removed from the atoms) by radiation, the liberated electrons neutralize the positive charge on the electrodes, which allows the fiber of the dosimeter to move closer to the other electrode. More exposure causes the creation of more ions, causing greater movement of the hair, which in turn shows a higher exposure on the reading scale. A pocket dosimeter is read either with a light on the charger or by holding the dosimeter to the light (Figure 3–15). The type read by holding to the light is called a *self-reading dosimeter*.

The advantages and disadvantages of a pocket dosimeter follow:

*Advantages*

- Can be used for short periods.
- Can give immediate readings.
- Useful for monitoring personnel who are not normally monitored.

*Disadvantages*

- The charge can leak on the dosimeter, causing a false reading.
- Mechanical trauma can change the reading.
- Easy to misread.

## SUMMARY

Radiation is energy in motion. Ionizing radiation causes the formation of negatively and positively charged ions in matter through which it passes. It can be particulate or part of the electromagnetic spectrum.

Alpha radiation and beta radiation are particulate radiations with low penetrating ability. X-radiation and gamma radiation are part of the electromagnetic spectrum and are more highly penetrating.

Four types of units are used to express the amount of radiation. The units of exposure in air are the roentgen (R; traditional unit) and coulombs per kilogram (C/kg; SI unit). The units of absorbed dose are the rad (traditional unit), an acronym for *r*adiation *a*bsorbed *d*ose, and the gray (Gy; SI unit). The units of occupational exposure or dose equivalent are the rem (traditional unit), an acronym for *r*adiation *e*quivalent *m*an, and the sievert (Sv; SI unit). The units of radioactivity are the curie (Ci) and the becquerel (Bq). The SI units are not in widespread use in the United States, but radiologic technologists are expected to be familiar with both traditional and SI units.

Radiation can be detected only indirectly by its effects on matter. The measurement of radiation dose is known as *dosimetry*. The two classes of instruments used to detect radiation are field survey instruments and personnel monitors. Types of field survey instruments include ionization chambers, Geiger-Mueller counters, and scintillation counters.

Personnel monitors should meet a set of desirable characteristics, including portability, ruggedness, sensitivity, reliability, and low cost. Types of personnel monitors include film badges, thermoluminescent dosimeters, and pocket dosimeters. The most common type is the film badge. The pocket dosimeter is most often used for visitors to the department or when a short-term second reading is required.

## Questions

1. Which of the following are particulate radiation?
   I. alpha
   II. beta
   III. gamma

a. I and II only  b. I and III only
c. II and III only  d. I, II, and III

2. The unit that measures exposure in air is the:

    a. roentgen.  b. rad.
    c. rem.  d. curie.

3. Which unit is used for personnel monitoring?

    a. roentgen  b. rad
    c. rem  d. curie

4. One rad is equal to how many grays?

    a. 10  b. 100
    c. 0.1  d. 0.01

5. The measurement of radiation by scientific means is:

    a. densitometry.  b. dosimetrist.
    c. dosimetry.  d. roentgenometry.

6. The field monitoring device that functions similarly to the automatic exposure control in an x-ray unit is the:

    a. ionization chamber.  b. Geiger-Mueller counter.
    c. scintillation counter.  d. film badge.

7. Which personnel monitor provides the best legal record?

    a. film badge  b. pocket
    c. thermoluminescent dosimeter  d. ring badge

8. Since ionization chambers measure the ionization of a gas, they report their units in:

    a. roentgens.  b. rads.
    c. rems.  d. curies.

9. Which type of personnel monitor is most sensitive to heat?

    a. film badge  b. pocket dosimeter
    c. thermoluminescent dosimeter  d. ring badge

10. A reading of M on a radiation dosimetry report indicates:

a. the badge could not be read.  b. minimal exposure.
c. maximum exposure.  d. mandatory exposure.

## Exercises

1. Define radiation, and differentiate this general term from *ionizing radiation.*

2. How does electromagnetic radiation differ from particulate radiation?

3. Ionizing radiation is not directly detectable. Describe how ionizing radiation is detected and measured.

4. What are desirable characteristics of personnel monitors? What is the most common monitor in current use?

5. Why are the SI units not in common use in the United States?

## Answers

Questions

| | |
|---|---|
| 1. a | 6. c |
| 2. a | 7. a |
| 3. c | 8. a |
| 4. d | 9. a |
| 5. c | 10. b |

Exercises

1. *Radiation* is a general term used to describe the process of emitting radiant energy in the form of waves or particles. It can also be defined as energy in transit. *Ionizing radiation* produces positively and negatively charged particles. Ionizing radiation can be man-made or natural; it can also be in the form of particulate or electromagnetic radiation.

2. Particulate radiation is ionizing radiation with mass and often a charge. Not all forms of electromagnetic radiation are ionizing radiation. X-radiation and gamma radiation are forms of electromagnetic radiation

that are also ionizing radiation. They have no mass or charge.

3. Ionizing radiation must be detected in terms of its effects on other media. This includes measuring its ionization in air, the basis for the roentgen, and its effects on photographic film, the basis for the film badge.

4. Personnel monitors should be, first, portable. They should also be rugged, or able to withstand stress. Sensitivity, or ability to detect low doses of radiation, is another desirable characteristic. Additionally, they should be reliable and have a low cost.

5. It is difficult to change long-term usage on the part of practitioners. Because they have used the traditional units for many years with success, they see little need for change, despite what some academic organization may say.

## CHAPTER 4

# Interactions of Radiation with Matter

**Steven B. Dowd • Elwin R. Tilson**

## Objectives

At the end of this chapter, the student
should be able to:

1. Describe the processes of attenuation,
   absorption, and transmission.

2. Describe the five basic effects for x-ray
   interaction.

3. Describe the interactions of particulate radiation with matter.

4. List the relative importance of each
   effect to diagnostic imaging and radiation therapy.

5. Define linear energy transfer and specific ionization.

6. Describe the relationship between linear energy transfer, specific ionization, and quality factor.

7. List the five means of measuring dose
   from x-ray exposure.

8. List the five factors that must be
   known in calculating the dose
   received from radionuclides.

## Important Terms

absorption
annihilation reaction
atomic density
attenuation
average dose

| | |
|---|---|
| binding energy | ion pairs |
| biodistribution | linear energy transfer (LET) |
| biologic half-life | mean marrow dose |
| coherent scatter | pair production |
| Compton electron | photodisintegration |
| Compton scatter | photoelectric effect |
| cumulative dose | photoelectron |
| characteristic cascade | organ dose |
| depth dose | potential energy |
| elastic interaction | scatter |
| entrance skin exposure (ESE) | skin dose |
| excitation | specific ionization (SI) |
| glandular dose | recoil electron |
| gonadal dose | transmission |
| inelastic interaction | source to image receptor distance (SID) |
| integral dose | |

## INTRODUCTION

The purpose of this chapter is to overview radiation attenuation and absorption, describe the five types of x-ray/matter interactions as well as particulate radiation interactions with matter, and, finally, determine radiation dose to the patient. As in the last two chapters, the physics information is a review for those who have already have had a physics course and gives enough information so those who have not had a physics course can understand the interactions.

In the information text boxes in the chapter, atomic number vs. K-shell binding energies, electron density vs. Z numbers, and the apparent contradiction between energy levels and the number of interactions are discussed.

## BASIC CONCEPTS OF INTERACTION: ABSORPTION AND ATTENUATION

When x-ray or gamma photons in the primary beam pass through matter, they undergo *absorption* or *scatter,* both of which are methods of *attenuation,* or they do not interact at all. That is, a certain number of photons in the beam are absorbed (all the radiation energy is lost) or scattered (some of the radiation energy is lost) in the patient, and others pass through unaltered. Attenuation is the reduction in the number of photons as they pass through matter.

In the x-ray beam, the relationship among primary radiation, the remnant or exit radiation, and attenuation can be expressed mathematically as follows:

Primary radiation – Attenuation
    = Remnant or exit radiation

### Gamma Radiation

Gamma radiation is produced inside the nucleus of atoms and consequently is monoenergetic (gives off only one energy level) for a given source such as radium. This is unlike x-radiation which is polyenergetic. An analogy is characteristic x-radiation production, in which a photon produced in a given atomic shell is monoenergetic as each shell/atom gives off a different but distinct photon. This means that the photon is emitted with a single energy. In monoenergetic radiation, attenuation is an exponential process. That is, assuming an equal thickness of the same absorber, photons are reduced in number by a certain percentage for each increment of thickness passed through. For example, if 1 cm of tissue removes 50% of the beam, then 50% of the primary beam remains after 1 cm; after 2 cm of tissue, 25% remains; after 3 cm, 12.5% remains, and so on. This is illustrated in Figure 4–1. Recall, the half-value layer (HVL) is the amount of attenuator necessary to

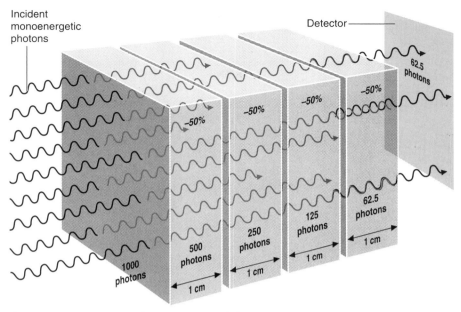

**Figure 4–1** Attenuation of a monoenergetic beam.

remove half of all the photons. With monoenergetic radiation the HVL of the beam is consistent no matter how much attenuation the beam has already passed through.

## X-Radiation

X-radiation is polyenergetic (photons with many different energies are emitted). Recall that x-rays are created by the interaction of high-speed electrons with a target material. Because these electrons lose their kinetic (motion) energy at different rates, the radiation produced is also of different energies. If 1 cm of an attenuator (say, bone) is the HVL for x-ray, it cannot be assumed that 2 cm of the same bone will form two HVLs. The percentage changes with each centimeter of tissue, as is shown in Figure 4–2. If we begin with 1000 photons and a mean energy of 50 kV, the first centimeter of tissue may reduce the number of photons by 30% to 700. This also increases the mean energy of the beam from 50 kV to 58 kV. This is similar to filtration of a tube, in which added thicknesses remove the lower energy photons and increase the average energy.

Another centimeter of tissue reduces the number of photons only by 23% to 539 and increases the average energy of the beam to 65 kV, and so forth. HVLs for diagnostic x-ray are shown in Figure 4–3 as 4 to 8 cm of tissue or about 3 to 5 cm of aluminum. If we begin again with 1000 photons with a mean energy of 50 kV, the first HVL of 4 cm of tissue removes 50% of the photons and increases the average energy to 58 kV. The second HVL (5.2 cm of tissue) again removes half of the remaining photons now leaving only 250 with an average energy of 69 kV, and so forth. Because the average energy, and consequently the penetration ability, of the beam increases as it passes through each successive HVL, it takes progressively thicker amounts of material to equal one HVL. However, after polyenergetic x-radiation passes through three to four HVLs, it is *functionally* monoenergetic at that point.

## General Concepts

Some photons will pass through matter and not interact. This is called *transmission*. Photons can interact with the entire atom, the nucleus, or

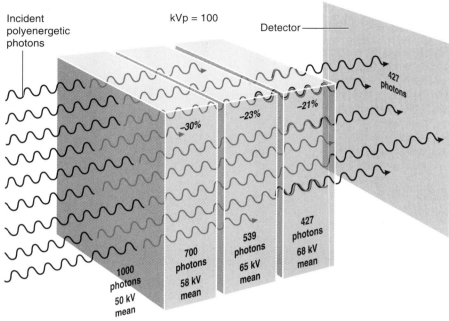

**Figure 4–2** A polyenergetic photon beam consists of high (H)–, medium (M)–, and low (L)–energy photons. As the beam passes through successive thicknesses of an absorber, more low- and medium-energy photons are removed from the beam, raising its average energy. It is also noted that as the average energy of the beam is raised, each successive thickness of the absorber attenuates less of the beam.

an orbital electron. A prime influencing factor is the energy of the x-ray photon. The photons with the lowest energies are likely to interact with the entire atom. Photons of middle energies usually interact with orbital electrons. These interactions are commonly seen in diagnostic x-rays and nuclear medicine. High-energy photons (e.g. those of MeV strength, as are seen in radiation therapy) interact with the nucleus. This is due to the fact that low-energy photons have a long wavelength, which is approximately equal to the size of a whole atom. As wavelength decreases, photons tend to interact with particles or groups of particles that match their wavelength in size.

As photons pass through matter, they transmit, scatter, or are absorbed. Thus, when a patient is irradiated, some x-rays pass through without interaction, some interact with the atom and transfer all their energy, and some interact with the atom and then lose some

energy while changing direction. This last process is called *scatter*. Photons that scatter continue on to again interact and scatter or be absorbed.

The atom was briefly reviewed in the previous chapter. An important concept of radiation interactions is the *binding energy* of the electron shells. K-shell electrons, which are the closest to the positively charged nucleus, possess the greatest force of attraction to the nucleus, or binding energy. The higher the atomic number of the element, the higher the binding energy of the electrons. Another concept that is important in the interaction of radiation and matter is that, although inner-shell electrons have a high binding energy, they have a low *potential energy*. Potential energy is the ability to do work and, for electrons, is relative to their position to the nucleus. This is similar to the idea that a rock on top of cliff has the ability to transfer a lot of energy if it

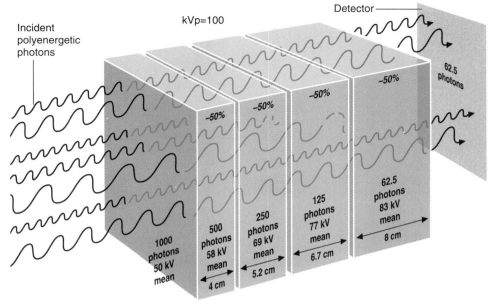

**Figure 4–3** As a polyenergetic beam passes through a series of absorbers, the average energy of the beam increases (see Figure 4–2). Consequently, each successive absorber must be thicker than the last in order to remove or absorb 50% of the remaining energy.

falls off but the same rock on a flat surface cannot fall and therefore cannot transfer energy. In atoms, the farther an electron is from the nucleus, the lower the binding energy and the higher the potential energy level.

Four factors affect attenuation. If the energy of the beam is increased (e.g. by increasing the kVp), more photons are transmitted. Thus, transmission is increased and attenuation is decreased with an increase in energy of the beam. Increasing the remaining three factors—*atomic density* (the amount of matter in a given area, which is closely related to Z number), atomic (Z) number, and electrons per gram—decreases transmission and increases attenuation.

There are five interactions of x-rays and gamma rays with matter:

- Photoelectric effect: very important in diagnostic radiology
- Compton scatter: very important in diagnostic radiology
- Coherent scatter: of little importance in diagnostic or therapeutic radiology
- Pair production: very important in therapeutic radiology
- Photodisintegration: important in therapeutic radiology

## PHOTOELECTRIC EFFECT

In the *photoelectric effect* (Figure 4–4), all of the energy of the incoming photon, usually referred to as the *incident photon,* is totally transferred to the atom. Following interaction, the photon no longer exists.

The incoming photon interacts with an orbital electron. This usually occurs in the innermost (K) shell but also occurs in the L- and M-shells. All of the photon's energy is transferred to the orbital electron, which causes that electron to be ejected from the atom. Because of the energy needed to overcome binding energy and eject the electron, the photon ceases to exist.

This is similar to a cue ball that hits another ball on a pool table, stops, and causes a target

***More Information:***
**Atomic Number and K-Shell Binding Energies for Elements Important in Radiology**

The atomic number and the K-edge binding energies (the amount of energy necessary to knock a K-shell electron out of orbit) follow. The atoms in soft tissues of the body are mostly carbon, oxygen, and hydrogen. The effective atomic (Z) number of human soft tissue about 7.4 and has a K-shell binding energy of approximately 0.5 keV. Magnesium, aluminum, copper, cadmium, and tin are used in filters. Magnesium has a Z number of 12 and a K-shell energy of 1.3 keV, aluminum has a Z number of 13 and a K-shell energy of 1.5 keV, copper has a Z number of 29 and a K-shell energy of 8.9 keV, cadmium has a Z number of 48 and a K-

shell energy of 26.7 keV, and tin has a Z number of 50 and a K-shell energy of 29.2 keV. Lead is used for shielding as well as in some filters. It has a Z number of 82 and a K-shell energy of 88.0 keV. Barium, used in GI and BE studies, has a Z number of 56 and a K-shell energy of 37.4 keV. Iodine, used in contrast studies of the kidneys and blood vessels has a Z number of 53 and a K-shell energy of 33.2 keV. Tungsten, used for target material in the x-ray tube, has a Z number of 74 and a K-shell binding energy of about 70 keV. The K-shell energy of tungsten is important in the production of characteristic radiation (discussed in Chapter 2).

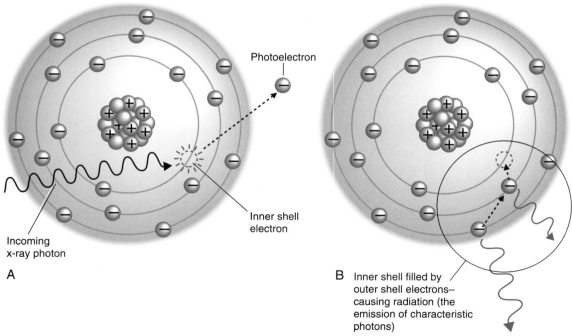

A

Photoelectron

Incoming
x-ray photon

Inner shell
electron

B  Inner shell filled by
outer shell electrons—
causing radiation (the
emission of characteristic
photons)

**Figure 4–4** Photoelectric effect.

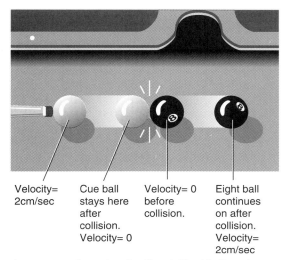

Velocity= 2cm/sec

Cue ball stays here after collision. Velocity= 0

Velocity= 0 before collision.

Eight ball continues on after collision. Velocity= 2cm/sec

**Figure 4–5** Photoelectric effect billiard ball analogy.

ball to move forward in the same direction and at the same approximate velocity of the cue ball (Figure 4–5).

The formula for the photoelectric effect is as follows:

---

Incident photon energy = Kinetic energy of the photoelectron + Binding energy, or

$$E_i = E_{ke} + E_b$$

---

**EXAMPLE**

If a 10 keV photon interacts with an electron with a binding energy (K-shell) of 9 keV, the kinetic energy of the photoelectron is:

$$10 - 9 = 1 \text{ keV}$$

---

Two basic rules about photoelectric interactions must be remembered:

1. Photoelectric interactions are more likely to occur if the x-ray photon's energy is greater than, but close to, the binding energy of the electron. Thus, a 38-keV photon is more likely to interact with an atom of barium used in contrast material (binding energy of the innermost shell of approximately 37 keV) than is a 100-keV photon. The probability of a photoelectric interaction decreases by the cube of the difference between the binding and photon energy. For example, if a 47-keV photon interacts with a barium atom, the difference between the two energies is $10^3 = 1000$, so the probability of a photoelectric interaction decreases by 1000 times.

   This may seem to go against what students have learned about using a high kVp for contrast studies involving barium, but consider that photon energy is emitted polyenergetically (with many energies) from the x-ray tube. The most common energies from a tube are emitted with about one third of the maximum energy (kVp). Thus, a 110-kVp setting will produce the greatest number of photons with energies of around 37 keV, with the average energy being about 44 keV. (Note: These numbers vary with the generator and tube type.) Thus, if 110 kVp is used, a much higher percentage of the photons will interact photoelectrically than at any other kVp setting.

2. Photoelectric interactions have a greater likelihood of occurrence when the electron is more tightly bound in its orbit. This is the basis for using lead aprons as a means of protection. Few x-ray photons possess sufficient energy to interact with the K-shell of lead, which has a binding energy of 88 keV. Most photons lose their energy through photoelectric interactions in the L- and M-shells of lead.

The likelihood of photoelectric interaction is approximately $Z^3$. Thus, if the atomic number is doubled, the likelihood of photoelectric interactions increases by a factor of 8 ($2^3 = 2 \times 2 \times 2 = 8$) because there are more total electrons with energies in the photon energy range when the L- and M-shells are considered. This can also be calculated in the form of a ratio:

$$\frac{Z^3 \text{ of second material}}{Z^3 \text{ of first material}} = \begin{array}{l} \text{Relative probability} \\ \text{of interaction of} \\ \text{second material.} \end{array}$$

This assumes that the conditions of rule #1 have been met.

This is also the basis for orthopedic radiography. Since bone has an higher effective Z number than soft tissue, photoelectric interaction is more likely to occur in bone than soft tissue. This is why bone tends to appear white and soft tissue gray on a radiograph. Bone has an atomic number about double that of soft tissue, so photoelectric interaction is about eight times more likely to occur in bone than in soft tissue.

In any interaction, such as a photoelectric one, the loss of an electron causes the atom to become ionized and have a positively charge. The atom (minus its electron) and the electron (minus its atom) are now known as an *ion pair*. Electrons ejected by the photoelectric process are known as *photoelectrons* or *recoil electrons*. Recoil electrons are absorbed within a few millimeters of soft tissue. What is important to remember is that, even though the ion is quickly absorbed, it will have interacted with the orbital electrons of other atoms. One photoelectric interaction causes many more ion pairs to be formed. For example, it takes about 34 eV to form one ion pair. With an initial kinetic energy of 68 keV (68,000 eV), a photoelectron causes 2000 more ion pairs to be formed (68,000 ÷ 34 = 2000). It is also important to remember how this process works in later chapters on the production of biologic effects, as the ionization process is important in creating biologic changes in tissue.

As the electron tries to reach equilibrium by refilling an empty K- or L-shell by moving electrons from orbits farther out, the kinetic energy of electrons gained as they "fall" from the outer to the inner orbit is given off as a form of characteristic radiation. This is due to the fact mentioned earlier that electrons more distant from the nucleus have a higher level of potential energy than those close to the nucleus. When the electron moves closer to the nucleus, the potential (position) energy is transformed into kinetic (motion) energy. This kinetic energy must be given off in the form of x-radiation when the electron is captured by the lower shell.

This shell-to-shell process is called a *characteristic cascade* (Figure 4–6). The energy of each photon produced is the difference in energy between the two shells. These characteristic photons are also called *secondary radiation*. This radiation is is called *secondary* because it is radiation other than that produced by the primary beam. Many other sources refer to secondary radiation and scatter radiation as *scatter* since secondary radiation behaves like scatter and has the same effect as scatter.

## COMPTON SCATTERING

*Compton scatter* production (Figure 4–7) is a process in which a photon is partially absorbed by an outer-shell electron, the electron absorbs enough energy to break the binding energy bond, and it is ejected while the remaining photon energy exits the atom. The ejected electron is called a *Compton* or *recoil electron*. The reason only part of the photon is absorbed is that the binding energy of outer orbital electrons is very low and not much energy is needed to release them from the binding-energy bond. The photon, now less energetic and more apt to be absorbed, continues on in a different direction as scatter radiation. Continuing the cue ball analogy, in this case the cue ball strikes a ball off-center so that the cue ball and the billiard ball move off in different directions (Figure 4–8). Thus, energy is shared rather than totally absorbed.

The formula for Compton scatter is:

Incident photon energy = Compton scatter photon energy + (Binding energy of orbital electron + Kinetic energy of Compton electron), or

$$E_i = E_s + (E_b + E_{ke})$$

The Compton photon has less energy than the incident photon, as just seen, as well as having a longer wavelength and lower frequency. This make it very likely that it will interact with another atom because, as the energy level goes down, the penetration ability of the photon also

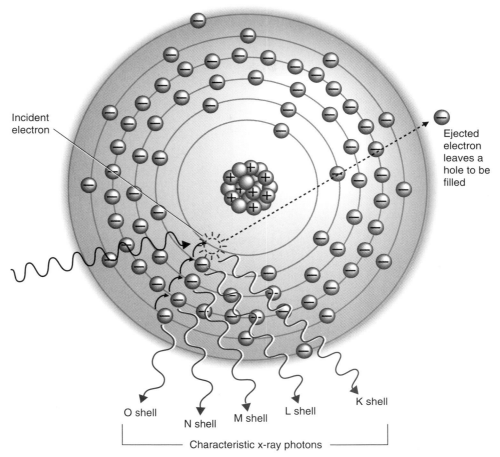

Incident electron

Ejected electron leaves a hole to be filled

O shell

N shell

M shell

L shell

K shell

Characteristic x-ray photons

**Figure 4–6** Example of characteristic cascade. Electrons have the ability to fall from any shell to any other shell, for example, O shell to L shell.

goes down. It becomes likely that the photon will ionize another atom. If the Compton photon exits the patient, one possible outcome is that it may reach the x-ray film and create scatter fog. Another possible outcome is that it may strike the radiographer. Scatter radiation is the primary source of occupational exposure for radiographers.

The amount of energy lost or retained depends on the initial photon energy and the angle of deflection. The angle of scatter can range from just above 0 (straight ahead) to 180 degrees (moving back the direction of the incident photon). Scatter deflected at a 180-degree angle is called *backscatter*. In diagnostic radiol-

**EXAMPLE**

If a 40-keV x-ray ionizes an atom of carbon, ejecting an O-shell (binding energy of 0.01) electron with 20 keV of kinetic energy, what is the energy of the scattered (Compton) photon?

$$40 = x + (0.01 + 20)$$
$$40 = x + 20.01$$

Subtract 20.01 from each side and x = 19.99; energy of Compton photon is 19.99 keV.

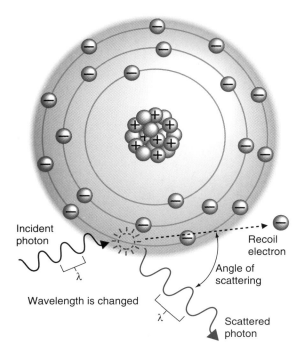

**Figure 4–7** Compton scatter.

Incident photon

λ

Wavelength is changed

λ

Recoil electron

Angle of scattering

Scattered photon

ogy, most scatter produced is forward rather than backscatter.

The Compton or recoil electron ionizes other atoms in the same manner as previously discussed under "Photoelectric Effect." Again, this is of importance in the biologic interactions between radiation and tissue.

In opposition to photoelectric effect, the probability of Compton scatter increases as photon energy increases. This is true only for x-ray energies in the diagnostic range (from around 20 to 150 keV). After 500 keV, the probability of Compton scatter decreases with an increase in photon energy. It must also be stated that the probability of interaction refers to the total percentage of interactions and not the total number of interactions, which tend to go down as the energy level goes up. Thus, at 50 kVp, the probability of scatter through Compton or coherent as opposed to photoelectric is about even at 50% of both categories. At 90 kVp, about 67% of interactions are Compton or coherent; 33% are photoelectric.

Compton scatter is also more prominent with greater electron densities. Elements with low Z numbers tend to have a high electron density, or compactness of electrons. Compton probability is increased for materials containing large amounts of hydrogen, such as soft tissue. As the

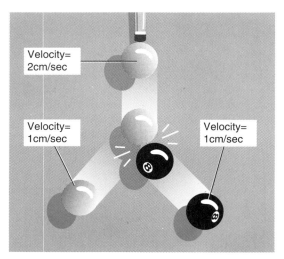

Velocity= 2cm/sec

Velocity= 1cm/sec

Velocity= 1cm/sec

**Figure 4–8** Compton scatter—billiard ball analogy.

Z number increases, the probability of Compton scatter decreases. See "More Information: Electron Density and Z Numbers."

## COHERENT SCATTERING

*Coherent scattering* (Figure 4–9), also called classic, Rayleigh, or Thompson scattering, occurs primarily with low-energy x-rays (below 10 keV). The photon causes *excitation* (an increase in the overall energy of an atom) rather than ionization of the target atom. This excess energy is given off as scatter in a different, but usually forward, direction in the form of an x-ray photon. The exiting photon has the same energy and wavelength as the incident photon and is considered by some to be the exact same photon. This interaction makes up only a small portion of the scattering that occurs in diagnostic radiology, as filters remove most of the radiation energy below 10 keV. Seeram reports that only about 5% of all interactions in diagnostic radiology are coherent in nature.

The formula for coherent scatter is:

Incident photon energy = Scatter photon energy, or

$$E_i = E_s$$

---

### More Information:
### Electron Density and Z Numbers

As stated in the text, the density of electrons is higher in atoms with fewer electrons (low Z number) such as oxygen or hydrogen. On the surface, this seems to be a contradiction. However, it is true. The reason that it is true has to do with the physical makeup of an atom. On average, more than 99.999% of the volume of an atom is empty space. Now, the trick here is the term *average*. The relative distance from the center of a hydrogen atom to the outermost electron (which, by the way is in the K-shell) is very, very much smaller than the relative distance from the center to the outermost electron in a uranium atom, in which those electrons are in the O-shell. Not only that, but the center–to–K-shell distance in hydrogen is less than the center–to–K-shell distance in uranium. What all that means is that even though there are more electrons in the uranium atom, they take up much more space per electron than does a hydrogen atom. In other words, the electron density of hydrogen is greater than the electron density of uranium.

An analogy would be the population of the United States compared to the population of the United Kingdom (England, Scotland, Wales, and Northern Ireland). According to 1996 figures, the United States had a population of 263.8 million and the United Kingdom has a population of 58.3 million. From those figures, it is apparent the United States has five time as many people and it might appear that the population density of the United States would be greater than that of the United Kingdom. However, the United States is a very large country, and its population density is only 72 people per square mile, whereas the United Kingdom is a small collection of islands with a population density of 619 people per square mile. Similarly, the number of electrons in low-Z-number atoms is small, but they are in a much smaller space, giving them a higher electron density.

In general, the higher the Z number, the lower the electron density and the less likely that element is to have a Compton interaction.

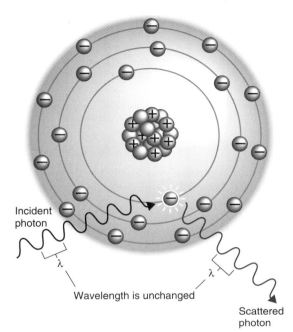

Incident photon

λ

Wavelength is unchanged

λ

Scattered photon

**Figure 4–9** Coherent scatter. The incident photon is momentarily absorbed by the atom and then is released with no change in energy but usually a change in direction.

## PAIR PRODUCTION AND PHOTODISINTEGRATION

### Pair Production

For *pair production* to occur (Figure 4–10), the incoming photon must have an energy of above 1.02 MeV. Even though the minimum energy necessary is 1.02 MeV, this interaction does not occur significantly until an energy of 10 MeV has been reached. This interaction is a good example of the conversion of energy into matter and matter back into energy: The photon approaches and interacts with the nucleus of an atom. The energy of the photon is then converted into two particles according to Einstein's formula, $E = mc^2$.

Two electrons are produced with this interaction. One has a negative charge and is called a *negatron*. It is readily absorbed by other atoms. The other particle is a positive electron, or

*positron*. Positrons are a form of antimatter and do not exist freely in nature. Positrons cannot exist near matter and will interact very quickly with the first electron they encounter. They interact with and destroy each other while converting all their matter back into energy in the process. Both particles disappear, releasing two photons with an energy of 0.51 meV. This is known as an *annihilation reaction*. These gamma photons then further interact with matter through either pair production or Compton scatter. As Z number increases, the probability of pair production increases.

The formula for pair production is as follows:

---

Incident electron energy = Energy in the mass of a negatron + Energy in the mass of a positron = Secondary photon energy + Secondary photon energy, or

$$E_i = E_{e-} + E_{e+} = E_s + E_s$$

---

### Photodisintegration

Photodisintegration (Figure 4–11) occurs above 10 MeV. In photodisintegration, a high-energy photon (as is found in radiation therapy) is absorbed by the nucleus. The nucleus undergoes excitation and becomes radioactive. To become stable again, the nucleus emits neutrons, protons, alpha particles, clusters of fragments and/or gamma rays.

The formula for photodisintegration is as follows:

---

Incident photon energy = Binding energy + Binding energy + ⋯ + Secondary photon + Secondary photon + ⋯ + Kinetic energy of particles + Kinetic energy of particles + ⋯ , or

$$E_i = E_b + E_b + \cdots + E_s + E_s + \cdots + E_{ke} + E_{ke} + \cdots$$

---

A summary of the five interactions is given in Table 4–1.

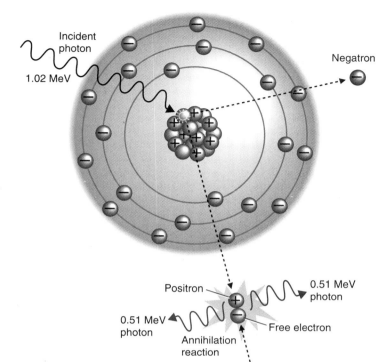

Figure 4–10 Pair production.

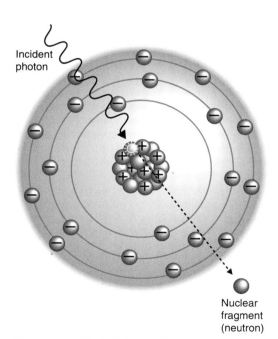

**Figure 4–11** Photodisintegration.

## INTERACTIONS OF PARTICULATE RADIATION WITH MATTER

Alpha radiation is monoenergetic; beta particles and positrons are polyenergetic. In general, charged particles such as alpha and beta particles and positrons tend to lose energy in matter through the production of ion pairs. Particles pass near or through a neutral atom and remove electrons through a force of attraction (if the particle is positive) or repulsion (if the particle is negative). This is illustrated in Figure 4–12.

The two main types of interactions of charged particles with matter are elastic and inelastic. In an *elastic interaction,* there is no change in the total kinetic energy of the interacting particles, as the kinetic energy is just transferred from one particle to another. With an *inelastic interaction,* however, the total kinetic energy is changed after the interaction because some of the kinetic energy is transformed into other types of energy such as x-rays.

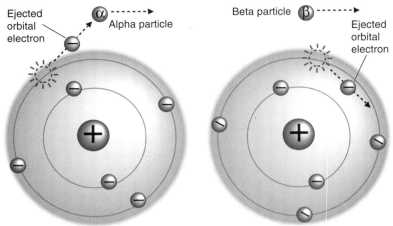

**Figure 4–12** Interactions of particulate radiations with matter. Alpha particles ionize by attracting an electron from the atom. Beta particles ionize by repelling an electron away from the atom. (Reprinted with permission from Thompson MA, Hall J, Hattaway P, Dowd S: Principles of Imaging Science and Protection. Philadelphia, WB Saunders, 1994.)

An example of an elastic interaction is alpha particles colliding with outer-shell orbital electrons. Although kinetic energy may have transferred as the alpha particle slows down and the electron speeds up, no kinetic energy is lost.

An example of an inelastic interaction is a beta particle interacting with an inner-orbit electron and slowing down. In this example, the inelastic process is known as *bremsstrahlung* and is similar to x-rays being produced inside an x-ray tube when electrons are slowed down and some of the kinetic energy is transformed into x-rays. It is for this reason that low-z-number materials such as plastic wood and cardboard are preferred for shielding from beta particles, as the interactions between the inner-shell electrons and the beta are weak and rarely produce x-rays. High-Z-number materials such as lead would produce x-rays because the interaction would be strong enough to significantly slow the beta particle.

## LINEAR ENERGY TRANSFER AND SPECIFIC IONIZATION

Two other important concepts to consider are *linear energy transfer* (LET) and *specific ionization* (SI; not to be confused with Système International units). LET is used extensively in radiobiology and focuses on the radiation absorption rate of an attenuator. SI is closely related to LET but is used when the focus of interest is the rate of energy loss by radiation. Specifically, LET is the rate at which energy is deposited in the form of a charged particle or ion pairs as it travels through matter. The number of ion pairs produced per unit of distance traveled (such as 1 cm) is known as the specific ionization (SI).

The unit for LET is keV/μm, the amount of energy (keV) transferred per unit path (μm). As stated before, LET and SI are closely related. As LET increases, the SI (number of ionizations per distance) also increases. X-radiation and gamma radiation are considered to be low-LET/low-SI radiations because they are very penetrating, do not give up energy quickly, do not cause a high rate of ionizations per centimeter, and do relatively little biologic damage. High-LET/high-SI radiations such as alpha and beta radiation do not penetrate very well, give up energy quickly, cause a large number of ionizations per centimeter, and cause greater amounts of damage. Thus, alpha and beta particles have a high LET and high SI; x-radiation and gamma radiation have a low LET and low SI. The relationship between LET, number of ionizations, and penetration

**Table 4–1** Photon/Matter Interactions Chart

| Name | Energy Level | Description | Secondary or Scatter | Where Important | Interaction |
|---|---|---|---|---|---|
| Classical, Thompson, Coherent | Under 10 KeV | Photon of low energy interacts with total atom. Atom absorbs photon and becomes excited. Atom gives off photon with same wavelength and energy. | Scatter | Not important | $E_i = E_s$ |
| Compton | Through diagnostic range | Photon interacts with outer-shell electron. Electron is ejected. Photon continues on with less energy, usually in different direction. Significant as major source of fog on film, patient dose, and technologist dose. | Scatter | Diagnostic radiology | $E_i = (E_b + E_{ke}) + E_s$ |
| Photoelectric | Through diagnostic range; must be about equal to or above binding energy. | Photon interacts with inner shell electron (usually K-shell). Ejects electron from K- or L-shell. Resultant cascading emits characteristic radiation. Significant because bone has more interactions then soft tissue, resulting in differential absorption. | Secondary | Diagnostic radiology | $E_i = (E_b + E_{ke})$ |
| Pair Production | 1.02 MeV; not significant below 10 MeV. | Photon interacts with nuclear field and converts energy into one electron and one positron. Positron quickly interacts with available electron with mutual inhalation resulting, giving off 1.02 MeV of energy in multiple photons | Secondary | Radiation therapy | $E_i = E_{e-} + E_{e+}$ $= + E_s + E_s$ |
| Photodisintegration | Over 10 MeV | Photon interacts with nucleus of atom. Nuclear field is disrupted by photon energy and nucleus is disassembled. Nuclear fragments are created and move away. | Secondary | Radiation therapy | $E_i = E_b + E_b + \cdots$ $+ E_s + E_s + \cdots$ $+ E_{ke} + E_{ke} \cdots$ |

of soft tissue is shown graphically in Figure 4–13.

As discussed in Chapter 3, we need a radiologic unit that allows us to compare the effects of all types of ionizing radiation on humans. This unit was described as the *rem*. Table 4–2 summarizes the relationship between SI, average LET, and the QF used to calculate rem from rad.

X-radiation, gamma radiation, and beta radiation with LETs of below 3 have QFs of 1, which means that all three do approximately the same damage rad per rad. The SI for x-radiation and gamma radiation is 1. The SI for beta radiation is 100. As this indicates, beta will cause about 100 times more ionizations per millimeter than either x- or gamma radiation. This does not

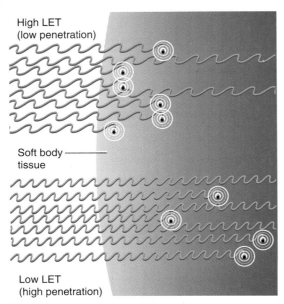

**Figure 4–13** Illustration of the number of ionizations and of penetration in soft tissue of high-penetration (low-LET) vs. low-penetration (high-LET) radiation.

mean that beta radiation has more energy than x-rays, beta particles just lose their energy into the tissue faster. Alpha radiation has an SI of 2500 and a QF of 10. That means that alpha radiation does about ten times as much damage rad per rad than x-rays and also cause about 2500 times more ionization per millimeter. Understanding the relationship between the number of ionizations produced is important in later understanding of biologic effects.

**Table 4–2** Relationship Between Specific Ionization (SI), Linear Energy Transfer (LET), and Quality Factor (QF)

| Average SI | Average LET | QF |
|---|---|---|
| ≤100 | ≤3.5 | 1 |
| 100–200 | 3.5–7.0 | 1–2 |
| 200–650 | 7.0–23 | 2–5 |
| 650–1500 | 23–53 | 5–10 |
| 1500–5000 | 53–175 | 10–20 |

## DETERMINING RADIATION DOSE

### X-Ray Exposure

In Chapter 3 we discussed the units used to determine radiation exposure and dose. Dose refers to the amount of radiation absorbed by the patient. However, calculating the radiation dose to the patient from an amount of radiation produced is a complex process. It is not difficult to determine the dose in air or the skin; it is much more difficult to calculate the dose to a specific organ. This will vary based on attenuation, absorption, and the production of scatter. See Figure 4–14 for an illustration of the difficulties involved. Dose to the patient from x-ray examinations is measured by one of five methods, which are illustrated in Figure 4–15.

*Skin dose* is an actual measure of radiation received by a portion of the patient's skin (Figure 4–15A). In the diagnostic range, this represents the maximum dose that any tissue will receive during this exposure. For this reason and because it is the easiest to measure, skin dose is used most often. TLDs are usually used to make the measurement and can be taped onto the patient's skin in the center of the beam. Radiographers should be familiar with common skin doses of procedures. These are

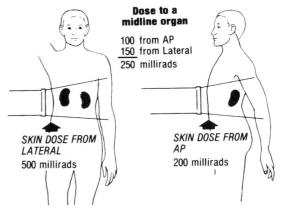

**Figure 4–14** Difficulty in measuring dose—anteroposterior and lateral x-ray projections. (Reprinted with permission from Whalen JP, Balter S: Radiation Risks in Medical Imaging. Chicago, Mosby-Year Book, 1984, Fig. 3–2.)

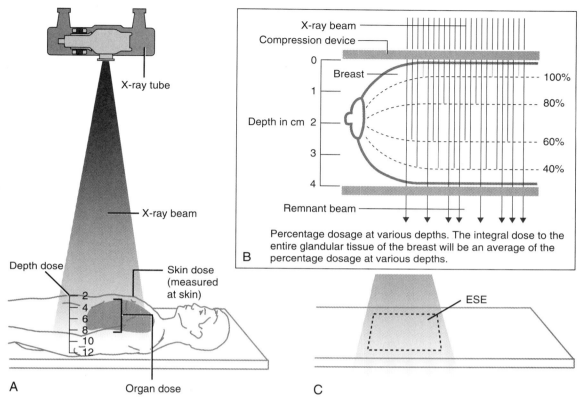

**A**

**B** Percentage dosage at various depths. The integral dose to the entire glandular tissue of the breast will be an average of the percentage dosage at various depths.

**C**

**Figure 4–15** Illustration of means of determining dose. Integral = dose to breast from mammography.

given in Chapter 11, although they vary somewhat between facilities. Students interested in more exact numbers should contact the radiation safety officer or medical radiation physicist at their affiliate institution for more accurate numbers.

*Entrance skin exposure* (ESE) is an estimated value used by some governmental agencies to regulate diagnostic x-ray exposures. It is determined without a patient or phantom by using the technical factors and geometry of an exposure such as body part, filtration, or SID (Figure 4–15C).

*Depth dose* measures the percentage of skin dose found at a certain depth within a patient. Because tissue acts as an attenuator, the deeper radiation passes into tissue, the fewer photons there will be left. Depth dose will be a certain fraction of the skin dose (Figure 4–15B).

*Organ dose* is the dose received by a particular organ. Because organs are not uniform in size, shape, and density, the dose to each part of an organ will differ. The *average dose* to the irradiated volume is a similar concept that averages the dose received by each portion of tissue contained within the x-ray beam. This is sometimes used instead of organ dose (Fig. 4–15A).

*Integral dose* refers to the total amount of energy absorbed by a specific mass of tissue. This may be an organ, a volume of tissue, or the entire patient (Figure 4–15A). Other examples of dose include the *mean marrow dose* (the dose to the entire bone marrow), the *gonadal dose,* the *glandular dose* in mammography, and the *cumulative dose* (all exposures received added together). According to Bushong (1982), bone marrow dose is an average of the dose received by the active bone marrow. Thus, if a dose of 20 mrad is received by 50% of the active bone marrow, the bone marrow dose is 10 mrad.

## Calculating X-Ray Exposure

The primary factor determining patient dose in radiography is the output intensity from the tube. This same factor is used to calculate the ESE. Output intensity varies directly with mAs, directly with the square of the kVp, and inversely with the square of distance from the focal spot. The formula for this is:

$$\text{Output intensity} = \frac{K(mAs)kVp^2}{d^2}$$

K is a constant determined by the characteristics of the x-ray tube. The measurement of K is taken at 70 kVp and 100 cm (40 inches). Bushong (1982) shows how this formula can be adapted to determine new intensities. Once K is known:

Output intensity (mR)
$$= K(mR/mAs) \ (mAs_2)\left(\frac{kVp_2}{70}\right)\left(\frac{100\ cm}{d_2}\right)$$

K = measured value at 70 kVp and 100 cm

$mAs_2$ = new technique

$kVp_2$ = new technique

$d_2$ = new SID

*SID* stands for source to image receptor distance, or the distance from the focal spot of the anode to the film (historically called the FFD).

### EXAMPLE

The calculated value for K is 25 mR/mAs at 70 kVp and 100 cm (40 inches) SID. For a abdomen, 40 mAs and 75 kVp are used. What is the intensity?

Output intensity (mR) = (25 mR/mAs)

$$(40\ mAs_2)\left(\frac{75}{70}\right)^2\left(\frac{100\ cm}{100\ cm}\right)$$

$$= 229.6\ mR$$

Further applications of this formula are described in Appendix A. We will also discuss three further applications of portions of this formula in Chapters 10 and 11—determining intensity with a change in distance, determining intensity with a change in mAs, and determining intensity with a change in kVp.

## Exposure from Radionuclides

To calculate the radiation dose from a radioactive substance in the body, five factors must be known:

* The amount of the radionuclide in curies
* The physical half-life of the radionuclide
* The mixture of radiation, such as alpha, beta, and emitted
* The fraction of the substance in each organ of the body, also called the *biodistribution*
* The *biologic half-life* of the material (the length of time the substance remains in each organ of the body)

This process is obviously complex. In most cases, dose can only be estimated and is well beyond the scope of this text.

## SUMMARY

When x-ray and gamma photons pass through matter, they may be absorbed, attenuated, or transmitted. *Attenuation* refers to the reduction in the number of photons as they pass through matter. *Transmission* describes that portion of the beam that passes through matter with no interactions.

The five interactions of x-rays and gamma rays with matter are photoelectric effect, coherent scatter, Compton scatter, pair production, and photodisintegration. The photoelectric effect and Compton scatter are the most common effects seen in diagnostic imaging, with coherent scatter occurring only at very low energies. Pair production and photodisintegration are seen with high-energy photons only.

Charged particles tend to lose energy in matter through the production of ion pairs. The two main types of interactions of charged particles with matter are elastic and inelastic.

Linear energy transfer (LET) is the rate at which energy is deposited in the form of a charged particle as radiation travels through matter. The unit for LET is keV/mm. X-radiation and gamma radiation are low-LET radiations; alpha and beta radiations are considered to be of high LET. Specific ionization (SI) is the number of ion pairs produced per unit of distance traveled. LET, SI, and the quality factor (QF) used for calculating the rem from the rad are interrelated.

Five methods are used to calculate patient dose from x-ray exposures: skin dose, entrance skin exposure (ESE), depth dose, organ dose, and integral dose. For exposure from radionuclides, five factors must be known to calculate dose: (1) the amount of the radionuclide in curies, (2) the physical half-life of the radionuclide, (3) the mixture of radiation emitted, (4) the biodistribution, and (5) the biologic half-life of the material.

---

## More Information:
## Energy Levels and the Number of Interactions. A Contradiction?

Recall from an earlier discussion in the text about increases in the energy of the beam (peak kilovoltage [kVp]) that:

1. As energy (kVp) increases, photoelectric effect decreases *greatly*.
2. As energy (kVp) increases, the percentage of Compton interactions decreases *slightly*.

Therefore, as kVp goes up, *fewer* scatter photons are created.

Also, recall from other texts or from your own experience that as the kVp goes up, more scatter is recorded on the film. Therefore, as the kVp goes up, we see *more* impact from Compton interactions.

Is this a contradiction? Surprisingly, no. Consider the hypothetical numbers* given below.

The total number of interactions has decreased. An increase in kVp has increased Compton scatter proportionally to photoelectric effect. However, there has been a decrease in the number of each type of interaction and the total number of interactions. Radiographers loosely use the term *increased scatter* to refer to the *increased appearance of scatter fog* on a radiograph. In actuality, as the kVp increases, fewer interactions occur, and therefore less scatter is creased. However, the scatter that is created has higher energy and is more likely to reach the film than to interact with the patient's body. This makes increased kVp a radiation protection tool that must be counterbalanced with image-quality concerns.

*These do not represent actual number of interactions but are provided as a point of clarification. Small numbers are used to facilitate understanding of the concept.

| kVp | Total Number of Interactions in 1 mm of Tissue | Number of Compton/Coherent Interactions | Number of Photoelectric Effects |
|-----|------------------------------------------------|-----------------------------------------|---------------------------------|
| 50  | 1000                                           | 500 (50%)                               | 500 (50%)                       |
| 90  | 500                                            | 335 (67%)                               | 165 (33%)                       |

## More Information:
## Other Types of Radiation

Radiologic technology students tend to be practical individuals who want to learn what they need to know to perform well at their chosen profession. Sometimes, learning about other types of radiation seems superfluous to students. Since they will not be using that type of radiation, it seems unnecessary to learn it.

However, it is important that, as educated professionals, technologists know about all types of radiation. There are several reasons why. First, technologists should be willing, according to their code of ethics, to educate other individuals, such as patients, other health care workers, and the general public about radiation, its potential benefits, and its potential hazards. To do this, technologists must have a basic understanding of other types of radiation.

For example, a nurse might ask a radiographer a question about a patient undergoing I-131 therapy. Compare the following responses:

1. I don't know. You had better call nuclear medicine.
2. I work only with x-ray and that's what I know the most about. I do know, however, that I-131 is a radioisotope that emits two different types of radiation, beta and gamma. Gamma is similar to x-ray, and the best protection from this type of radiation is combining time, distance, and shielding. If you need to know more, talk to a nuclear medicine technologist or the radiation safety officer.

Both of these statements indicate that the radiographer does not have a strong knowledge about other types of radiation, but the first statement is so negative that the radiographer appears less educated and less professional. The second statement is positive but does not give the pretense of great knowledge. Don't make up what you don't know, and don't be afraid to say "I don't know," but do it in a way that doesn't minimize your profession.

Second, technologists should have a basic understanding of imaging and therapeutic uses of radiation other than what they use on a daily basis. Also, in some smaller institutions, a technologist may be asked to serve as a radiation safety officer. This individual must understand all types of radiation, their interactions, and the potential hazards associated with radiation.

Finally, many state regulations call for a nuclear medicine technologist to be present in the hospital emergency department if a radiation accident victim is brought to the hospital. If the hospital does not employ a nuclear medicine technologist or one is not present, the usual backup is a radiographer. This is similar to the amount of knowledge a radiography student must have about x-ray equipment. Again, one sometimes hears the statement from students, "I'm going to be running the equipment, not fixing it!" Students do not learn nearly as much about equipment as repair personnel do. Instead, they need to know how to explain a suspected malfunction to the supervising technologist or service representative. Students learn about other types of radiation to better understand radiation.

## Questions

1. Which of the following are polyenergetic for a given atom?

I. x-radiation
II. gamma radiation
III. beta radiation

a. I and II only
b. I and III only
c. II and III only
d. I, II, and III

222.

2. The half-value layer of gamma radiation from a given atom is the same, no matter how many thicknesses of material the radiation has passed through.

   a. true
   b. false

3. If the initial energy of a beam is 51 keV, then _____ ion pairs are produced with a photoelectric effect.

   a. 1000
   b. 1500
   c. 2000
   d. 3000

4. The rate at which energy is deposited in matter describes:

   a. linear energy transfer.
   b. specific ionization.
   c. relative biologic effect.
   d. quality factor.

5. As Z number increases, the probability of Compton scatter

   a. increases.
   b. decreases.
   c. does not change.

6. Which of the following measures of patient dose is most often used?

   a. organ dose
   b. skin dose
   c. entrance skin exposure
   d. depth dose

7. When electrons strive to fill shells and give off x-rays in the process, it is known as:

   a. pair production.
   b. photodisintegration.
   c. coherent scatter.
   d. characteristic cascade.

8. Which of the following causes excitation rather than ionization?

   a. photoelectric effect
   b. Compton scatter
   c. coherent scatter
   d. photodisintegration

9. Which of the following is most likely an outer-orbit interaction?

   a. photoelectric effect
   b. Compton scatter
   c. coherent scatter
   d. photodisintegration

10. Which of the following is the basis for using lead aprons?

    a. photoelectric effect
    b. Compton scatter
    c. coherent scatter
    d. photodisintegration

## Exercises

1. Compare LET, SI, and QF.

2. Why is high kVp used with contrast studies such as barium enemas?

3. Compare absorption, attenuation, and transmission.

4. Describe how increases in energy affect Compton scattering.

5. Describe monoenergetic and polyenergetic radiation, and how they relate to attenuation.

## Answers

Questions

| | |
|---|---|
| 1. b | 6. b |
| 2. a | 7. d |
| 3. b | 8. c |
| 4. a | 9. b |
| 5. b | 10. a |

Exercises

1. LET stands for linear energy transfer, the rate of absorption in tissue. The number of ion pairs produced per unit of distance traveled is specific ionization, or SI. Quality factor (QF) is the multiplier for rad to rem conversions. Increases in LET and SI are associated with increases in QF.

2. High kVp (100 and above) produces beams with energies close to the binding energy of the innermost shell of barium. This promotes the production of the photoelectric effect and maximizes contrast.

3. With absorption, photons no longer exist. Attenuation is the reduction in the number

of photons as they pass through matter. This can be due to absorption or deflection of the beam. Transmission describes the portion of the primary beam that passes through the patient in x-ray. This is also called the *remnant beam*. In the x-ray beam, the relationship between primary radiation, the remnant beam, and attenuation can be expressed mathematically as:

Primary – Remnant = Attenuation

4. Increases in energy increase the relative probability of Compton scatter over photoelectric effect. Numerically, scatter interactions decrease as photon energy increases, but there is an appearance of greater scatter on an x-ray film as more scatter reaches the film.

5. *Monoenergetic* refers to radiations emitted with one energy. *Polyenergetic* refers to radiations emitted with many energies, or from 0 to maximum. Monoenergetic radiations have a consistent half-value layer (HVL) and thus a consistent absorption percentage in tissue. Polyenergetic radiations have varying HVLs and do not have a consistent absorption percentage in tissue.

## CHAPTER 5

# Cellular Biology and History of Radiobiology

Steven B. Dowd • Elwin R. Tilson

## Chapter Outline

I. The Cell
  A. Properties of a Cell
  B. Chemical Components of the Cell
    1. Proteins
    2. Lipids
    3. Carbohydrates
    4. Nucleic Acids
  C. Cell Structure
    1. Nucleus
    2. Cytoplasm
  D. Cell Division and the Cell Cycle
    1. Somatic Cells
    2. Germ Cells
    3. Malignant Cells
II. History of Radiobiology and Protection
  A. Discovery of Radiation and Radioactivity
  B. Law of Bergonie and Tribondeau
III. Summary

## Chapter Objectives

At the end of this chapter, the student should be able to:

1. List the properties of the cell.
2. Discuss the chemical components of the cell.
3. List the parts of the cell.
4. Name the main function of each organelle.
5. Outline the structure and function of DNA.
6. List the types of RNA with their functions.
7. Describe the steps of mitosis.
8. Contrast meiosis with mitosis.
9. Differentiate normal and malignant cells.

## Important Terms

adenine
agranular
alleles
amino acid
anabolism
anaphase
autosome
biology
catabolic
catabolism
catalysts
centromere
chromatid
chromosome

| | |
|---|---|
| cytoplasm | mitotic |
| cytosine | monomers |
| deoxyribonucleic acid (DNA) | monosaccharide |
| diploid number | nuclear envelope or membrane |
| direct effects | nuclear pores |
| disaccharides | nucleolus |
| dominant | nucleus |
| double helix | oncogene |
| *Drosophila* | organelles |
| endoplasmic reticulum | organic |
| enzymes | organism |
| extrapolation | organs |
| fat | osmotic pressure |
| fractionation | polymers |
| $G_1$ | polysaccharide |
| $G_2$ | prophase |
| gametes | protoplasm |
| genes | purine |
| germ cell | radioactivity |
| Golgi apparatus | radiobiology |
| granular | radiologic physics |
| guanine | radiosensitive |
| haploid number | radiosensitivity |
| heterozygous | radioresistant |
| homozygous | radiounique |
| indirect effects | recessive |
| inorganic compounds | ribonucleic acid (RNA) |
| interphase | ribosomal RNA (rRNA) |
| isomotic | ribosomes |
| isotonic | roentgen martyrs |
| Law of Bergonie and Tribondeau | rough ER |
| lysosome | S-phase |
| macromolecule | selectively permeable |
| malignant | smooth ER |
| meiosis | system |
| messenger RNA (mRNA) | telophase |
| metaphase | tetrad |
| metastasize | thymine |
| mitochondria | tissue |
| mitosis | transfer RNA (tRNA) |

## THE CELL

### Properties of a Cell

All living things are made up of protoplasm. The term *protoplasm* comes from the Greek *pro-* *tos,* which means "first," and *plasm,* which means a "thing formed." Protoplasm is defined as a thick, viscous colloidal (suspension) substance that constitutes the physical basis of all living activities. It exhibits the properties of:

- assimilation—it takes things such as water or food from the environment.
- growth—it increases in size or mass.
- motility—it has the ability to move itself or parts of itself.
- secretion—it discharges chemical compounds and/or waste.
- irritability—it responds to the environment.
- reproduction—it produces offspring.

Just as the smallest component of matter is the atom, the smallest unit of protoplasm capable of independent existence is the cell. Simple life forms consist of one cell. More complex life forms such as human beings are made up of many types of cells. These cells are modified and specialized for specific activities. For example, muscle cells are designed for contraction; nerve cells send and receive electrical impulses; and red blood cells carry oxygen to body tissues.

Groups of cells that perform the same basic activity are called *tissues*. These include epithelial, connective, muscular, and nervous tissue. Groups of tissues that work in close association and perform a specialized function are called *organs*. The stomach, for example, is an organ composed primarily of muscle and epithelial tissue.

A *system* is the next higher level of organization and consists of a group of organs that work together to perform a common function, such as the gastrointestinal or reproductive system. The *organism*, such as a person or a bird, is the highest level of organization.

Although we are interested in the effect of radiation on the organism, it is important to have a good background in cell biology to understand radiation effects at their most basic level. This is so because all radiation damage is at the cellular or subcellular level.

## Chemical Components of the Cell

Protoplasm consists of *organic* compounds (made of carbon, hydrogen and oxygen) and *inorganic compounds* such as salts, water, and minerals. Both are either suspended or dissolved in water ($H_2O$). Water, the most common substance inside the cell, makes up 70% to 85% of all its contents. One of the main

functions of water is as a dispersion medium that helps hold and transport substances in the cell. Also, cell-related chemical activities occur primarily in water, and water serves as a temperature buffer. Without water, the cell would be vulnerable to extreme changes in temperature, which it could not survive. Water both absorbs and conducts heat, so a constant temperature can be maintained.

Water alone is not enough. Mineral salts, one of the other inorganic compounds of the cell, must also be present. To compare the cell to a balloon, too much air in the balloon can rupture it and too little air means that the balloon collapses. The balloon is at the optimum point when the pressure on the inside of the balloon is slightly higher than the pressure outside of the balloon. At this pressure, the balloon holds its shape but is not in danger of rupturing. Cells have a similar situation but use water instead of air. If a cell has too little water inside it, it will collapse and will not be able to carry on normal biologic functions. If the cell has too much water in it, the cell is likely to rupture. So, maintaining the correct amount of water in the cell is very important. Moving water in or out of the cell is done through *osmosis*, which is defined as substances being pushed or pulled through a membrane because there is more pressure on one side than the other. Whether water moves into or out of the cell is determined by the *osmotic pressure,* which is determined by the concentration of mineral salts inside and outside the cell. If too little sodium is present inside the cell or if too much potassium is outside the cell, the water will be pulled outside the cell and the cell will collapse. A solution causing a cell to shrink is *hypertonic.* Contrarily, if too much sodium is inside the cell or if not enough potassium is inside the cell, an excessive amount of water will be absorbed by the cell and it is then at risk of rupturing. A solution causing a cell to swell is *hypotonic.* A correct balance of mineral salts both inside and outside the cell maintains the correct osmotic pressure. Animal cells have an osmotic pressure equal to that of the circulating blood and are called *isotonic* or *isomotic.* Mineral compounds also prevent cramping, and salts aid in the production of energy as well as in the conduction of nerve impulses. Plant cells have much higher internal pressures because they are encased in a rigid wall of cellulose against which the cell can push without rupturing.

Organic compounds in the cell are divided into four major classes:

- proteins
- lipids
- carbohydrates
- nucleic acids

## Proteins

*Proteins* are macromolecules or *polymers,* large molecules formed by joining together simple units known as *monomers* into a long chain (monomer + monomer + monomer = polymer or macromolecule). Making up about 15% of the content of the cell, proteins are considered to be the basic building block of the cell. They are also the building blocks of some materials, such as hair, that are not made of cells. The functions of protein include:

- building of new tissue.
- repair of injured or broken-down tissue.
- intercellular messengers.
- composition of *enzymes,* large protein molecules that control the speed of most chemical reactions inside the cell.

Proteins are integral to the structure of such tissues as skin, bones, tendons, ligaments, hair, silk, and collagen. Proteins also protect the organism as they make up antibodies, which protect the organism from infections and are essential to clotting and wound repair. Proteins transfer information from one cell to surrounding cells to help maintain the well-being of the organism. Finally, proteins are made of enzymes, which are essential to the chemical release of energy from food.

The basic building blocks of proteins are amino acids. About 80 amino acids are found in nature, but only 20 are essential to humans. They are believed to have first been formed in the earth's early atmosphere when lightning interacted with gases such as ammonia, methane, water, and hydrogen. Amino acids consist of a carbon atom surrounded by an amino group ($NH_2$), a carboxyl group (COOH), and a side group (R), which varies from amino acid to amino acid and determines the type of

the acid it is and consequently its chemical activity. The following is a typical amino acid:

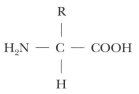

## Lipids

*Lipids* or *fats* make up about 2% of a cell on the average. When a cell takes in more energy than it needs for current use, it stores that excess energy for later use. The sugar molecules from which the cell usually gets its energy are converted into lipids for storage. Lipids are not soluble in water but are soluble in certain solvents such as alcohol, ether, oil, and chloroform. There are four classifications of lipids: (1) those that are stored inside the cell for energy; (2) those that are used to form the cell membranes and as a thermal cushion for the cell as well as in the production of steroids, cholesterol, testosterone, and estrogen; (3) long-chain lipids, which are important in pigmentation, such as eye color and chlorophyll in plants; and (4) a type of fatty acid that is involved with muscle contraction, blood vessel constriction, cell reproduction, and the inflammatory response. Lipids have these functions:

- Storage of energy
- Integral component of cell membrane
- Protection against cold and heat
- Assistance in digestive processes
- Components of substances such as hormones

## Carbohydrates

*Carbohydrates* make up about 1% of the cell, provide most of the cell's energy, and are composed of carbon, hydrogen, and oxygen. Sugars and starches are typical carbohydrates. They are stored throughout the body but primarily in the liver and muscles. Usually, a carbohydrate contains carbon, hydrogen, and oxygen in the ratio 1:2:1. Because carbohydrates have a large number of carbon–hydrogen bonds, they release large amounts of energy when the bonds are broken through metabolism.

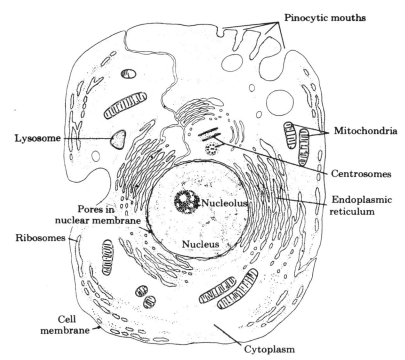

**Figure 5–1** The cell. (Reprinted with permission from Dorland's Illustrated Medical Dictionary, 27th ed. Philadelphia, WB Saunders, 1988, p 290.)

TYPICAL ANIMAL CELL

Carbohydrates are classified as follows:

- *Monosaccharides* such as glucose or fructose are the primary source of energy for the cell.
- *Disaccharides* such as sucrose, lactose, and maltose are not easily metabolized and are a storage form of energy that can readily be converted into glucose and used for energy requirements.
- *polysaccharides,* such as starch, dextrin, cellulose, and glycogen, consist of monosaccharides that are joined (polymerized) into a long chain. Some, like starch, are used by organisms as an energy source. Others, like cellulose, are used for structural purposes.

## Nucleic Acids

*Nucleic acids* are macromolecules that serve several purposes. They are the blueprint for reproduction of the cell, a template used in protein synthesis, a transport mechanism to bring together materials necessary to build proteins, and a control mechanism to regulate the cell's metabolism and reproduction. There are two types of nucleic acids, DNA and RNA, which are discussed below.

## Cell Structure

The two major sections of the cell are the *cytoplasm* and the *nucleus*, both of which are filled with protoplasm. The protoplasm is described as inside the nucleus (nucleoplasm) or outside the nucleus (cytoplasm). Structures within the protoplasm of the cell are called *organelles* (see Figure 5–1 for a diagram of the cell). Table 5–1 summarizes functions of the organelles of the cell. In nature, any idea or process that is successful (i.e. helps the organism survive) is not abandoned. It is modified and passed along in a more complex form to future generations. For example, one of the ways in which human cells

Table 5–1   Location and Function of Cellular Organelles

| Organelle | Function | |
|---|---|---|
| **Cytoplasm** | | |
| Cell membrane | A limiting structure; it actively and passively regulates the flow of all substances into and out of the cell. | |
| Endoplasmic reticulum | | |
|    Granular | Produces protein for export outside cell. | |
|    Agranular | Synthesizes carbohydrates and lipids and is involved in detoxification. | |
| Golgi body | Divides cell into subunits; concentrates and packages secretory products; participates in carbohydrate synthesis and the binding of other organic compounds to proteins. | |
| Lysosome | Contains enzymes capable of recycling old organelles by breaking down proteins, carbohydrates, and lipids. | |
| Mitochondria | Provides energy to cell through oxidation; also involved in protein synthesis. | |
| Ribosome | Synthesizes and releases protein in response to messenger RNA. | |
| **Nucleoplasm** | | |
| DNA | Directs cellular activity; also transmits genetic information. | |
| Chromosome | Is linear thread that contains DNA. | |
| Gene | Is basic unit of heredity; located on chromosomes. | |
| Nuclear membrane | Contains nuclear material and allows only some proteins and RNA to pass through. | |
| Nucleolus | Contains most of the RNA. | |
| RNA | Controls protein synthesis (mRNA), transfers amino acids to ribosome for protein synthesis (tRNA), assists in RNA reproduction (rRNA). | |

break down sugars to release energy is very inefficient and adds little to cell function. That very same process is found in the most primitive, single-cell life forms on Earth. Because the process was successful in keeping cells alive, it was never abandoned but was incorporated into more and more complex systems. Likewise, many of the organelles found in a cell can also be seen in some form at the organism level. The skin is analogous or similar to the cell membrane, the nucleus is analogous to the brain, and so forth. Therefore, some of the functions of the organelles can be more easily understood if they are compared to the systems of the organism.

## Nucleus

The function of the nucleus is to contain the genetic and metabolic information of the cell. The nucleus is similar to the brain of an organism, which controls how that organism functions in its environment. The nucleus contains the following components:

- nuclear envelope
- chromosomes
- nucleolus
- nuclear sap, the liquid portion of a cell nucleus

The nucleus is separated from the cytoplasm by the *nuclear envelope* or *membrane*. The nuclear membrane is a double-walled structure with a space between the walls. This space is contiguous or connected to the space between the membranes of the endoplastic reticulum (discussed below). At points all over the nuclear envelope, there are areas where the two walls of the membrane are pinched together into *nuclear pores*, which look like dimples on a golf ball. These pores are filled with proteins that allow some materials to pass between the cytoplasm and nucleus while they prevent other materials from passing. The only known materials that can pass through the nuclear envelope are proteins moving into the nucleus to be incorporated into the nuclear structure and various RNAs (discussed below), which move from the nucleus into the cytoplasm.

*Chromosomes* are linear threads in the nucleus of a cell. Chromosomes are composed of protein and *deoxyribonucleic acid (DNA)*. By the use of four organic nitrogenous bases, DNA encodes the information necessary to control the metabolism and reproduction of the cell. These bases are similar to the letters on this page in that sequences have meaning. On this page, the letter sequences make words that have meaning. In DNA, the bases make up sequences that have specific functions such as turning on the production of a specific substance or controlling the rate of cell division. Because DNA can also serve as a template to produce an exact copy of itself used in cell division, it is considered the genetic material. DNA consists of:

- deoxyribose—a sugar in the backbone.
- phosphoric acid—a phosphate in the backbone.
- four nitrogenous bases—the actual genetic code.

The four nitrogenous bases are *adenine, guanine, thymine,* and *cytosine*. Adenine and guanine are considered *purines;* thymine and cytosine are *pyrimidines*. See Figure 5–2 for an illustration. More specifically, adenine must always bond with thymine because both of them have a two-hydrogen bonding mechanism. Guanine must always bond with cytosine because they both have a three-hydrogen bonding mechanism. (As an aid in remembering which base matches with which base, keep in mind the two rounded first letters [Guanine and Cytosine] go together.) DNA looks like a twisted ladder. The bases are the rungs of the ladder and are attached to two very long backbones (sides of the ladder). The backbones are make up of the sugar, deoxyribose, and phosphoric acid. The backbones are twisted around each other, forming a *double helix* as shown in Figure 5–2.

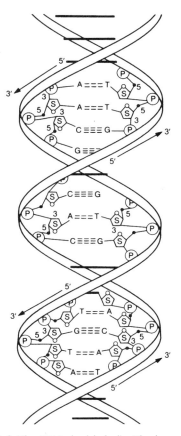

**Figure 5–2** The DNA double helix. The base pairs are perpendicular to the long axis and lie stacked on one another. A = adenine, G = guanine, C = cytosine, T = thymine. (Reprinted with permission from Dorland's Illustrated Medical Dictionary, 27th ed. Philadelphia, WB Saunders, 1988, p 448.)

*Genes* are the basic unit of heredity and are made up of a long sequence of DNA on a chromosome. Genes are found in pairs (*alleles*) and determine the characters of the organism in one of two ways. Normally, the DNA sequences for characteristics such as the number of organs and limbs, and so on, are the same for both parents, so offsprings have a matched pair of these genes. However, some gene pairs are mixed through sexual reproduction and determine characteristics such as skin color, height, gender, and so forth. The nature of the characteristic is determined by whether the DNA sequences on both genes match. Gene pairs that match are termed *homozygous*. Gene pairs that do not match are called *heterozygous*. Genes may also be *dominant* or *recessive* in the expression of a trait. If the gene pairs consist of one dominant and one recessive gene, a dominant gene expresses itself without assistance from its matching allele. A recessive gene can express itself (be seen in an offspring) only if it is homozygous, but a dominant gene will be expressed even if heterozygous. Yet other gene sets are neither dominant nor recessive but give a mixture of the two traits in offsprings.

As stated above, the genes are contained within the chromosomes. The normal number of chromosomes is constant for each species but varies from species to species from one or two up to over a thousand chromosomes. Humans have 46 chromosomes (23 pairs in all somatic or non-reproductive cells). This is called the *2n* or *diploid number*. This number of chromosomes is reduced to half that in *gametes* or reproductive cells such as ova (eggs) and spermatozoa (sperm) and is called the *haploid number*. Twenty two of these diploids are considered *autosome* (any chromosome other than a sex chromosome), and one is either an X or Y sex chromosome.

The *nucleolus* is a single spherical structure usually found in the nucleus. However, at times, there may be several or no nucleolus in the nucleus depending on the phase of reproduction. The nucleolus is composed of *ribonucleic acid* (RNA), which controls protein synthesis in all living cells and is similar to DNA in structure. It differs from DNA in that all its sugar is ribose (the R in RNA) as opposed to deoxyribose (the D in DNA), the base uracil replaces thymine, and it is a single helix. RNA occurs in several forms:

1. *Messenger RNA (mRNA)* carries the code for specific amino acid sequences from the DNA to structures in the cytoplasm for protein synthesis.
2. *Transfer RNA (tRNA)* transfers amino acid groups to the ribosome for protein synthesis.
3. *Ribosomal RNA (rRNA)* exists in the ribosomes and is thought to assist in protein synthesis.

## Cytoplasm

All metabolic functions occur in the cytoplasm. The processes of *anabolism* (*anabole* is Greek for "building up") and *catabolism* ("breaking down") both occur in the cytoplasm. Examples of anabolism are duplication of DNA, production of hormones, and converting sugars into starches. An example of catabolism is the breaking of the carbon–hydrogen bond to release the energy of glucose. Keep in mind that all activities inside the cell are either building or breaking processes used to convert substances from one form to another. The purpose of this is to store or release energy.

**Cell Membrane.** There are still many mysteries about the structure and function of the *cell membrane*. It is composed of lipids and proteins in a flexible structure. It is the limiting structure of the cell and is analogous to the skin of an organism.

The lipid molecules form a two-walled structure with the long "tails" of the lipids touching each other between the layers. This arrangement of lipids normally prevents passage of other molecules through the membrane. Both inside the layers and between them are proteins that have various functions that help the cell to interact with its environment. Transport proteins help substances pass though the cell membrane either into or out of the cell or between areas within the cell. This allows the membrane to regulate the flow of all substances and is termed *selectively permeable*. Receptor proteins on the outside of the membrane trigger a reaction inside the cell when it comes into contact with a specific molecule such as a hormone. Marker proteins on the outside identify the cell as being a specific type.

**Ribosomes.** *Ribosomes* are extremely small portions of the submicroscopic structure of a cell that function to synthesize proteins. Ribosomes are made up of several forms of *ribosomal RNA* (rRNA) and numerous proteins. The information on when and how to produce proteins is given by the DNA and sent to the ribosomes by *messenger RNA* (mRNA). Ribosomes are similar to growth area of the organism which when turned on by a chemical message will build a tissue such as bone.

**Endoplasmic Reticulum.** The *endoplasmic reticulum* (ER) is a connecting network of microcanals or tubules that interconnect throughout the nucleus and cytoplasm of the cell, and at times to the exterior of the cell. They can be seen only with the electron microscope. When a cell is observed using a light microscope, the inside of the cytoplasm appears to be a large, single container holding all the organelles of the cell. When viewed using an electron microscope, it can be seen that the ER divides the cell into many smaller units and also acts as a transport system within the cell. The endoplastic reticulum is made up of a lipid bilayer with embedded proteins similar to the cell membrane. Similar processes at the organism level would be either the tissue that divides the body into parts such as the abdominal lining or a transport system such as blood vessels (both of which are made up of connective tissue).

Endoplasmic reticula are divided into two categories which have different functions. When ribosome particles are attached, it is termed *granular* or *rough ER*. When the ER is free of ribosomes, it is called agranular or smooth ER. Rough ER is covered with ribosomes and is devoted to the production of proteins. Because of the density of the ribosomes in rough ER, it looks as if it is covered with pebbles giving it the distinction of "rough." Proteins produced in the rough ER are thought to be exported outside the cell as signal proteins. Parts of the ER that are free of ribosomes are considered smooth. Smooth ER has many types of enzymes embedded into the membrane that are used to build carbohydrates and lipids and to detoxify some substances found inside the cell.

**Mitochondria.** *Mitochondria* are the source of energy in the cell. They are slender, double-walled, microscopic filaments with a tubular or sausage shape. One interesting aspect of mitochondria is that they contain their own DNA. It is thought that this DNA is used by mitochondria to produce the proteins necessary to release energy from sugars. This energy is provided through a *catabolic* process known as *oxidation*, which breaks the carbon–hydrogen bonds of sugars to release the energy that the cell needs to survive and grow.

Cardiac muscle cells have the greatest number of mitochondria because of their need for large amounts of energy. Other cells have mitochondria in proportion to their need for energy.

**Golgi Apparatus.** Named for the Italian histologist Camillo Golgi, the *Golgi apparatus* is a lamellar (arranged in thin plates or scales) membranous structure located near the nucleus and contains a curved parallel series of flattened saccules often expanded at the ends. The function of the Golgi apparatus is to collect molecules produced in one part of the cell, modify or synthesize new molecules, package them, and distribute them to different parts of the cell. Lipids and proteins manufactured in the endoplastic reticulum are transported to the Golgi apparatus. There they are collected and modified by having sugar molecules added to them and are stored at the expanded ends of the apparatus. When enough modified lipids and proteins have been collected, the apparatus surrounds them with a membrane, which is then "pinched" off from the apparatus so that they can be transported to the needed location. An analogy to the organism level would be the digestive system, which collects and modifies molecules, then transfers them to a transport mechanism to be used where needed.

**Lysosomes.** *Lysosomes* are part of the intracellular digestive system and break down proteins, carbohydrates, lipids, and nucleic acids from old organelles so that they can be recycled. A lysosome is a membrane-lined sac filled with a concentrated solution of enzymes. Sometimes they are called "suicide sacs" because they can lyse or destroy the cell if ruptured (a rare occurrence). It is thought that lysosome are another example of how the Golgi apparatus divides the cell into compartments. An organism analogy to lysosome would be the stomach, which is filled with a concentrated solution of acid used to break down lipids, proteins, and carbohydrates. Like the lysosome, if the stomach is ruptured, its contents can kill the organism.

## Cell Division and the Cell Cycle

### Somatic Cells

**Mitosis.** *Mitosis* (Figure 5–3) is a type of cell division of somatic (nonreproduction) cells wherein each daughter cell contains the same number of chromosomes as the parent cell. Mitosis is part of the total cell cycle, which has five phases, four of which are mitosis or the cell-reproduction phases. The five phases are described below. This is the process by which the body grows and by which somatic cells are replaced.

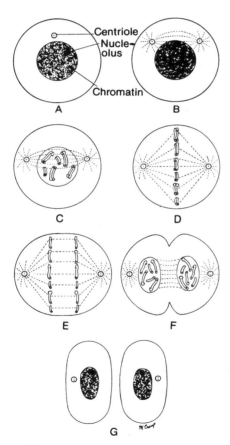

**Figure 5–3** Mitosis. A = resting stage (interphase), B = early prophase, C = later prophase, D = metaphase, E = anaphase, F = telophase, G = daughter cells. "G" refers to a gap. (Reprinted with permission from Dorland's Illustrated Medical Dictionary, 27th ed. Philadelphia, WB Saunders, 1988, p 1044.)

INTERPHASE: The period between the division is known as *interphase* and has three subphases. $G_1$ is the first subphase in which the cell spends most of its life and where the cell primarily grows. (See Figure 5–4.) The next subphase is the *S-phase,* in which the DNA is replicated but stays attached to the *centromere,* a clear region in the middle of each chromosome. In the S-phase, the number of chromosomes in the cell is doubled and is called a *tetrad.* $G_2$ is the final subphase, in which the organelles are reproduced, spiral filaments called *chromatids* reproduce, and the DNA starts to tightly coil and become visible under a light microscope.

PROPHASE: Prophase begins when the chromosomes become visible with a light microscope. During this phase, the chromatin granules of the nucleus become organized into chromosomes that first appear as long, delicate, spiral structures, each consisting of two chromatids. As prophase progresses, the chromosomes become shorter and more compact. The nuclear membrane and the nucleoli disappear. At the same time, the centriole divides and the two daughter centrioles move to opposite poles of the cell.

METAPHASE: The paired chromatids arrange themselves in an equatorial plane midway between the two centrioles forming this plane.

ANAPHASE: The chromatids are now called daughter chromosomes and diverge and move toward their respective centrosomes. The end of their migration marks the beginning of the next phase.

TELOPHASE: The chromosomes at each end of the spindle undergo changes that are the reverse of prophase. Each becomes a long, loosely spiraled thread. The nuclear membrane re-forms and nucleoli reappear. Outlines of chromosomes disappear, and chromatin appears as granules scattered throughout the nucleus and connected by a net. Two complete cells result from the cytoplasm's becoming separated into two parts.

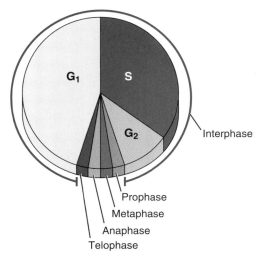

**Figure 5–4** The cell cycle. Note that cells spend most of the cycle in interphase.

## Germ Cells

**Meiosis.** *Meiosis* (Figure 5–5) is a type of cell division that produces *germ cells* or reproductive cells (sperm or ova). Meiosis consists of two successive divisions of the mother cell, producing four daughter or granddaughter cells that each contain only half the number of chromosomes present in somatic cells. The first division produces two cells with the normal diploid somatic number, and these divide again to produce cells with a haploid number.

## Malignant Cells

*Malignant* or cancer cells are those which are dividing abnormally (usually much more often than normal cells) and differ physically from normal cells in two ways:

- an increased amount of chromatin.
- an increased ratio of nuclear material to cytoplasm.

Although malignant cell may remain unchanged in size from the normal cell from which they derive, cancer cells can also vary greatly in size and shape. In normal tissue, cells usually stick together. Some types of cancers *metastasize* or spread to other portions of the body by allowing cells to break free of the tumor site. Also, as stated above, most malignant cells show an increase in mitotic activity, which often leads to bizarre mitotic divisions.

## HISTORY OF RADIOBIOLOGY AND PROTECTION

*Radiobiology* is basically a marriage of two disciplines: *radiologic physics,* which studies the spread of energy through space (a precise definition of radiation) and its absorption in living matter, and *biology,* the study of living organisms. Radiobiology is a branch of science that deals with the modes of action and the effects of ionizing radiation on living matter. In radiobiology we study cell biology, since most effects of radiation occur at the cellular level. The responses to radiation of organs, tissues, embryo, fetus, and the whole body all grow out of injury to the cells.

### Discovery of Radiation and Radioactivity

Radiology's birth is the result of three events. First, in 1895, Wilhelm Conrad Roentgen discovered x-rays. He observed the action of these invisible rays on a barium platinocyanide screen. In 1896, Henri Becquerel observed the emission of rays from a uranium containing mineral. This phenomenon was later named *radioactivity* by Marie Curie. The third event was Pierre and Marie Curie's discovery of radium in 1898.

Becquerel is often cited as the first individual to notice that ionizing radiation had certain biologic effects. He noted a skin reaction (a reddening and irritation of skin known as *erythema*) 2 weeks after carrying a tube of radium in his pocket. In 1896, J. Daniel first noted the loss of hair (epilation) due to radiation exposure. Pierre Curie experimented on himself by exposing an area of his own skin to radium and observing the reactions.

In 1904, the first x-ray fatality occurred in the United States. A man named Clarence Dally, who worked for Thomas Edison in the development of the fluoroscope and fluorescent screens, was the first victim. Although it was known that radiation had certain localized effects on skin, its potential for fatality was not known. The radiologist Rollins had set the first "safe" intensity in 1902 at an exposure of less

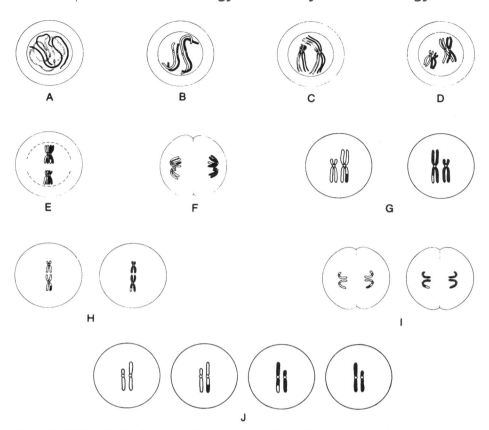

**Figure 5–5** Meiosis. A = leptotene, B = zygotene, C = pachytene, D = diplotene, E = metaphase, F = anaphase, G = telophase, H = metaphase, I = anaphase, J = telophase. (Adapted from Thompson MW, et al: Genetics in Medicine, 4th ed. Philadelphia, WB Saunders, 1986, in Dorland's Illustrated Medical Dictionary, 27th ed. Philadelphia, WB Saunders, 1988, p 997.)

than 7 minutes, but this was only to prevent erythema. Edison often worked 20 hours per day, sleeping at his bench, and he demanded the same type of routine from his assistants. Thus, Dally was exposed every day to doses far in excess of today's lifetime limits. Tubes and workers were rarely shielded.

The most common short-term effects noted in those days were skin damage, loss of hair, and anemia. Operators of equipment often had to expose themselves to the beam to show patients that it did not hurt. Radiologists often had multiple amputations of fingers from unshielded fluoroscopy devices and had increased inci-

dence of leukemia over other physicians. An entire group of individuals died because of overuse of radiation. They sacrificed themselves for us to determine the safe uses of radiation and are known as the *roentgen martyrs*. We have these individuals to thank for safety developments such as lead gloves, aprons, and personnel monitoring devices such as film badges.

### Law of Bergonie and Tribondeau

In 1906, one of the most important discoveries for radiobiology was made—the Law of Bergonie and Tribondeau. These individuals exposed rabbit testes to x-rays and observed the effects of radiation on testicular reproductive cells. Simply put, this law states that *radiosensitivity* (how much damage radiation does to a particular cell) is a function of the metabolic state of the cell being irradiated. The level of metabolism is directly related to the reproductive (*mitotic*) rate and indirectly related to the specialization of the cell. More specifically, it states that:

1. A high metabolic rate increases the radiosensitivity of cells.
2. With increased cell maturity, cells are more resistant to radiation (*radioresistant*). Mature cells have lower metabolic rates generally.
3. Younger cells and tissues are more radiosensitive.
4. An increased mitotic rate for cells and an increased growth rate for tissues increase the radiosensitivity of cells.
5. Stem cells are *radiosensitive*. Stem cells are the precursors of specialized cells such as muscle or neuro cells, and these cells have very high mitotic rates and are not yet specialized.

A good solid understanding of the *law of Bergonie and Tribondeau* will be helpful when learning about the various biologic effects of radiation in this and the next three chapters.

In the 1920s, a variety of researchers found that biologic effects were due primarily to ionization processes in tissues. Two different processes were identified:

- *Direct effects,* in which the radiation directly ionized a *macromolecule* (a large *molecule* made by joining together a number of simpler molecules) such as DNA or proteins. Physical or chemical changes result.
- *Indirect effects,* in which the radiation interacts with *water* in the cell, causing the formation of free radicals (a chemical compound that damages the cell) though the radiolysis of water (discussed in Chapter 6). This formed the basis for much research in the 1930s through the 1950s.

Radiation was used somewhat indiscriminately on patients for many years. For example, a radiologist in New York City irradiated women in the 1920s to cure infertility. The treatment worked, and many of the women bore apparently healthy children, although the long-term effect over many generations cannot be determined. Most of what we can say about radiation comes from a statistical technique known as *extrapolation,* in which we make predictions about low doses from high doses. There is, of course, some potential for error in such a technique.

*Fractionation* is the process of dividing a radiation dose into several small doses given over time. The concept of fractionation for radiation therapy came from French experiments in the 1920s and 1930s. Ram testes were exposed to x-rays. It was found that the animals could not be sterilized with one large dose without also causing skin reactions at the scrotum. However, if the dose were fractionated over time, the animals could be sterilized without causing much skin damage.

In 1927, a scientist named H.J. Miller experimented with *Drosophila* (fruit flies) and is credited with the discovery of radiation mutagenesis (the induction of mutation with ionizing radiation). One important discovery he made was that mutations resulting from radiation were the same as those found in nature. Radiation increased the frequency of mutation but did not cause any unique effects. For this reason, it is often stated that there are no *radiounique* effects: any type of damage caused by ionizing radiation can also be caused by such things as heat, chemical, or mechanical trauma. Miller later received the Nobel Prize for his discovery.

The definition of the roentgen (R) in the 1930s led to a greater attention to personnel protection but protection remained fairly lax until the 1960s. As late as the 1930s, it was accepted that there was a tolerance dose of about 1 rem/day below which no effects would be seen.

In the 1940s and 1950s, the oxygen effect was also studied. First stated in 1912, it states that the lack of oxygen inhibits the formation of free radicals, which are chemical compounds that damage the cell. In 1956, Puck successfully cultured mammalian cells (from a mammal) in artificial media. These cells were derived from a carcinoma (cancer) of the uterine cervix from a human patient. They received the name HeLa, the He and the La standing for the first two letters of the patient's first and last names.

The following, in review, can be considered significant historical events in the development of radiobiology. It is not the intent of this text to have students memorize the following but, instead, this chronology is to show how radiobiology and protection have developed over time.

Today, the main thrust of radiobiology is the study of very low levels of radiation such as those received by radiation workers and by people living around nuclear sites. You will note from the chronology given that as more has been learned about radiobiology, exposure limits have consistently gone down. One of the major assumptions in the protection arena is

that low levels of radiation have the same *proportional* effect as higher levels of radiation. For example, the damage done by a single mrad of a 1-mrad dose is the same as the damage done by a single mrad in a 5000-mrad dose. As current radiation protection guidelines are based on this assumption, determining if it is correct may have a significant impact on future limits. Another area of significant research is the impact of prolonged low levels of radiation such as those found in technologists on organ-specific cancers. At the time of this writing, a major study of over 100,000 technologists in the United States was being completed. This study may shed some light on the relationship (if any) between working in a radiation field and the development of specific types of cancer.

## Chronology of Radiation Protection and Radiobiology

### *Pioneer Era*

1895
- Discovery of x-rays by W. Roentgen.

1896
- Discovery of radioactivity by H. Becquerel.
- First reports of possible x-ray injury; damage to eyes by T.A. Edison and W.J. Morton.
- Concern expressed over possibility of x-ray injury by F. Battelli.
- Epilation (loss of hair) noted from x-ray exposure by J. Daniel.
- Skin effects first noted by L.G. Stevens.
- First x-ray protective device: a heavy glass plate to protect the eyes during dental radiography by W.H. Rollins.
- Reports of accidental injury (burns) by H.D. Hawks.

1898
- Aluminum filter used as protective device by E. Thomson.
- Leaded x-ray tube housing; collimators developed by W.H. Rollins.

- Radium discovered by P. and M. Curie.
- Gamma rays discovered by P. Villard.

1899
- Radiographer licensure recommended to protect public by J. Dennis.
- First malpractice award for x-ray burns.
- Listing of protective devices (gloves, aprons, etc.) in x-ray catalog by R. Friedlander Co.

1900
- Increased target to skin distance recommended by M.K. Kassabian to reduce skin dose.

1901
- Several reports of alleged x-ray deaths (lethality).
- Skin burn caused by radium carried on person reported by H. Becquerel.
- X-ray lethality to mammals demonstrated experimentally by W.H. Rollins.

1903
- Protection committee within American Roentgen Ray Society (ARRS) proposed by S.H. Monell.

## Chronology of Radiation Protection and Radiobiology *(Continued)*

1904
- First x-ray pioneer death attributed to cumulative overexposure of C.M. Dally.

### Dormant Era

1905
- Radiation unit based on ionization first proposed by M. Franklin.

1906
- Law of radiosensitivity of tissues put forth by J. Bergonie and R. Tribondeau.

1907
- Mutation by x-ray reported in toads by C.R. Bardeen.
- Photographic plate carried in pocket for monitoring x-ray exposure reported by R.V. Wagner.
- Use of gas-filled tubes for detection of radiation by E. Rutherford.

1911
- International radium standard and Curie unit devised.

1912
- Half-value layer concept proposed by T. Christan.

1913
- Hot cathode x-ray tubes and tungsten targets permitting higher voltages developed by W.D. Coolidge.

1915
- British Roentgen Society adopts radiation protection recommendations.

1920
- First standing x-ray protection committee by American Roentgen Ray Society.
- Ionization processes officially defined.

1920s
- Concept of fractionation is developed.

1921
- British X-Ray and Radium Protection Committee issues first memorandum.

1922
- American Roentgen Ray Society adopts radiation protection rules.
- Film badges for personnel monitoring developed by G. Pfahler.
- Compton demonstrates scattering of x-rays.

### Era of Progress

1925
- First "tolerance dose" proposed by A. Mutscheller.

1927
- Genetic effects of x-ray shown by H.J. Muller.

1928
- Roentgen unit formally adopted.
- Operator exposure comes under greater scrutiny.
- International X-Ray and Radium Protection Committee formed (forerunner of International Committee on Radiation Protection [ICRP]).

1929
- U.S. Advisory committee on X-Ray and Radium Protection (USACXRP) formed (forerunner of National Council on Radiation Protection and a Measurement [NCRP]).

1931
- USACXRP publishes first recommendations—0.2 R/day.

1932
- Concept of greater permissible dose for partial body irradiation (hands) introduced by G. Failla.

## Chronology of Radiation Protection and Radiobiology *(Continued)*

**1934**
- International Committee on X-ray Protection (ICXRP) recommends permissible dose of 0.2 R/day.

**1936**
- USACXRP recommends reduction in permissible dose to 0.1 R/day.

**1937**
- Roentgen accepted internationally.

**1940s**
- Oxygen effect is defined.

**1941**
- Suggested maximum permissible dose (MPD) of 0.02 R/day given by L.S. Taylor.

**1943**
- 4 R/week shown to cause injury by H.M. Parker.

**1944**
- Rem introduced by H.M. Parker.

### Postwar Era

**1950**
- ICRP adopts basic MPD of 0.3 R/week for radiation workers.

**1953**
- Rad officially adopted as unit of absorbed dose.
- Dose limit of 1.5 rem/yr to individual members of the general public set by Third Tri-Partite Conference on Internal Dosimetry.

**1956**
- MPD of 5 rad/year recommended by National Academy of Sciences and ICRP.

**1957**
- Age prorating concept of 5(age – 18 yrs)

rad for occupational exposure and 0.5 rad/year general public introduces by NCRP.

**1960**
- Pamphlet from American College of Radiology states that effects from x-radiation may be more severe than nuclear testing; patient protection is increasingly emphasized.

**1961**
- U.S. Federal Regulations on radiation protection and safety adopted in Title 10 Code of Federal Regulations, Part 20 (10 CFR 20).

### Current Era

**1962**
- Operator Maximal Permissible Dose (MPD) set at 5 rem/year.

**1964**
- Average annual limits of 170 mrem/year to general population set by CFR.

**1987**
- 1.5 rem per year for workers set by NRPB (Britain).
- NCRP reconfirms 50 mSv (5 rem) as annual permissible dose and redefines lifetime (cumulative) allowable dose as 10 rad × age of operator.

**1991**
- New version of 10 CFR 20 (Code of Federal Regulations) published. Combines internal and external doses, redefines extremities to include knees and elbows. Concept of MPD abandoned and replaced by Dose Limits (DLs).
- ICRP sets annual dose limit to 20 mSv, but standard not adopted in United States

## SUMMARY

Radiobiology is a branch of science that deals with the modes of action and the effects of ionizing radiation on living matter. It is a combination of two disciplines, radiologic physics and biology. A variety of early developments including the discovery of radioactivity, the law of Bergonie and Tribondeau, oxygenation, fractionation, and Miller experiments with fruit flies were all instrumental in the establishment of radiobiology.

Cells are made up of a variety of organic and inorganic components. The cell is made mostly of water, a fact of great significance in the study of radiation effects. The organelles of the cell are the endoplasmic reticulum, ribosomes, mitochondria, lysosomes, and the Golgi apparatus. The nucleus contains DNA, RNA, genes, and chromosomes. It directs the reproductive activity of the cell. Somatic cells divide by a process known as *mitosis,* germ cells by a process known as *meiosis.*

## Questions

1. About what percentage of the cell is water?
   a. 28             b. 37
   c. 66             d. 75

2. About 15% of the cell is:
   a. salts.              b. protein.
   c. carbohydrates.      d. lipids.

3. Animal cells that have an osmotic pressure equal to that of the circulating blood are called:
   a. isotonic.           b. hypertonic.
   c. hypotonic.          d. monotonic.

4. Gene pairs are also known as:
   a. alleles.            b. homozygous.
   c. dominant.           d. heteroxygous.

5. The 2n number in cells is also known as the _____ number.
   a. autosomal           b. gametal
   c. haploid             d. diploid

6. What is the function of the mitochondria?
   a. transportation system for the cell
   b. produce enzymes and hormones
   c. break down nutrients to produce energy
   d. none of the above

7. The primary function of carbohydrates in the cell is to:
   a. build enzymes.
   b. fill membranes.
   c. supply energy.

8. Which of the following organelles is associated with dividing the cell into compartments?
   a. lysosomes
   b. mitochondria
   c. endoplasmic reticulum
   d. ribosomes

9. At which phase of the cell cycle is the DNA replicated?
   a. anaphase
   b. prophase
   c. metaphase
   d. interphase

10. If a radiation dose is delivered continuously, but at a lower dose rate, it is referred as what kind of dose?
    a. protracted
    b. undivided
    c. unenhanced
    d. retarded

## Exercises

1. Describe the Law of Bergonie and Tribondeau.

2. Discuss the concept of fractionation of dose.

3. Relate physical activity to cell cycle stages.

## Answers .

### Questions

| | |
|---|---|
| 1. d | 6. c |
| 2. b | 7. c |
| 3. a | 8. b |
| 4. a | 9. d |
| 5. d | 10. a |

### Exercises

1.  Essentially, the law of Bergonie and Tribondeau states that radiosensitivity is a function of the metabolic state of the cell being irradiated.

2.  The concept of fractionation came from French experiments in the 1920s and 1930s. It was found that rams could not be sterilized with one large dose without also causing skin reactions at the scrotum. However, if the dose were fractionated, or split into smaller amounts over time, the animals could be sterilized without causing much skin damage.

3.  The physical activity of the cell is highest during mitosis, when the cell goes through duplication and division.

## CHAPTER 6

# Principles of Radiobiology

### Steven B. Dowd • Elwin R. Tilson

Chapter Objectives

At the end of this chapter, the student should be able to:

1. Define radiobiology.

2. Outline the Law of Bergonie and Tribondeau.

3. Differentiate direct and indirect effects.

4. Outline the process of water radiolysis.

5. Differentiate between linear energy transfer and relative biologic effectiveness.

6. Apply the formula for relative biologic effectiveness.

7. List the four types of dose–response curves and summarize each in terms of important concepts.

8. Define stochastic and deterministic effects and construct a comparison between them.

9. Relate dose and rate to radiation effects.

10. Discuss the oxygen effect.

11. Relate age to radiation responses.

12. Diagram the most common types of chromosomal effects.

13. Describe what impact each type of chromosomal effect has on cell function/survival.

14. Overview the four target theories and relate each to radiosensitivity.

15. Discuss cell survival curves and their implication for protection and therapy.

**Important Terms**

acentric
carcinogen
certainty effect
curvilinear
deletion
deterministic effect
dicentric
division delay

dose–response curve
dose-rate effect
duplication
free radical
hypoxic
interphase death
interstitial deletion
inversion
latent period
linear dose–response curve
linear quadratic
malignant
nonstochastic
nonthreshold
one-break effect
oxygen enhancement ratio (OER)
point mutation
radiologic physics
radiolysis
radiounique
relative biologic effectiveness (RBE)
reproductive failure
ring chromosome
sigmoid
statistical response
stochastic
sublethal
terminal deletion
threshold
translocation
two-break effects

## INTRODUCTION

This chapter deals with the major concepts or principles that determine how sensitive cells are to radiation, the mechanisms that damage cells that are exposed to radiation, and how much impact radiation has in a given environment. The role chromosomal damage has on cell function and survival will be investigated, including common chromosomal aberrations found after radiation doses. Finally, this chap-

ter will relate the target theory to the survival rate of colonies of cells. For the advanced student, the impact of oxygen, fractionation, and protraction will be discussed.

## PRINCIPLES OF RADIOBIOLOGY

Radiobiology, like all sciences, functions around a group of principles that determine the processes that are studied. Radiobiology principles revolve around the random nature of radiation interactions, how radiation interacts at the cellular level, and factors that alter these interactions. Several generalizations about radiation interactions with cells have important ramifications in the study of radiobiology.

It is very important to keep in mind that all radiation damage is done at the cellular or subcellular level. The visible effects of radiation damage are due to the impact of cellular damage to millions of cells in an organ, system, or body part. Because all damage is cellular or subcellular, understanding the impact of radiation on cells is essential to understanding the impact of radiation on a person or a population.

- All radiation interactions are probability functions. That means that we can predict what an overall effect will be but there is no way to predict individual events such as a particular cell or DNA sequence will be struck by radiation. However, in probability functions, the percentages and trends are well documented and understood. For example, if we have 1,000,000 squares or targets and expose them to 1,000,000 photons of x-radiation, we have no way of knowing which specific squares will be hit by the radiation, which ones will have not be hit, and which will have multiple hits. However, we do know the average percentage of squares that will be hit will be 63%, we just don't know which ones. (See Figure 6–1.) That is because these interactions are nonselective or random in nature. This is similar to saying that average lifetime earnings will be so many dollars. Although we know the average earnings, we have no way of knowing how much specific people will earn in their lives because education, gender, location, and many other factors influence that amount.
- Another issue is time frame. Energy is transferred from the photon to matter in $10^{-17}$ to $10^{-5}$ second. That is very fast. So fast, in fact, that it is difficult to measure exactly what is happening in the process at any given point in time. When you read that A happens inside a cell, causing B to happen, which then causes C to occur, which then causes D, keep in mind that these things are happening in a very short

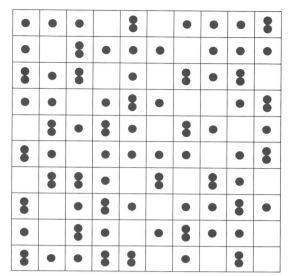

**Figure 6–1** Radiation interactions are random in nature. If 100 x-ray photons interacted with a surface divided into 100 squares, some squares would be struck once (single dot) and a few would be struck multiple times (two dots). On average, 37% of the squares would not be struck at all (empty). If another 100 photons interacted with the same 100 squares, the number of squares left empty would be 37% of the squares left empty after the first 100 photons ($100 \times 0.37 \times 0.37$ or 14 squares left empty).

time frame. Observing that when A happens, we see D isn't too difficult, but defining the steps in between is hard, because such chains of events appear to be almost simultaneous.

- Radiation interaction with cells can be either ionization, in which an electron is removed from an atom, or excitation, in which one or more electrons are pushed into a higher energy state (suborbit) from which the q.
- Most interaction inside cells occurs in water, which constitutes 70% to 85% of cell contents. These are called *indirect interactions*. Some interactions occur in biologic macromolecules such as DNA or proteins. These are called *direct interactions*.
- Radiation damage to the cell cannot be distinguished from damage caused by other sources such as chemicals, heat, or trauma.

This makes it very hard to determine exactly what caused specific minor damage to a cell. This is an issue when studying effects of low-level radiation exposure. Any cell or DNA damage seen cannot clearly be determined to be radiation induced.

- Finally, biologic changes occur only after a *latent period* during which no evidence of damage is present. This latent period can be as brief as a few minutes or as long as several decades. The length of the latent period is determined by the amount of the dose and the types of cells involved.

## BIOLOGIC INTERACTIONS AND MEASUREMENT OF EFFECTS

Ionizing radiation causes biologic damage. To understand how the damage occurs, the mechanism involved must also be understood. The specific mechanisms of importance are (1) direct and indirect actions of radiation, (2) linear energy transfer (LET), and (3) *relative biologic effectiveness* (RBE).

### Direct and Indirect Action

When interactions occurs as a result of ionization, they occur either in critical biologic macromolecules (e.g. DNA) or in their suspension (water). This classifies the interaction as direct or indirect. In a direct action, the radiation ionizes a molecule or atom inside a macromolecule such as a protein or RNA. Because of the break in bond of an electron, there is a change in the chemical or biologic function of that macromolecule. In some cases, this damage is not fatal to the cell and can be repaired. In other cases, the damage is fatal to the cell. If the damage happens to be on a DNA molecule, that damage may also be genetic and passed on to the future generations of cells. Direct action occurs primarily with high-linear-energy-transfer (LET) radiations such as fast neutrons.

### Radiolysis of Water

The primary mechanism for indirect action is the *radiolysis* (breakdown by radiation) of water. Although DNA is the most sensitive target, radiolysis of water is the primary effect from radiation exposure to the cell. For every molecule of DNA in the cell, there are $1.2 \times 10^7$ molecules of water. When radiation interacts with water, the water is ionized, producing an ion pair of $HOH^+$ and $e^-$.

$$HOH \xrightarrow{\text{Radiation}} HOH^+ + e^-$$

The electron produced may reconnect with the $HOH^+$ ion or it may attach itself to another uncharged water molecule creating a *free radical*. Free radicals (denoted by the $^\bullet$ symbol) contain a single unpaired electron piggybacking in their outer shell, making them chemically unstable. The $HOH^\bullet$ tends to break down into hydroxyl, $OH^-$, and a hydrogen free radical, $H^\bullet$. These free radicals tend to combine with oxygen, creating hydroperoxyl radicals. The hydroperoxyl radicals may cause biologic damage directly or break down to form hydrogen peroxide and oxygen:

$$H^\bullet + O_2 \longrightarrow HO_2^\bullet$$
$$HO_2^\bullet \longrightarrow H_2O_2 + O_2$$

The $HOH^+$ may interact with another HOH molecule, creating a hydroxyl radical, $OH^\bullet$, and $H_3O$, or it may break down into a hydrogen ion, $H^+$, and a hydroxyl radical:

$$HOH^+ + HOH \longrightarrow OH^\bullet + H_3O$$
$$HOH^+ \longrightarrow H^+ + OH^\bullet$$

In both of these cases, the hydroxyl radicals can combine with other hydroxyl radicals to form $H_2O_2$, hydrogen peroxide. About two thirds of all biologic damage is caused by the hydrogen peroxide from these two processes.

### Linear Energy Transfer and Relative Biologic Effectiveness

As you will recall from Chapter 4, linear energy transfer was defined as the rate at which the energy of the radiation was transferred to tissue and was related to specific ionizations because as the LET goes up, the number of specific ionizations also goes up. Recall also from Chapter

Table 6–1   Comparison of Low- and High-LET Radiations

| Low LET | High LET |
|---|---|
| <10 keV/μm | >10 keV/μm |
| Sparsely ionizing | Densely ionizing |
| Random interactions | Uniform energy deposition |
| Penetrating radiation | Superficial penetration |
| External radiation hazard | Internal radiation hazard |
| Indirect damage | Direct damage |
| Single strand break | Double strand break |
| Repair not error-prone | Highly error-prone repair |
| Damage to one side of DNA backbone—usually repairable | Damage to both sides of DNA backbone—not usually repairable |
| Sublethal | More likely lethal |
| Dependent oxygen concentration (maximum OER*) | Independent of oxygen concentration (minimum OER*) |
| Example: x-ray photon | Examples: fission fragments, charged particles |

*OER is the oxygen enhancement ratio; this is called the *oxygen effect* in the chapter.

4 that we talked about high-LET radiation such as alpha particles and low-LET or sparsely ionizing radiation such as x-rays or gamma rays. Table 6–1 compares low- and high-LET radiations in terms of physical and biologic effects. Although radiations do fall into such general categories as high and low LET, it is not correct to assume that a given type of radiation has a specific LET because the LET of a given radiation is determined by the energy of that beam. As you know, no type of radiation is monoenergetic in all cases—there is always a range of energies associated with a given type of radiation. When an LET value is given, it must be kept in mind that the value is the average LET for all energies of that radiation. Table 6–2 gives average LET values for several types of radiation.

LET is important in that it is closely related to the amount of biologic damage done by different types of radiation. Figure 6–2 shows the relationship of LET and ion pair formation inside tissue for gamma rays, high-energy x-rays, low-energy x-rays, and alpha particles. When the energy is transferred in the form of ionizations in a small area (high LET), more damage is done to tissue than when less energy is transferred in the same area. Because LET is so closely related to the amount of biologic damage, it is also closely related to the unit of measurement of biologic damage: the relative biologic effectiveness (RBE).

Table 6–2   LETs of Various Types of Radiation

| Type of Radiation | LET in keV/μm |
|---|---|
| Gamma rays | ~0.1–0.3 |
| 10-MeV x-rays | ~0.4–0.7 |
| Diagnostic x-rays | 1–3 |
| Fast neutrons | ~65 |
| 5-MeV alpha particles | 100 |
| Heavy nuclei | 1000 |

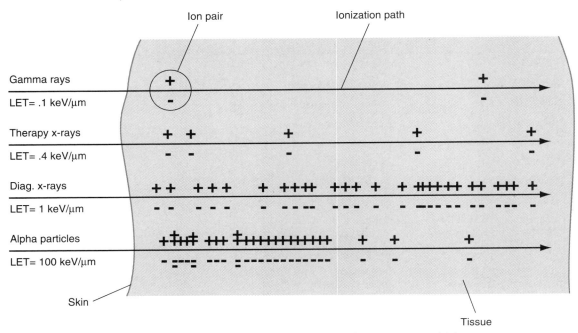

**Figure 6–2** Relationship of LET and ion pair formation inside tissue for gamma rays, high-energy x-rays, low-energy x-rays, and alpha particles. Arrows show ionization paths as straight lines for illustration purposes. Paths are normally very contorted.

The concept of comparing how much biologic damage one type of radiation does compared to another type of radiation was already introduced in Chapter 3 as the quality factor (QF). Essentially, a QF is a rounded estimate of the RBE for any type of radiation. RBE compares how much of one type of radiation (the test radiation) is needed to do the same amount of damage as a known dose of 250-keV x-rays. Thus, the 250-keV x-ray is a standard to which all other radiations are compared. RBE varies not only with the type of radiation but also because of the type of cell or tissue, the physiologic status of the cells, and the dose rate.

The formula for RBE is as follows:

$$\frac{\text{Dose of 250-keV x-rays to produce the same effect}}{\text{Dose of test radiation to produce an effect}}$$

Remember the key word is *relative,* which means we are comparing types of radiation.

---

**EXAMPLE 1**

It takes 40 rad (40 cGy) of a test radiation to produce an effect, and 120 rad (120 cGy) of 250-keV x-rays produces the same effect. What is the RBE of the test radiation?

120/40 = 3     The RBE is 3.0.

---

**EXAMPLE 2**

It takes 50 rad (50 cGy) of a test radiation to produce an effect and 210 rad (210 cGy) of 250-keV x-rays to produce the same effect. What is the RBE of the test radiation?

210/50 = 4.2     The RBE is 4.2.

*In general*, as LET increases, so does RBE. Thus, high-LET radiations such as alpha and beta particles also have a high RBE. Low-LET radiations such as x-rays and gamma rays have a low RBE. The obvious question is, "Why are alpha and beta seen as relatively 'benign' radiations?" The answer lies in the fact that they are also not highly penetrating and can cause damage for only a few millimeters. Thus, they are absorbed in clothing or within the first few millimeters of skin and do little damage. One of the functions of the skin is to protect the internal environment of the body from the external environment, including radiation (see Chapter 13).

## DOSE–RESPONSE CURVES

### General Concepts of Dose–Response Curves

A dose–response curve is a graphic representation of the relationship between the amount of radiation absorbed by a cell or organism (dose) and the amount of damage (response) seen. Authorities are not in complete agreement on the shape(s) of dose–response curves. Generally, as the dose increases, so does the response, but that response may or may not be a straight line, and there may be some doses below which no response is seen.

Dose–response curves vary in two basic ways (Figure 6–3):

1. Response curves are either linear or nonlinear. In linear responses there is a proportional relationship between the dose and response, and the curve forms a straight line when graphed. Nonlinear responses are those in which there is no fixed proportional response between dose and response and form a curved line when graphed. Nonlinear curves are also called *curvilinear, sigmoid,* or *linear–quadratic* based on their exact shape.
2. Response curves are either *threshold* or *nonthreshold*. A response that has a threshold is one in which a level is reached below which no effect (damage) is observed. An example of a threshold is eye damage and light levels. Normally, light does not damage the human eye, but at some point (the

threshold), a bright enough light will cause blindness. At levels below the threshold, the eye responds to the light but is not damaged. If there is a radiation-dose threshold, cells respond to the radiation but no damage is done. A nonthreshold response is one in which theoretically even the smallest dose could cause an effect. With a nonthreshold response, some damage is always done if any dose at all is given.

These two characteristics give the possibility for four types of dose–response curves: linear threshold, linear nonthreshold, nonlinear threshold, and nonlinear nonthreshold (see Figure 6–3). Although there is no absolute consensus on which type of curve best describes human interactions with radiation, the following are generally accepted as most accurate: (1) the linear nonthreshold for low to moderate dose levels as used for regulatory purposes; (2) the sigmoid threshold for high dose levels associated with radiation therapy; and (3) the linear-quadratic, which is the model for overall human reponse to a radiation dose.

### Linear Nonthreshold Dose–Response Curve

A linear nonthreshold dose–response curve exhibits some effect, no matter how small

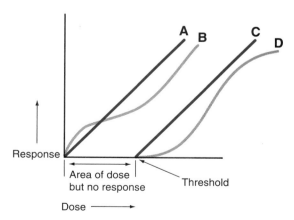

**Figure 6–3** Types of dose response curves. *(A)* linear, nonthreshold. *(B)* nonlinear (linear quadratic), nonthreshold. *(C)* linear, threshold. *(D)* nonlinear (sigmoid), nonthreshold.

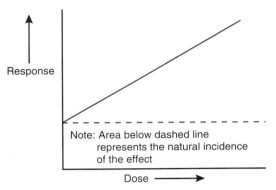

**Figure 6–4** Linear nonthreshold–dose response curve. (Reprinted with permission from Thompson MA: Principles of Radiation Protection for Nurses and Other Medical Facility Personnel. Birmingham, AL, University of Alabama at Birmingham, 1986.)

the dose. Theoretically, even one photon could cause an effect to occur. Unlike threshold curves, the observed effects are seen even if no radiation is absorbed because there is usually a natural incidence of the effect. For example, leukemia is often seen as responding to the linear dose–response curve. It occurs naturally to a certain extent in the population, and radiation serves to increase the incidence. The radiation impact is known as a *stochastic effect* (see below), which means it is random in nature.

A direct proportion is observed between dose and response for the linear nonthreshold curve (Figure 6–4). Besides leukemia, breast cancer (at low radiation doses) and genetic damage are assumed to follow this curve. Because these types of effects are assumed to follow a linear curve and the curve lacks a threshold, we focus much of our radiation protection efforts on these effects. In fact, this is the model used by many regulatory agencies to set standards and dose limits. This is why we spend so much time studying the potential effects of mammography on breast cancer, even though the doses are low. We also focus strongly on having individuals wear lead aprons, since lead aprons cover most of the active blood-forming organs in the body. Finally, we provide gonadal shielding because genetic effects follow the linear curve: we can never know if it was one stray photon that caused a genetic effect. If we knew, for example, that

genetic effects followed a threshold curve, and thus did not exhibit any effects on future generations until a dose of, say, 5 rad (5 cGy), we could afford to be lax in gonadal protection. As it stands, we cannot. If we are lax, we jeopardize the future health of unborn children.

The linear nonthreshold dose–response curve can be summarized as follows:

1. There is no threshold.
2. The response to radiation in terms of frequency or severity of effects is directly proportional to the dose.
3. There is no dose rate effect (see below), which means that there is no reduced effect at small dose rates.
4. The curve exhibits a stochastic or statistical response (see below).

### Sigmoid Threshold Dose–Response Curve

The term *sigmoid* means "S-shaped," a term probably familiar to radiologic technology students from the sigmoid colon. This dose–response curve applies primarily to the high-dose effects seen in radiation therapy. There is usually a threshold, a level (minimum dose) below which no observable effects occur. This minimum dose varies for different effects. For example, changes are seen in the formation of blood components such as platelets and white blood cells with doses as low as 25 rad (25 cGy), but damage to kidneys may not be seen without several hundred rad of dose.

Because the curve is S-shaped, there is a nonlinear relationship between effect and dose (Figure 6–5), which means that the frequency or intensity of an effect is not proportional to dose. There is a partial recovery at low doses, reflected in the tail of the curve. The curve will eventually level off and then turn downward at the highest doses because the affected animal or tissue will die before the effect is manifest (appears).

The following are characteristics of a sigmoid dose–response curve:

1. There is usually a threshold.
2. There is a partial recovery from lower doses.
3. There is a decreased response at lower doses; this is called the *dose rate effect* (discussed in more detail below).

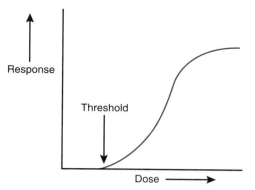

**Figure 6–5** Sigmoid threshold dose–response curve. (Reprinted with permission from Thompson MA: Principles of Radiation Protection for Nurses and Other Medical Facility Personnel. Birmingham, AL, University of Alabama at Birmingham, 1986.)

4. There is at least a plateau and probably a turning downward at the highest doses.
5. The curve exhibits nonstochastic behavior, or the certainty effect (see below).

## Linear–Quadratic Nonthreshold Dose–Response Curve

The linear and quadratic curves do not hold true for all types of radiation responses. In 1980 the Committee on Biologic Effects of Ionizing Radiation (also called the BEIR Committee) proposed a model for certain types of responses. This curve is linear or proportional at low dose levels and becomes curvilinear at higher doses (Figure 6–6). This curve has no threshold and is stochastic, since it is linear at the lowest levels.

The danger in this model is that it can underestimate the low-dose effects of radiation, since the linear portion of the curve is somewhat "flattened." For this reason, some opt for the linear model to err on the side of safety rather than to be too liberal. Dose limits (DLs), for example, assume that the linear curve holds for all effects, even though the effects of many cancers probably hold for the linear quadratic curve.

The linear–quadratic dose response curve can be summarized as follows:

1. There is no threshold.
2. There is a linear response at low dose levels.
3. There is a quadratic response at high dose levels.
4. The curve exhibits the stochastic or statistical effect.

## STOCHASTIC AND DETERMINISTIC EFFECTS

### Stochastic Effects

The term *stochastic* literally means "random in nature." This is also called the *statistical response*, which means that the probability of occurrence of effects increases in proportion to radiation dose of the entire population. It is assumed that stochastic effects do not exhibit a threshold. They are associated with the linear and the linear–quadratic dose–response curves.

An analogy that may help the student to remember this concept is investing money (Figure 6–7). If this money (radiation dose) is invested in the lottery, there is only a small chance that any return will be seen. There is no threshold in that someone or some amount of people will absolutely receive a payoff (have a radiation effect). As the amount of money invested increases, the individuals investing that money have a greater (though still remote)

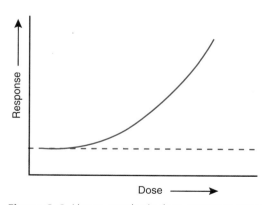

**Figure 6–6** Linear–quadratic dose–response curve. (Reprinted with permission from Thompson, MA: Principles of Radiation Protection for Nurses and Other Medical Facility Personnel. Birmingham, AL, University of Alabama at Birmingham, 1986.)

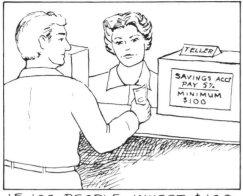

IF 100 PEOPLE INVEST $100 IN A BANK AT 5% INTEREST...

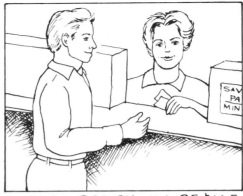

...THEIR RETURN WILL BE $105 ($100 PLUS $5). THIS IS AN EXAMPLE OF A NONSTOCHASTIC EFFECT. THE RETURN IS CERTAIN.

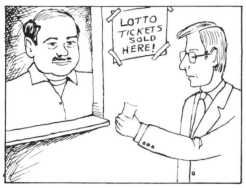

IF 100 PEOPLE BUY A LOTTERY TICKET FOR $1.00 EACH, THAT PUTS $100 IN THE POT TO BE WON BY ONE PERSON.

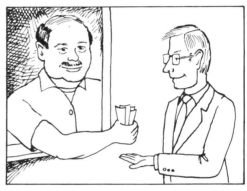

99 PEOPLE WILL WIN NOTHING IN THIS CASE, AND ONE PERSON WILL WIN $100. THIS IS AN EXAMPLE OF A STOCHASTIC EFFECT.

**Figure 6–7** Illustration of stochastic and deterministic effects.

chance of winning, and the overall cash pot (number of effects) increases.

Thus, a stochastic effect, especially at diagnostic levels, where doses are low, puts the odds heavily in one's favor that no effect will occur. An unlucky few (who cannot be predicted because it is random chance) will experience an effect. Radiation risks from diagnostic imaging, with the exception of in utero exposure of a viable fetus, are considered to be stochastic. Heredity effects and carcinogenesis are considered to be stochastic.

## Deterministic Effects

Since the ICRP changed the terminology in 1991, the term *deterministic effect* has been used rather than *nonstochastic* or *certainty effect*. Deterministic effects increase in severity with dose, and a threshold is assumed. They are also sometimes called *certainty effects* because at high doses such as in radiotherapy, it is assumed that certain effects will occur, such as skin erythema or cataracts. They are associated with the sigmoid dose–response curve.

Our investment analogy holds here also. Here, the money would be invested in a savings account, and we are certain of some kind of return unless the amount invested is too low (threshold). Most banks, for example, would not accept a deposit of 50 cents to open an interest-bearing account. Thus, below a certain amount, no effect would occur.

Cataract induction, nonmalignant damage to skin, hematologic deficiencies, and impairment to fertility are considered nonstochastic effects. The dose must be high enough to begin the effect, at which point the probability of an effect occurring is fairly high.

## RADIATION EFFECT FACTORS

### Dose and Rate Effects

The type and amount of biologic damage done by any type of radiation is determined in part by both the total dose to the cells and the rate at which the dose is delivered. As might be expected, there is a direct relationship between dose and effect. In general, the higher the dose, the greater the biologic impact. However, this effect is not necessarily linear in nature. In other words, doubling the dose may or may not double the biologic effect. As an example, the rate of leukemia in nuclear bomb survivors in Hiroshima and Nagasaki shows an increase in the rate up to a given point (about 4 Gy to the marrow-forming organs) and then a drop-off with doses higher than that. At the levels of radiation used in diagnostic procedures, most biologic effects are approximately linear in nature.

The rate at which radiation is absorbed by the cell has a major impact on the effect of the dose. This concept can be seen in the example of having pressure applied to, say, one's hand. If 1000 kilograms of pressure were applied to someone's hand for 1 second, it is reasonable to assume that some damage was done. Not only that, it probably hurt, too. In this case, 1000 kilogram-seconds of pressure were used. On the other hand (no pun intended), if 1 kilogram of pressure were applied to a hand for 1000 seconds (about 16 minutes), 1000 kilogram-seconds of pressure were also used but it is unlikely that the amount of damage to the hand (if any) was as great as in the first case.

Similarly, if a radiation dose is given over an

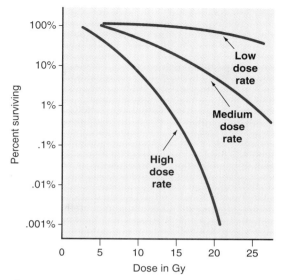

**Figure 6–8** Dose–response curves for mammalian cells irradiated with varying rates of radiation dose. (Redrawn from Bedford JS, Mitchell JB: Dose-rate effects in synchronous mammalian cells in culture. Radiat Res 1973; 54:316–327. Used by permission.)

extended time, such as several months, it will have less biologic impact than if that same dose of radiation was given quickly (see Figure 6–8) because the dose is *sublethal*. This means that the dose of radiation is not enough to kill a cell and the cell has a chance to recover from the damage. In the above example, the pressure on the hand for the extended period might by uncomfortable but no significant injury occurs. After the weight is removed, the hand quickly recovers.

The dose-rate effect states that in some situations, there is less damage cGy for cGy at lower doses than at higher doses. For example, the damage done by 10 Gy is more than 10 times greater than the damage of 1 Gy. This effect is most often seen in the kill rate of cells. At diagnostic levels of radiation, the concept of dose rate has no practical implications. However, dose rate is important in radiation therapy and also when dealing with strong radioactive sources such as nuclear reactors. The cause of the dose-rate effect is discussed in the section on target theories.

## Oxygen Effect

The concentration of oxygen in a cell or tissue has an important effect on the amount of biologic impact from radiation. The oxygen effect is not important in diagnostic procedures for two reasons. First, only when high radiation doses are used does the oxygen state of the cell become important. Second, cells that generally have a very low oxygen state are less responsive to radiation than are cells at a high oxygen state. As the blood supply in the human body provides enough oxygen to the cells for metabolic requirements, normal tissue is well oxygenated. The impact of the oxygen state becomes important only in the radiation treatment of some solid or nonvascular tumors, which can be hypoxic or nonoxygenated. One approach used to try to overcome this hypoxic state is the use of hyperbaric chambers, which subject the patient to pure oxygen environments at high pressures. The theory behind such a process is that this will increase the radiosensitivity of the tumors.

The concept used to describe the impact of oxygen on radiation effects is called the *oxygen enhancement ratio* (OER). It is nothing more than the ratio of the amount of radiation damage done when oxygen is present compared to the amount when oxygen is not present.

Some radiations, such as alpha particles, seem to be insensitive to the presence of oxygen. Others, such as x- and gamma rays, have OERs as high as 3 and above. Current thinking about this process is that the presence of oxygen is necessary for the formation of free radicals when radiolysis occurs. Without the free radicals, no hydrogen peroxide is formed and the damage to the cell from that process is reduced.

## Age Effects

In any organism, age has an impact on the amount of biologic damage. This is consistent with the law of Bergonie and Tribondeau. The human embryo/fetus begins in an extremely radiosensitive state; this sensitivity decreases with increased development. A fetus is more sensitive than a newborn, who is more sensitive than a young child. Radiosensitivity continues to decrease into the late teens, stabilizes until old age, and then begins to increase. It will not increase, however, to the levels found in children. It must be noted that, as with all effects, these depend on other factors, including systemic factors. Thus, *radiosensitivity* is a very broad and almost meaningless term unless you answer the question, "radiosensitive to what?"

Various studies have shown age effects—growing children have been shown to be two to three times more radiosensitive than adults in the development of leukemia. Breast cancer rates are increased if individuals are exposed as children (with the greatest incidents occurring if the individual was exposed at a time when breast tissue was developing). Thyroid cancer susceptibility appears to be increased if one was exposed as a child, a fact that appears to be reconfirmed with exposure to children from the Chernobyl accident. Not only children are at risk—the A-bomb survivor studies showed an increased incidence of stomach cancer with increased age at time of exposure.

The primary implication of age-related effects is that radiation protection efforts are often concentrated on the fetus and young children. However, it should be noted that complete inattention to the radiation protection of older individuals is not warranted based on this information.

Because the dose levels used in diagnostic radiology are far lower than those associated with most types of cancer, age is not a major concern for the average patient. However, it is a significant concern when irradiating the fetus in utero or in newborns, and in therapy. This will be discussed more in Chapter 10.

## Chromosomal Effects

Most biologic damage occurs as result of breakage of the chromosomal backbone made up of the phosphates and sugars. Changes to the DNA, rather than the backbones, are called *point mutations* (single break in a base) and *frameshift mutations* (double backbone breaks). Point mutations, common with low LET radiations, are associated with a greater chance for repair.

There are two subtypes of chromosomal mutations (Figures 6–10 and 6–11):

## More Information:
## LET, RBE, and OER

The relationship among LET, RBE, and OER is complex. At the radiation levels used in diagnostic procedures, this relationship is not important. However, in radiation therapy it is. Figure 6–9 shows this relationship. Note that a low-LET radiation such as used in many therapeutic approaches has a low RBE because RBE is based on 250-keV x-rays. However, the OER for these low-LET radiations is quite high and can be used in the therapeutic process (see above). When

radiation sources such as electrons (beta particles) or neutrons are used for therapeutic purposes, the RBE goes up and the OER goes down. One of the major problems with using high-LET radiation, besides the complications of producing and/or storing it, is that LETs above about 100 have a significant fall-off in RBE. These types of radiation are hard to produce and are not as effective as high-energy x-rays, neutrons, or beta particles.

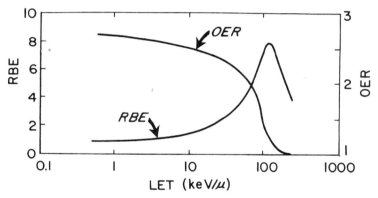

**Figure 6–9** Relationship among RBE, LET, and OER. Note that as the LET increases, the RBE also increases up to about 100 keV/μm but then drops off significantly. Also note that the OER decreases as LET increases until it has no impact. (Used with permission from Hall, EJ: Radiobiology for the Radiologist, 2nd ed. New York, Harper & Row, 1978.)

## More Information:
## Cancer in Cells from Radiation

It is well known that the rate of cancer increases with exposure to radiation. This is known as a *carcinogen* effect. Unfortunately, the mechanism of cancer induction by ionizing radiation is still not well understood even though ionizing radiation has been described as "the most thoroughly studied human car-

cinogen." Most studies have been epidemiologic in nature; that is, they have analyzed the factors that affect the frequency and distribution of disease by studying the relationships between a population and a disease rather than analyzing directly how radiation causes cancer. The problem with this approach is

---

**Cancer in Cells from Radiation (Continued)**

that we know exposing a fetus to a certain amount of radiation just prior to birth will increase the rate of leukemia threefold but we don't know exactly why. One common theory is that cancer might be inducted through structural changes in chromosomes. This theory is not well accepted because it is doubtful that any one change could cause malignancy. Another theory is that ionizing radiation might activate dormant *oncogenes* in

the cell. Oncogenes are genes that are believed to originally been implanted inside human cell chromosome by a virus. Oncogenes are thought to influence the rate of mitosis and have the ability to cause a cell to become malignant. This is also not proven. Until more basic research is completed on the actual mechanism of cancer induction in cells by radiation, we will not be able to fully understand this process.

---

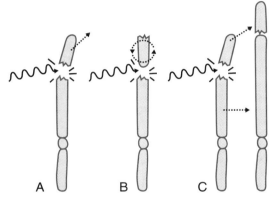

**Figure 6–10** One-break effects. (*A*) Terminal deletion. (*B*) Inversion. (*C*) Duplication.

1. *One-break effect:* This involves a portion of the arm of the chromosome being cleared off. Large *deletions* usually are expressed fatally in the next generation.
   If the deletion does not reattach, it is called *terminal deletion.*
   If it inverts and reattaches, it is called *inversion.*
   If it attaches to another chromosome, it is called *duplication.*
2. There are several types of *two-break effects:*
   *Interstitial* deletion is similar to terminal deletion, except that two segments are produced.
   *Inversion* is similar to inversion in one-break effects, except that two segments break off, invert, and reattach to the chromosomal arm.

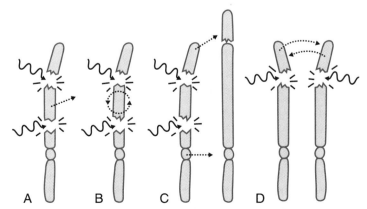

**Figure 6–11** (*A*) Interstitial deletion. (*B*) Inversion. (*C*) Duplication. (*D*) Translocation.

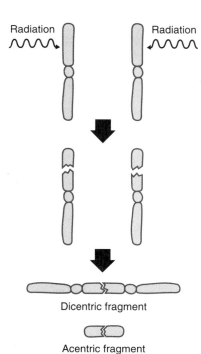

**Figure 6–12** Formation of acentric and dicentric fragments.

In *duplication,* one or both segments attach to another chromosome.

Two chromosomes exchange segments in translocation.

Also possible is the formation of acentric (no centromere) and dicentric (two centromeres) fragments (Figure 6–12). Acentric fragments are a loss of genetic information that can lead to cell alteration or death. Another possibility is that the arms may break off and attach to each other, forming an acentric fragment and a ring chromosome (Figure 6–13).

The characteristics of radiation mutation can be summarized as follows:

1. If the mutation is genetic (germ cell), it has an effect on the gametes of one or both parents. It will possibly be expressed in future generations. A somatic mutation will have possible consequences for the exposed individual *only.*

2. Radiation effects are nonspecific (as stated earlier, there are no *radiounique* effects).
3. Most mutations are undesirable.
4. Mutagenic effects are probably cumulative.
5. Straight line proportionality probably does not extend down to the very lowest doses. (A threshold exists.)

## TARGET THEORIES AND CELL SURVIVAL CURVES

### Target Theories

As discussed above, radiation can cause a number of types of damage to the chromosomes, and the damage can be either lethal or sublethal. When we look at damage that is lethal to the cell, it is necessary to understand target theories. Basically, a target theory states that there are areas on the DNA chain that, if damaged, are lethal to the cell. However, there are a number of variations to this theory that have an impact on the survival rate of cells. Studies of cellular sensitivity first became possible in the 1950s when Puck and Marcus (1956) first used HeLa cells derived from a human patient for in vitro studies. The first study was of reproductive

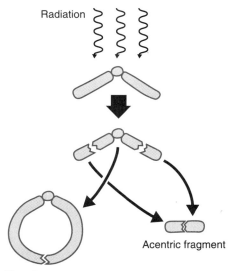

**Figure 6–13** Formation of a ring chromosome.

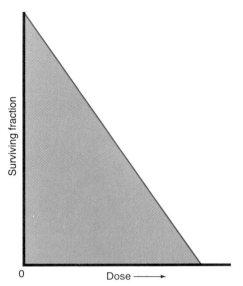

**Figure 6–14** Graphic representation of survival curve for simple cells.

target/multiple-hit theory or the multiple-target/single-hit theory, and the third is the multiple-target/multiple-hit theory.

The implications of each of these theories regarding cell survival are significant. At one extreme is the single-target/single-hit theory, which means the cell is the most sensitive to radiation. On the other extreme is the multiple-target/multiple-hit theory, which means the cell is least likely to be fatally damaged by radiation and has a linear–quadratic cell survival curve. This relationship can be shown by the following:

| Single target/ single hit | Single target/ multiple hit *or* Multiple target/ single hit | Multiple target/ multiple hit |
|---|---|---|
| Easily damaged. Simple cells. Linear survival curve. | Less easily damaged. Shouldered, steep linear survival curve. | Least damaged by radiation. Shouldered, shallow linear linear survival curve. |

## Cell Survival Curves

Cell survival curves deal with the percentage of cells not killed by various doses of radiation. Cell survival curves can be represented on a graph by plotting the dose on a linear scale on the x-axis and plotting the surviving fraction on a logarithmic scale on the y-axis. This gives a description of the relationship between dose and proportion of surviving cells. For simple cells, the survival curve is linear (Figure 6–14). When looking at a cell survival curve for humans (Figure 6–15), you will note that the curve is quadratic at the top and linear thereafter. This means that when the radiation dose is small, the number cells killed *per cGy or rad* is less than the number of cells killed *per cGy or rad* when the dose is higher. This shoulder is best explained by the multiple-target, single-hit theory and is an example of the dose-rate effect.

Figure 6–14 is a straight line in nature. In simple cells, which abide with the single-target/single-hit theory, once a cells's target is hit, any additional hits make no difference. This all or none effect makes the response linear or deterministic in nature. The curve in Figure 6–15 exhibits a shouldered or flattened area of the

failure. The experimental method involved exposing HeLa cells to various doses of radiation and then counting the number of cells that survived.

If you will recall the discussion about chromosomal damage, the types of damage that could occur were point lesions, which were usually repaired or became recessive traits, one-backbone breaks, which are usually repairable, and two-backbone breaks, which cause massive damage to the cell. Also recall that genes come in pairs (alleles) so that there are usually two identical sequences of important DNA. These facts give rise to the target ideas. Two general distinctions in target theories give rise to four distinct possibilities. The first states that some DNA sequences are so important to the cell that damage to any of these targets will kill the cell; the contrary view is that no single sequence is that important and that two or more of these targets must he hit or damaged to kill the cell. The other distinction is that a target need only be hit once to damage it; the opposite states that targets need to be hit twice or more to cause fatal damage. These two possibilities give rise to three functional target theories: the first is a single-target/single-hit theory, the second is the single-

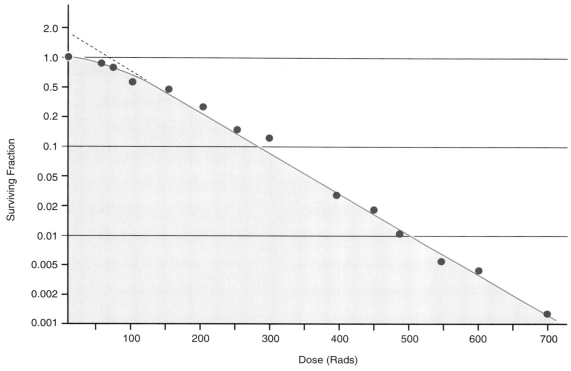

**Figure 6–15** Graphic representation of survival curve for complex cells based on data from Puck and Marcus. (Used with permission from Puck TT, Marcus, TI: Action of x-rays on mammalian cells. J Exp Med 103:653, 1956.)

curve in which lethality is not evident until some of the targets have sustained enough multiple hits to be killed. In complex cells like those found in humans, it is thought that at least one hit to at least two targets is needed to kill the cell.

Because humans have two of each chromosome, it is believed that both of these chromosomes or targets must be damaged in order for the damage to kill the cell. The cell survival curve for humans has a shoulder at low doses, which would be expected to be seen with the multiple-target (two chromosomes)/single-hit theory. Recall from Figure 6–1 that there is a random distribution of radiation across cells or targets. What that means is that even at very low levels, at which there are about as many hits as targets, some cells will have two targets

hit and will be killed, many will have only one target hit and will not be killed, and 37% will not be hit at all. As the amount of radiation increases, the number of cells with no targets hit will decrease until, for all practical purposes, all cells have at least one target hit. Up to that point, the response curve would be quadratic or flattened. From that point on, the curve would be linear. Another reason why it is believed that human cells usually abide by the two-target/single-hit model has to do with extrapolation the linear portion of the curve up to the y-axis of the curve, which gives some idea of the number of targets in the cells. See Figure 6–15 for extrapolation of n, or the target number. For more information, see "More Information: Cell Survival Curves."

## More Information:
## Cell Survival Curves

As mentioned earlier, simple cells have linear survival curves. Simple cells exhibit the same response to the same dose in terms of percentage of cells killed. That is, if 5 rad (5 cGy) of ionizing radiation kills 10% of a population, then 5 rad will always kill 10% of that population. It does not matter if it is the first or second or third 5-rad dose. Complex cells have a curvilinear response curve, and the first 5 rads will not kill 10% of the cells but the next 5 rads might.

The multiple-target/single-hit theory best explains the shoulders of the curve seen in complex cells. There are n targets in a cell, where n represents the number of critical targets that must be hit to kill a cell. If fewer than n targets are hit, the cell can repair itself and will not die. The shoulder of the curve is the region in which the number of hits is less than the number necessary to hit each target of each cell at least once. Note in Figure 6–15 that the linear portion of the curve is projected back up to the y-axis of the graph. In humans, n is usually extrapolated as two. This agrees with the idea that cells have two sets of chromosomes.

However, there is some slope in the very initial portion of the shoulder, which cannot be explained by the random distribution of radiation. Since these low doses probably do not cause enough multiple-target damage to produce the amount of lethal damage seen, there must be some cells in humans that act like simple cells and are killed off by single-target, single-hit models. Exactly which cells, if any, behave this way is not clear.

## RADIATION EFFECTS ON THE CELL

Three things can happen to a cell after being irradiated. The first is division delay. Low doses (under 1 Gy) of radiation delay mitosis in humans. In this process, the mitotic rate goes down, increases to a rate higher than normal, and finally levels off again near normal. The cause of division delay is not known. There are three theories: (1) a chemical involved in mitosis is altered; (2) proteins necessary for mitosis are not yet synthesized; and (3) DNA synthesis slows down. At doses up to about 0.5 Gy, this effect is not usually seen. With doses of up to about 3 Gy, the mitotic rate returns back to normal. With doses above this, the mitotic rate may never fully recover.

Small mature lymphocytes are especially prone to an effect known as *interphase death*. The dose for interphase death depends on the type of cell and varies from 0.5 Gy up to 30 Gy. In general, rapidly dividing, undifferentiated cells exhibit interphase death at lower doses than nondividing, differentiated cells. Cytoplasmic organelles remain intact while cells break down and condense. It is theorized that this effect is due to changes in the cell membrane, resulting in an imbalance of electrolytes.

Any cell that does not divide repeatedly or that divides many times, giving dead progeny, is said to have undergone reproductive failure. This effect is seen in some cells after irradiation. The percentage of cells undergoing reproductive failure is based on the dose. Up to about 1.5 Gy, the rate is random and nonlinear in nature. However, at doses above that, there is a linear relationship between the rate and the effect.

## RELATIVE TISSUE AND ORGAN RADIOSENSITIVITY

### Tissue Makeup Based on Cell Type

Cells make up tissues, and tissue radiosensitivity is essentially a function of the cell type(s) that make up that tissue. The simplest classification of cell types is as follows:

Table 6–3  Comparison of Tissue Types

| Tissue Type | Description | Sensitivity |
|---|---|---|
| Vegetative intermitotic tissue cells (VIMs) | Undifferentiated, highly mitotic | Very radiosensitive |
| Differentiating intermitotic cells (DIMs) | More differentiated, highly mitotic | Less radiosensitive |
| Multipotential connective tissue cells (MCTs) | Differentiated, occasionally mitotic | Moderately radiosensitive |
| Reverting postmitotic cells (RPMs) | Highly differentiated, divide rarely | Moderately radioresistant |
| Fixed postmitotic cells (FPMs) | Highly differentiated, do not divide | Radioresistant |

*Stem cells* exist to self-perpetuate and produce cells for another population, for example, spermatogonia.

*Transit cells* are cells in movement to another population, for example, a reticulocyte, which is in transit to becoming an erythrocyte.

*Static cells* are cells that are fully differentiated and do not exhibit mitotic activity, for example, adult muscle cells.

In reality cell typing is more complex that than. A more complex typing of cells from most to least radiosensitive is as follows (see Table 6–3):

*Vegetative intermitotic tissue cells* (VIMs) are rapidly dividing, undifferentiated, and have a short lifetime. These are the most radiosensitive of all tissue types because of their level of biological activity. Examples are basal cells of epidermis and crypt cells of intestines.

*Differentiating intermitotic cells* (DIMs) are produced by division of VIMs. They are still very actively mitotic and relatively undifferentiated but are more differentiated than VIM cells. An example is Type B spermatogonia.

*Multipotential connective tissue cells* (MCTs) are highly differentiated cells that still divide but do so irregularly. Examples are endothelial cells (blood vessels) and fibroblasts (connective tissue).

*Reverting postmitotic cells* (RPMs) are cells that do not normally divide but can do so under some situations. RPMs are very highly differentiated and long lived. Liver cells are an example.

*Fixed postmitotic cells* (FPMs) are very highly differentiated and do not divide at all. Nerve cells are an example.

## The Composition of Organs

Organs are a combination of various tissues organized into a given structure and function relationship. Organs are composed of parenchyma and stroma. The parenchyma of an organ is the functional tissue. The stroma is a more broadly defined component of the connective tissue and vasculature that supports the organ parenchyma for its structure and function.

## Tissue and Organ Radiosensitivity

Organ and tissue radiosensitivity can be subdivided into the radiosensitivity of the individual components of tissues and cells; that is, in general, tissues and organs that contain radiosensitive cells also are sensitive to radiation. Conversely, tissues and organs that contain radioresistant cells are resistant to radiation.

Some organs are highly dependent on having a high degree of cellular proliferation. In these organs, radiation injury becomes quickly evident shortly after exposure due to the loss of dividing cell components. The greater the number of dividing cells affected, the shorter the time to evidence of injury. Examples of organs that respond in this way are bone marrow, the gastrointestinal tract, skin, and testes. These are called *acutely responding organs.*

Other organs are more dependent on the integrity of stromal elements. This includes the lungs and kidneys, which depend on an intact microvasculature. Cellular division occurs at a greatly reduced rate in comparison to the previously mentioned organs. Organs such as the lungs and kidneys show an initial presentation of clinical symptoms that are relatively nonspecific. What may occur over time following exposure is that, as slowly dividing cells begin to divide to replenish their numbers, latent damage to DNA may impair this ability to meet the organ's need for new cells. Organ responses in this group may take 6 to 9 months to manifest (show the evidence of injury). They are called *late-responding organs.*

The effect of radiation effects on small blood vessels is important. Radiation-induced injury of small blood vessels following high doses of radiation is seen as swelling of endothelial and smooth muscle cells in the vessel wall. This leads to restricted blood flow in the vessel. This increases the possibility of focal tissue alterations and blood clot occlusion, which are not usually seen with low doses of radiation.

This thickening of the vessel wall can lead to areas of altered vessel architecture. This can lead to telangiectasis, a vascular lesion caused by dilation of a group of small blood vessels that can impair blood flow and nutrition of an organ. This impairment of organ function can lead to organ failure. This is what may be seen following irradiation of the spinal cord at high doses. Students may sometimes wonder why, in radiation therapy, there is a concern that the spinal cord will be damaged by radiation. It consists of individual nerve fibers that are nondividing and hence should be considered radio-resistant. However, the spinal cord has a continuous need for oxygen and nutrients. This maintains normal cellular function.

With a thickening of the surrounding vasculature, the delivery of oxygen and nutrients becomes restricted. This leads to a decrease in the ability of the nerve fiber to maintain a polarized membrane. Nerve conduction can then become impaired, showing as weakness in the lower extremities, tingling sensations in the fingers, and so on. This depends on the level at which nerve fibers have been affected and is known as transection of the spinal cord. It is believed that damage within the microvasculature and connective tissue, as well as damage to the parenchyma, is what gives rise to the late effects of radiation as seen after radiation therapy.

## Tissue Type/Dose Relationship

The relative radiosensitivity to tissues and organs following high doses can be summarized as follows. More data exist for high doses of radiation than low doses. Tissues and organs considered highly radiosensitive, such as lymphoid tissue, show hypoplasia following doses of 200 to 1000 rad (2–10 Gy). Intermediately radiosensitive organs and tissues such as the cornea of the eye (cataracts) and the liver (ascites) demonstrate effects with doses of 1000 to 5000 (10–50 Gy) rad. Radioresistant organs and tissues such as muscle (fibrosis), brain (necrosis), and spinal cord (transection) show effects at 5000 rad (50 Gy).

## Advanced Information: Protraction and Fractionation

Both protraction and fractionation are important concepts in the use to radiation to treat cancers. In the normal radiation therapy protocol, the patient is given a sublethal dose of radiation on a daily basis for up to several weeks. The idea behind this process is to give the skin and other organs in the path of the radiation beam time to recover from the daily radiation dose enough so as to not be killed. Because tumors are normally very fast growing, and hence highly mitotic, they are more radiosensitive, and what is a sublethal dose to other, normal organs hopefully is a lethal dose to the tumor.

## Protraction and Fractionation *(Continued)*

### The Four R's

There are four processes that make fractionated radiation therapy useful. The first is the ability to *recover* from sublethal damage. Many tumors are hypoxic and, based on research with mammalian cells, have a reduced ability to repair damage. As noted above, almost all healthy tissue in the human body is well oxygenated. Consequently, any normal tissue that the radiation beam passed through has a greater ability to repair any damage done by the dose. Many tumors, on the other hand, are not able to sufficiently repair the radiation damage and, over time, are killed off by the fractionated doses.

The second is *repopulation*. Generally, both normal and cancer cells repopulate at about the same rate, but some normal cells do repopulate faster than cancer cells. If tumors were only made up of cancerous cells, then repopulation would have no impact. However, estimates are that as little as 0.1% of a tumor is made up of cancer cells. So, even though the tumor cells will repopulate, they do not do so as quickly as some types of health cells. If the fractionation is optimal, the result will be that the number of cancer cells will be constantly reduced while the number of normal cells will not be reduced significantly.

The third is *reoxygenation*. In tumors that have hypoxic cells, irradiation will reduce the number of these cells because of improved blood circulation after shrinkage of the tumor and also due to increased availability of oxygen not being used by cells already killed. Over time, the percentage of hypoxic cells will return to the preexposure level, but if the dose is fractionated so that additional radiation is given when the number of hypoxic cells is lowest, the tumor will continue to be reduced. In practice, this is seldom taken into consideration in radiation therapy treatment planning.

Finally, *redistribution* deals with forcing more cells to a mitotic state at the same time. As noted by the Law of Bergonie and Tribondeau, cells are most radiosensitive when they are biologically active. Cell division (mitosis) is a very radiosensitive period for that very reason. Cells that have been irradiated during the mitotic phase tend to die off more than other cells. This means that there is a redistribution of cells in the mitotic cycle and that a higher percentage of cells will be dividing at some times than otherwise would be observed. If the fractionated dose can be timed to match this cycle in the tumor, significant kill-off will occur. As with timing for reoxygenation, timing for redistribution is seldom taken into consideration in radiation therapy planning.

### SUMMARY

LET is a measure of the rate at which energy is transferred from radiation to the cells. High-LET radiation, such as alpha particles and neutrons, transfers energy in a limited area. Low-LET radiation, such as x-rays and beta particles, transfers energy over a greater area. RBE is a ratio describing how much biologic damage a type of radiation does when compared to 250-keV x-rays.

There is a general correlation between LET and RBE—as one goes up, so does the other. At very high LETs (over 100 keV/μm), this correlation breaks down.

When radiation interacts with a cell, one of two types of effects happens. In a direct effect, the energy of the radiation is directly transferred to a macromolecule that is ionized. This direct effect can injure or kill a cell. A indirect effect is when the radiation interacts with water by radiolysis. In this process, water is ionized, a free radical is formed, and the end by-products of that ionization can include hydrogen peroxide, which does damage to the cell. The vast majority of interactions in the cell are indirect, as the cell is mostly made up of water.

Sigmoid dose–response curves are usually associated with a threshold, exhibit a partial recovery from lower doses, show a decreased response at lower doses, have at least a plateau and probably a downward turn at the highest doses, and exhibit the nonstochastic or certainty effect. Nonstochastic effects increase in severity with dose.

The linear dose–response curve is not usually associated with a threshold, the response to radiation in terms of frequency or severity of effects is proportional to the dose, there is no reduced effect at small dose rates, and the curve exhibits a stochastic or statistical response. The term *stochastic* literally means "random in nature," which implies that the probability of occurrence of effects increases in proportion to radiation dose of the entire population. Radiation risks from diagnostic imaging (with the exception of in utero exposure of a viable fetus, heredity effects, and carcinogenesis) are stochastic.

There is a direct relationship between the amount of the dose and the impact of that dose. The rate of the dose also impacts the effect. If the radiation is given over a longer time, the amount of damage is less. The level of oxygen in a cell also affects the amount of damage done by radiation. If the cell is hypoxic, less damage is done. If the cell is highly oxygenated, more than the normal level of damage will occur.

The age of the person being exposed affects the amount and type of damage. A fetus is the most radiosensitive, with children being the next most sensitive. When a person becomes elderly, sensitivity to radiation increases somewhat over that of early adulthood.

Cell survival curves graphically represent the survival of cells in relationship to dose. Complex cells show a shoulder, or area of lessened effects, at low doses; simple cells show a straight line proportional relationship between dose and effect.

There are two subtypes of chromosomal mutations: one-break effects and two-break

effects. Also possible are the formation of acentric and dicentric fragments.

Groups of cells show varying levels of radiosensitivity based on their level of differentiation and mitotic rate. The most radiosensitive are the vegetative intermitotic cells (VIMs). VIMs are often precursor cells and are highly mitotic and undifferentiated. Differentiating intermitotic cells (DIMs) are a more specialized version of VIMs and are less mitotic and radiosensitive. Multipotential connective tissue cells (MCTs), such as endothelial cells, are of medium radiosensitivity. Reverting postmitotic cells (RPMs), such as liver cells, are very specialized, occasionally mitotic, and somewhat radioresistant. The last category is fixed postmitotic cells (FPMs), such as nerve cells, which are also highly specialized, do not divide except under unusual conditions and are radio resistant.

## Questions

1. If a one-break effect to a chromosome does not reattach, it is called:

   a. inversion.          b. duplication.
   c. terminal deletion.  d. translocation.

2. Low-LET radiations such as x-radiation and gamma radiation are also:

   a. sparsely ionizing.  b. highly
                            ionizing.
   c. high RBE.           d. particulate.

3. Another name for a stochastic effect is the:

   a. certainty effect.   b. statistical
                            response.
   c. linear sigmoid effect.  d. nonrandom
                                 effect.

4. No threshold, no dose rate effect, and a stochastic response best define the _____ curve.

   a. linear threshold
   b. linear nonthreshold
   c. sigmoid threshold
   d. sigmoid nonthreshold

5. A partial recovery from lower doses, decreased response at lower doses, and a

certainty effect best describe the _____ curve.

a. linear threshold
b. linear nonthreshold
c. sigmoid threshold
d. sigmoid nonthreshold

6. Deterministic is the term used by the ICRP for the _____ effect.

   I. certainty
   II. nonstochastic
   III. stochastic

   a. I only
   b. II only
   c. I and II only
   d. I and III only

7. A retired technologist tells you she is certain that her recent diagnosis of cataracts is due to her many years of working in Doctor Jones' outpatient clinic, performing primarily chest and extremity exams. Which of the following is the most accurate statement regarding her belief?

   a. Since radiation can cause cataracts, the statement is probably correct.
   b. Since radiation can't cause cataracts, the statement is incorrect.
   c. Since cataract formation is a stochastic effect, the statement is probably correct.
   d. Since cataract formation is a nonstochastic effect, the statement is probably incorrect.

8. A shouldered, shallow linear survival curve best describes the _____ theory.

   a. single-target/single-hit
   b. single-target/multiple-hit
   c. multiple-target/single-hit
   d. multiple-target/multiple-hit

9. Which of the following have an impact on the effect on a cell?

   a. the amount of radiation delivered
   b. the rate of radiation delivered
   c. the oxygenation of the cell
   d. all of the above

10. Which of the following is the proper probable ranking of radiosensitivity to leukemia induction from most to least radiosensitive?

    a. fetus, 85-year-old woman, 6-year-old child, 25-year-old man
    b. fetus, 6-year-old child, 25-year-old man, 85-year-old woman
    c. fetus, 6-year-old child, 85-year-old woman, 25-year-old man
    d. fetus, 25-year-old man, 85-year-old woman, 6-year-old child

## Exercises

1. Compare LET and RBE.

2. Describe the mechanisms of indirect action.

3. Describe fractionation and explain where it is used.

4. Contrast deterministic and stochastic effects. Which effect pertains most directly to diagnostic uses of radiation?

5. What is the rationale behind use of the linear quadratic dose–response curve?

## Answers

Questions

| | |
|---|---|
| 1. c | 6. c |
| 2. a | 7. d |
| 3. b | 8. d |
| 4. b | 9. d |
| 5. c | 10. c |

Exercises

1. In general, as LET increases, so does RBE. Thus, high-LET radiations such as alpha and beta particles also have a high RBE. Low-LET radiations such as x- and gamma radiation have a low RBE.

2. The primary mechanism for indirect action is the radiolysis of water. When radiation interacts with water, the water is ionized, producing a free radical. Free radicals contain a single unpaired electron in their outer shell, making them chemically unsta-

ble. There are a variety of possible reactions. The water molecules may then recombine to form a normal water molecule, or they may form hydrogen peroxide, which may damage cellular macromolecule.

3. If a dose is fractionated, or split into smaller amounts over time, the damage done to healthy tissue is usually less than if the same dose were given in a single dose. Fractionation is used in radiation therapy because this process can help kill tumor cells while sparing healthy cells.

4. The term *stochastic* literally means "random in nature" and is associated with the linear dose–response curve and diagnostic levels of dose. This means that the probability of occurrence of effects is "all or none" for each individual, and the likelihood of an effect increases in proportion to the radiation dose of the entire population.

   The nonstochastic or certainty effects are associated with thresholds, the sigmoid dose-response curve, and high doses such as are found in radiation therapy. Once the dose reaches the threshold, almost all individuals will have a response.

   Radiation risks from diagnostic imaging (with the exception of in utero exposure of a viable fetus, heredity effects, and carcinogenesis) are considered to be stochastic. Thus, for the most part, stochastic effects are the most important in terms of diagnostic imaging.

5. Neither the linear or quadratic curves hold true for all types of radiation responses. The Committee on Biologic Effects of Ionizing Radiation proposed the linear-quadratic model for certain types of responses. This curve is linear or proportional at low doses, becoming curvilinear at higher doses. It best describes the response of human cells to radiation.

## CHAPTER 7

# Early Effects of Radiation

Steven B. Dowd  •  Elwin R. Tilson

## Chapter Outline

## Chapter Objectives

At the end of this chapter, the student should be able to:

1. Define $LD_{50/30}$

2. Describe the radiation syndromes in terms of dose and effects.

3. Describe radiation effects to the skin

4. Cite radiation effects to germ cells.

5. Describe the induction of radiodermatitis at high doses to the extremities.

6. Describe possible hematologic effects.

7. Define karyotype.

8. Formulate a list of limitations to chromosomal studies at low doses.

## Important Terms

aberration
acute radiation syndrome
ataxia
basal cell
biologic dosimetry
central nervous system syndrome
dermis
desquamation
epidermis
epilation
erythrocyte
gastrointestinal syndrome
granulocyte
Grenz ray therapy
hematologic syndrome
$LD_{50/30}$
$LD_{100}$
latent period
lymphocyte
malaise

| | |
|---|---|
| manifest illness | pluripotential stem cell |
| maturation depletion | prodromal radiation syndrome |
| oogonia | radiodermatitis |
| pancytopenia | spermatogonia |
| phenotype | thrombocyte |

## INTRODUCTION

Early effects such as the acute radiation syndromes are of more than academic interest to the radiologic technologist. Technologists learn these syndromes to be fully informed about the effects of ionizing radiation—the hallmark of a true professional. Professionals are interested in all aspects of the science of their profession. Sometimes patients still ask about the possibility of "x-ray burns," for example, which is a holdover from the early days of radiology. It is certainly important that a radiographer knows *why* this cannot occur at today's dose levels, for example, and that a radiation therapist can describe the type of skin effects that can occur as a result of therapeutic radiation to patients.

*Early effects* refers to effects that occur soon after radiation exposure. The time to onset of early effects is measured in terms of minutes, hours, days, and weeks as opposed to that for late effects, which can take many years to develop.

## ACUTE RADIATION SYNDROMES

Acute radiation syndromes involve a total body exposure, an acute exposure of a few minutes, and many hundreds or thousands of rad. An important concept is the $LD_{50/30}$—the lethal dose required to kill 50% of a population in 30 days. The $LD_{50/30}$ is often used in animal studies; for humans the $LD_{50/30}$ is not often used as humans tend to survive beyond the 30-day period. Table 7–1 summarizes some $LD_{50/30}$ values. The $LD_{50/30}$ is under investigation because of the nuclear power plant explosion at Chernobyl, where more humans survived than would have been expected under current $LD_{50/30}$ expectations.

Mammals exposed from 200 to 1000 rad sur-

**Table 7–1** $LD_{50/30}$ Values

| Species | $LD_{50/30}$ (rad) |
|---|---|
| Human | 250–450* |
| Dog | 300 |
| Monkey | 400 |
| Rat | 900 |
| Turtle | 1500 |
| Newt | 3000 |

*Varies depending on source. Figure is higher if clinical support (medical treatment) is available.

vive a few weeks at the lower dose levels. From 1000 to 10,000 rad, this survival decreases to 3 to 4 days. Above 10,000 rad, this survival rate decreases to hours or minutes.

Besides the three lethal syndromes to be discussed, two other events occur in total body irradiation. The first is the prodromal radiation syndrome. The term *prodromal* means "running before." It refers to the initial stage of a disease. The prodromal syndrome can occur with a dose as low as 50 rad and occurs within a matter of minutes at high dose levels (in excess of 1000 rad). It consists of nausea, vomiting, and diarrhea and is also called the NVD syndrome.

There is usually a latent period following the prodromal syndrome. During this period, the individual appears to be symptom-free; in reality, the lethal effects or recovery is beginning. This period is a matter of hours at higher doses and weeks at lower doses. There are four basic stages: prodromal, latent, manifest, and recovery or death. This staging process is illustrated in Table 7–2.

**Table 7–2  Staging of Acute Radiation Syndromes**

| Stage 1 | Stage 2 | Stage 3 | Stage 4 |
|---------|---------|---------|---------|
| Prodromal  →  | Latent  →  | Manifest illness  →  Three possibilities:  ■ Hematologic syndrome  ■ Gastrointestinal syndrome  ■ CNS syndrome | Recovery or death* |

*Recovery is dose dependent and is seen only in the hematologic syndrome; this can take 3 weeks to 6 months, and many individuals do not survive.

Reprinted with permission from Thompson MA, Hall J, Hattaway D, Dowd S: Principles of Imaging Science and Protection. Philadelphia, WB Saunders, 1994.

## Hematologic Syndrome

Also called the bone marrow or hematopoietic syndrome, the hematologic syndrome occurs at lower dose levels because of the extremely sensitive nature of the blood-forming cells of the bone marrow. This effect occurs from 100 to 1000 rad; some texts cite the range as 200 to 600 and still others as 200 to 1000. Different types of radiation produce different effects even when the dosage in rad is the same (e.g. 500 rad of neutrons will have a greater effect than 500 rad of x-ray), and this is one of the reasons why texts do not fully agree on the dosage needed to produce a syndrome.

Sensitive individuals die within 6 to 8 weeks following a dose of 200 rad. No one has ever lived following a dose of 1000 rad (also called the $LD_{100}$ because it is the lethal dose for 100% of the population). An individual exposed to this dose will die within 2 weeks.

The first stage of manifest illness involves the prodromal effects of nausea, vomiting, and diarrhea. There then appears a latent period in a matter of a few hours that can extend up to 4 weeks. During the latent period, the only sign of the disease is in the declining numbers of red and white blood cells and platelets in the circulating blood.

The mitotic stem cells that produce the above components have been sterilized in this syndrome. This diminished supply of blood cells is called *pancytopenia,* the term *pan* meaning "all." Symptoms observed include fever, a generalized malaise, anemia, hemorrhage, and infection due to a lack of white blood cells. Death may occur as a result of dehydration, an imbalance in electrolytes, or generalized infections.

## Gastrointestinal Syndrome

The range of effect for the gastrointestinal syndrome holds the least agreement among authorities. The ranges are:

- 600 to 1000 rad—Selman
- 1000 to 5000 rad—Bushong
- "Some symptoms" at 600 rad, the "full syndrome" after 1000 rad—Travis

After the prodromal syndrome, which last up to 1 day, a latent period of 3 to 5 days results. A second wave of nausea and vomiting results in the manifest illness stage, along with prolonged diarrhea. The lining of the gastrointestinal tract is being depopulated (removed), which results in dehydration. Lethargy and anorexia may also result. Medical intervention cannot prevent progression of the syndrome, and death can result in 3 to 4 days.

## Central Nervous System (CNS) Syndrome

After about 5000 rad to the whole body, the central nervous system syndrome results. Death usually occurs within hours, although it may take several days. The hematopoietic and gastrointestinal syndromes are occurring simultaneously, and there is not sufficient time for them to manifest.

Nausea and vomiting occur within minutes, and the exposed individual usually becomes nervous and confused. Consciousness may be lost. The latent period is extremely short at 6 to 12 hours. Ataxia (loss of muscle coordination), convulsions, difficulty in breathing, loss of coordination, lethargy, and coma may ensue before the individual dies. The cause of death in the central nervous system syndrome is not known, but it has been suggested that it is increased pressure in the cranial vault.

## LOCAL TISSUE DAMAGE

Local tissue damage results from high doses to parts of the body. Following such exposure, cell death results, leading to atrophy (shrinkage) of that organ. Recovery of the organ may be full, partial, or nonexistent, depending on dose and cell type. In the event of nonrecovery, necrosis (death) of the organ results.

### Skin

Because of radiation therapy and early uses of radiation, we have a good deal of information on skin effects. Many of the early x-ray pioneers suffered x-ray burns to the skin. Patients also often suffered x-ray burns as a result of exposures that used low kilovoltages, unshielded tubes, and several minutes of exposure time.

Radiodermatitis in the form of what were then called "roentgen-ray burns" were the cause of many lawsuits against untrained operators, including physicians. Thousands of dollars were awarded to individuals burned by x-ray. This led to certification of radiographers and to the creation of physicians specializing in the use of x-ray for diagnosis and treatment.

A review of the following techniques recommended by Borden in 1900 shows why x-ray burns could easily occur. At a distance of 10 inches, the following techniques were recommended:

*Hand and forearm*—1 to 2 minutes
*Shoulder and chest*—10 minutes
*Knee*—9 minutes
*Hip, head, and pelvis*—20 minutes

Also, operators would, for example, determine how well a fluoroscopic tube was working by seeing if the shadow of a watch was visible through their own skull. The development of intensifying screens (used fairly commonly after World War I) and beam-restricting devices lowered the above doses somewhat, although good radiation protection was not mandated in any form.

The skin consists of three layers and some accessory structures (Figure 7–1):

● Subcutaneous layer of fat and connective tissue
● Middle layer of connective tissue, the true skin or dermis
● The outer layer, or epidermis
● Accessory structures—sensory receptors, hair follicles, sebaceous glands, and sweat

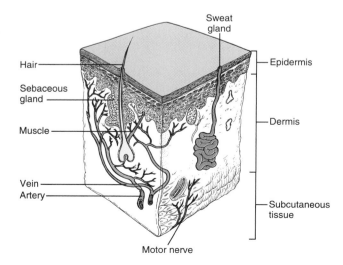

**Figure 7–1** The skin. The epidermis, the thin outer layer, is composed of four to five layers. Underneath the epidermis is the thicker dermis, composed of connective tissue containing lymphatics, nerves, blood vessels, hair follicles, sebaceous glands, and sweat glands. Beneath the dermis is a layer of subcutaneous adipose tissue. (From Leonard, PC: Building a Medical Vocabulary, 4th ed., 1997.)

glands (the final two of which are relatively radioresistant).

Skin is sensitive because it represents a continually renewing system of cells. About 2% of the skin is replaced each day. Damage to the germ cells of skin, the basal cells, causes most of the damage to the skin from radiation. A single dose of 100 to 300 rad (1–3 Gy) can cause a mild erythema or reddening of the skin within 1 or 2 days. Another more severe skin reddening occurs in about 2 weeks. Before radiation units were developed, the skin erythema dose (SED) was used as a measurement of the amount of radiation received by an individual.

Skin effects follow a nonlinear, threshold dose–response relationship. Erythema is not noted with small doses of radiation. Erythema depends on three factors: size of field irradiated, dose rate, and the individual's radiosensitivity. Other acute changes in the skin that can occur as a result of moderate to high doses of radiation include a general inflammation and a dry or moist desquamation or removal of the surface of skin.

At one time, radiation therapy was associated with producing dramatic necrotic effects in skin. Today's high-energy units and fractionation of doses may lead to an atrophy of the irradiated area, but severe necrotic effects are rare.

Radiation can also result in the loss of hair, known as epilation. This was associated with a type of radiotherapy known as Grenz ray therapy, formerly used for ringworm treatments (see Chapter 8), which used very low kVp levels of 10 to 20 kVp. This loss of hair was fairly long-term (several months) in these patients,

**CASE STUDY**

The following case study shows how early effects such as radiodermatitis can lead to late effects such as cancer. As a teenager and young woman, the patient had atopic dermatitis that was treated by local radiation and by many doctors. From repeated exposure to radiation, the patient developed severe radiodermatitis. During the previous 10 years, several basal cell carcinomas had appeared and had been treated by curettage or excision. Figure 7–2 shows that

a new tumor has developed and that necrotic facial bone is visible.

The patient's history illustrates many points:

1. It is dangerous to treat benign conditions with radiation, particularly in young people.
2. A patient can go from one physician to another, each being unaware of the treatment administered by the others. It was estimated that parts of this patient's face had received a total dose of over 11,000 cGy (11,000 rad). This is two to three times the dose commonly given to treat a malignant tumor.
3. Chronic ulceration is a feature of radiodermatitis.
4. Healing of radiation ulcers is slow, and skin grafting is often unsatisfactory because of the local ischemia.
5. Multiple tumors can develop in radiation-damaged tissue.

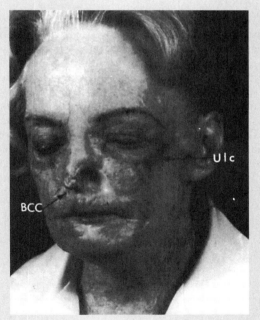

**Figure 7–2** Radiodermatitis and its complications.

(Reprinted with permission from Walter JB: An Introduction to the Principles of Disease, 3rd ed. Philadelphia: WB Saunders, 1992, p 248.)

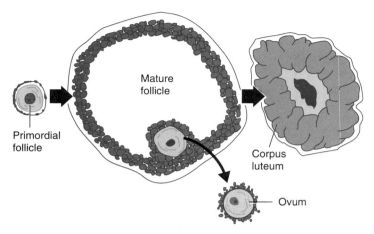

**Figure 7–3** Life cycle of oogonia.

and it was permanent in cases in which the doses were very high.

**Gonads**

The human gonads are extremely sensitive to radiation, and, because they contain the human germ cells that potentially pass on effects to future generations, it is extremely important to have well-documented information on the effects of radiation on them. Unfortunately, most of our information comes from animal studies. Some information does come from radiation accident victims, radiotherapy patients, and studies conducted on volunteer convicts. For example, some of our knowledge of the radiosensitivity of the male testes comes from convicts who agreed to be irradiated in exchange for earlier release time.

The means by which germ cells are produced in male and female gonads is, of course, different. The stem cells of the ovaries, the oogonia, multiply only in the fetus, after which their number steadily declines throughout life (Figure 7–3). On the other hand, the testes stem cells, the spermatogonia, are continually renewing (Figure 7–4).

**Testes**

A dose of 10 rad (10 cGy) can lead to a reduction in the number of spermatozoa. This reduction increases and lengthens the time of effect as the dose is increased. Since there is a 3- to 5-week period for maturation of spermatozoa, a dose of 200 to 250 rad (2–2.5 Gy) results in temporary sterility that takes 2 months to become fully manifest. This eventual depletion of mature sperm is called *maturation depletion*. Although fertility returns, there may be chromosomal damage in functional sperm. This sterility lasts up to 1 year. Perma-

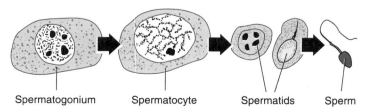

Spermatogonium    Spermatocyte    Spermatids    Sperm

**Figure 7–4** Life cycle of spermatogonia.

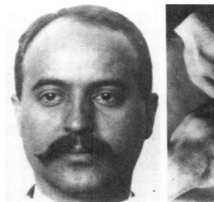 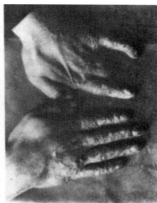

**Figure 7–5** Radiodermatitis of Dr. M.K. Kassabian. (Reprinted with permission from Grigg EN: Kassabian and his hands. *In* The Trail of the Invisible Light. Springfield, IL, Charles C Thomas, 1965, p 679. Courtesy of Charles C Thomas, Publisher.)

nent sterility is produced with a dose of 500 to 600 rad (5–6 Gy).

## Ovaries

In the female, a dose of 10 rad (10 cGy) can suppress and delay menstruation. The ovaries are especially radiosensitive in the fetus and child. This lessens with age until about age 30, when radiosensitivity again gradually increases with age. As in the male, 200 rad (2 Gy) produces a temporary sterility; 500 to 625 rad (5–6.25 Gy) causes permanent sterility. After temporary sterility has ended, the possibility of chromosomal damage cannot be discounted.

## Extremities

We discussed previously the effects of radiation on skin. Wolfram Fuchs, one of the x-ray pioneers, noted that the hair on his hand fell out after fluoroscopy, but he also stated that the hair grew back "with no apparent ill effects."

The majority of effects to the extremities were noted in the hands of early radiologists, who often had multiple amputations of their fingers as a result of being (unknowingly) careless with fluoroscopy. Often, operators had to put their hands in the beam to "prove" to the patient that the "x-ray light" did not hurt.

These operators contracted radiodermatitis, which often metastasized and resulted in death. Dr. M.K. Kassabian documented the deterioration of his hands due to radiodermatitis. These photographs are shown in Figure 7–5. Dr. Kassabian formulated a number of radiation protection measures based on his experiences, some of which are still used in modified form today (see the insert). He died in 1910 of a metastatic malignancy to the axilla.

Many years ago, shoe fluoroscopes were popular additions to shoe stores. The customer could observe how well the shoes fit under a fluoroscopic device. There were often no restrictions on their operation, and schoolchildren would rush to the shoe store after school to play with the machine. Their use was outlawed in the late 1950s and early 1960s.

Today, the group of individuals who must be most careful about the potential effects of radiation to the extremities are nuclear medicine technologists. Although no skin changes have been observed on the hands of nuclear medicine technologists, hand doses are increasing as a result of the number of procedures performed and the amounts of certain radionuclides being used, such as $^{99m}$Tc.

## HEMATOLOGIC DEPRESSION

The dose needed to produce a hematologic depression is about 25 rad (25 cGy), much higher than doses sustained today by radiation workers. At one time, hematologic depression was used as a measure of biologic dosimetry for radiation workers. Today's doses make the use of blood tests for dosimetry invalid.

---

### Radiation Protection Guidelines of Dr. M.K. Kassabian

*Patient Protection*

1. Only small interrupted doses should be given.
2. High-gas tubes produce less radiodermatitis than low-gas tubes.
3. The more distance from the tube, the less danger of burning the patient.
4. Screen surrounding parts of the body with thin sheets of lead.
5. The soft and unnecessary x-rays should be filtered by leather or aluminum.

*Operator Protection*

1. Never use the hands to test the intensity of x-ray.
2. The operator should be in a communi-cating room while the patient is undergo-ing treatment or examination; he or she should be behind lead and be able to observe the fluorescence of the tube.
3. The best place for lead protection is behind the anode.
4. Wherever x-rays may be detected (Kass-abian recommended using an electro-scope or photographic plate to do so) is unsafe for the operator.
5. Opaque lead rubber gloves, aprons to pre-vent injury to the gonads, and lead glass spectacles should be word for added pro-tection.

Although some of these are obsolete, they represent a philosophy of radiation protec-tion that still holds true today.

---

Cells of the hematopoietic system all develop from a single cell known as a *pluripotential stem cell*. From this one cell, the lymphocytes, granu-locytes, thrombocytes, and erythrocytes are produced (Figure 7–6). Constantly being pro-duced, these cells have life spans that vary from a few days to about 4 months. Some lym-phocytes have life spans of only a few hours. Along with spermatogonia, lymphocytes are considered to be the body cells most sensitive to radiation.

Erythrocytes, with a life span of about 4 months, are among the least radiosensitive cells. They are considered to be differentiated cells in opposition to their stem cells, the ery-throblasts. In fact, even with higher doses, injury to erythrocytes may not be apparent for several weeks.

## CYTOGENETIC DEPRESSION

Some of the mechanics of chromosomal aber-rations were discussed in Chapter 6. It is known that both low and high doses of radia-tion can cause chromosomal damage that does not manifest itself for some time.

A chromosome "map" is also known as a *karyotype*. This map is used in cytogenetic analy-sis. It consists of a photograph (photomicro-graph) of the human cell nucleus taken at metaphase that shows each chromosome dis-tinctly. The karyotype is made by cutting and pasting it with its sister into a map. Analysis of single- and double-hit aberrations does *not* require a karyotype to be constructed; recipro-cal translocations do. A point mutation cannot be detected even with a karyotype.

Recently, specific types of mutations for long- and short-term effects have been identi-fied by various scientists. For example, the p53 protein has been identified as the mutation associated with lung cancer in smoking and non-smoking radon miners (see Chapter 8). A robertsonian translocation (review Chap-ter 5 for a discussion of translocations) involves two acrocentric chromosomes. If chromosomes 14 and 21, the individual will have a complete chromosomal complement, although only 45 chromosomes exist in addi-tion to the translocation chromosome. This individual is normal according to phenotype (genetic expression) but has an increased risk

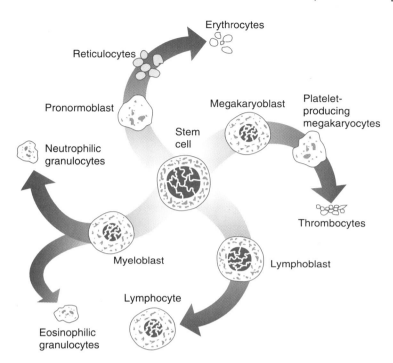

**Figure 7–6** Cells of the hematopoietic system.

of producing offspring with trisomy 21 (Down syndrome).

## Chromosomal Aberrations of Radiologic Technologists

A variety of reports have stated that chromosomal aberrations are higher in those exposed to low doses of radiation, especially over long periods, as opposed to unexposed controls. A study of radiologic technologists in Japan compared 53 radiologic technologists with 36 controls, finding an aberration rate in somatic chromosomes of 2.5% in the technologists and 1.6% in the controls. Although small, it was of statistical significance. Aberrations increased with age in both groups, but more were seen in the radiologic technologists. Most of the aberrations observed in both groups were translocations or deletions. Figure 7–7 shows a metaphase photograph for one of the technologists; Figure 7–8 is a karyotype of a 50-year-old technologist.

Such studies are interesting, but the significance to practice is not clear. For example, older technologists had higher doses than younger technologists, because of a greater laxity in radiation protection practices in earlier years. Also, the exact doses for some of the older technologists could not be documented because film badges were not in common use until 1963 in the area studied. The damage to chromosomes could be due to exposure to various types of illness. Also, the significance of the effects is not known. That is, is the doubling of damage, even though "statistically significant," going to make a significant difference? Today, we cannot answer either yes or no to the question. The term *statistically significant* means that the damage observed can be, with a reasonable assurance (e.g. 95% assurance) attributed to radiation. It does not mean that the damage causes observable effects in humans. Some of this will be discussed in the next chapter in terms of expected late effects.

A variety of new chromosomal tests were developed in the past decade. Today, we can observe somatic mutation of four genes and two cell types, the peripheral blood lymphocyte and the red blood cell. It is conceivable that in the near future we will be able to

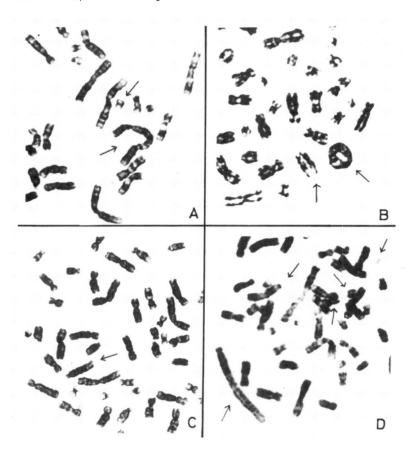

**Figure 7–7** Metaphase photograph from a technologist. (Reprinted with permission from Kumagai E, Tanaka R, Kumagai T, et al: Effects of long-term radiation exposure on chromosomal aberrations in radiologic technologists. J Radiat Res 31:270–279, 1990.)

observe these effects in the epithelial cells of skin and mucous membranes, other blood cells, subcutaneous cells, and possibly colon, bladder, and semen cells. This will allow us to better observe potential radiation effects. It has been suggested by some authors that lymphocyte monitoring be used as a form of biologic dosimetry, although this has found little favor. Table 7–3 shows chromosomal defects found after various examinations.

## SUMMARY

Radiologic technologists learn about early effects, although they are not common in diagnostic imaging, to be fully informed about the effects of ionizing radiation. The acute radiation syndromes involve a total body exposure, an acute exposure of a few minutes, and many

hundreds or thousands of rads. Besides the three lethal syndromes, two other events occur in total body irradiation, the prodromal radiation syndrome and the latent period that may follow the prodromal stage. The three lethal syndromes are the hematopoietic syndrome (100 to 1000 rad), the gastrointestinal syndrome (assigned a range by various authors of 600 to 5000 rad), and the central nervous system syndrome (over 5000 rad). The lethal dose for all exposed individuals is 1000 rad to the whole body.

Local tissue damage can result from high doses to parts of the body. Following this dosage, cell death results, leading to atrophy of that organ. Recovery can be full, partial, or nonoccurring, leading to death of the tissue. Skin effects (primarily erythema) follow a nonlinear, threshold dose–response relationship. The

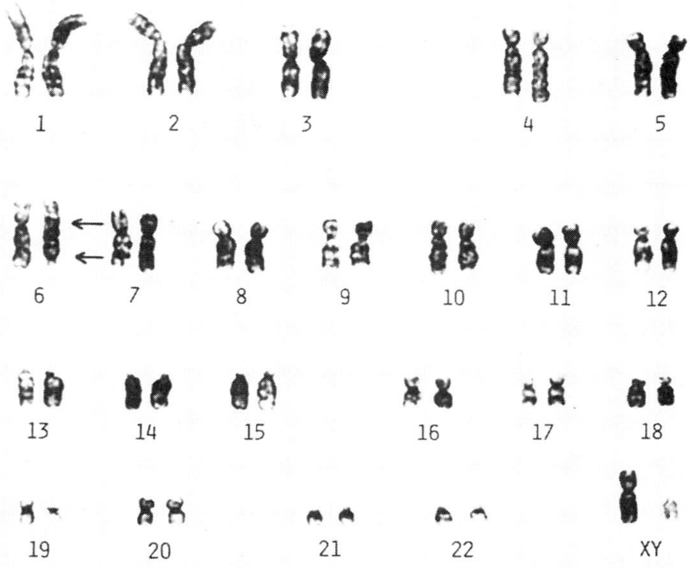

**Figure 7–8** Karyotype of a 50-year-old technologist. (Reprinted with permission from Kumagai E, Tanaka R, Kumago T, et al: Effects of long-term radiation exposure on chromosomal aberrations in radiologic technologists. J Radiat Res 31:270–279, 1990.)

**Table 7–3  Chromosomal Defects Found After Various Examinations**

| Examination | Dose | Defect |
|---|---|---|
| Chest | 20 mR | None |
| Intravenous pyelogram | 3 R | None |
| Cardiac catheterization | 4–12 R | Fragments; gaps |
| Gastrointestinal series | 1.2–3.9 R | Fragments; dicentrics; rings (adults) |
| | | Deletions, dicentrics (fetal exposure; 6-week fetal age) |
| [131]I therapy | 5 mCi (5 rad whole body; 2 rad ovary) | 6% aberration rate (control, 0.7%) |

human gonads are extremely sensitive to radiation. In males, 10 rad can lead to a reduction in the number of spermatozoa, a dose of 200 to 250 rad results in temporary sterility, and permanent sterility is produced with a dose of 500 to 600 rad. In females, 200 rad produces a temporary sterility, and 500 to 600 rad produces a permanent sterility.

The dose needed to produce a hematologic depression is about 25 rad. Along with spermatogonia, lymphocytes are considered to be the most sensitive cells in the body to radiation. Erthyrocytes are not considered to be especially radiosensitive.

Mapping of chromosomes is also known as karyotyping. This map can be used to detect chromosomal aberrations. Reports have indicated that chromosomal aberrations are higher in those exposed to low doses of radiation, especially over longer periods, than in unexposed controls. New chromosomal tests will help in determining somatic and genetic mutations.

## Questions

1. The term that refers to the initial stage of a disease is:

   a. manifest illness.
   c. development.
   b. prodomal.
   d. latent.

2. After about 5000 rad, the _____ syndrome will occur.

   a. NVD
   c. gastrointestinal
   b. hematologic
   d. CNS

3. Since chromosomal aberrations were found to be statistically significant in one study of radiologic technologists, it can be assumed that observable effects will manifest from the aberrations.

   a. true
   b. false

4. The dose for temporary sterility in either sex is:

   a. 10 rad.
   c. 200 rad.
   b. 100 rad.
   d. 400 rad.

5. Erythema is dependent on which of the following factors?

   I. size of field irradiated
   II. dose rate
   III. individual radiosensitivity

   a. I and II only
   c. II and III only
   b. I and III only
   d. I, II, and III

6. *Epilation* refers to the loss of _____ due to radiation.

   a. blood cells
   c. hair
   b. lymphocytes
   d. skin

7. Which of the following are considered to be relatively radiosensitive?

   I. spermatogonia
   II. erythrocytes
   III. lymphocytes

   a. I and II only
   c. II and III only
   b. I and III only
   d. I, II, and III

8. A chromosome map is also known as a:

   a. photochronograph.
   c. chromogram.
   b. karyotype.
   d. film badge.

9. The ovaries:

   a. are very radiosensitive throughout life.
   b. are not very radiosensitive.
   c. are very radiosensitive in early life, decline in radiosensitivity until age 30, and then increase in radiosensitivity.
   d. are not very radiosensitive in early life, increase in radiosensitivity until age 30, and then decrease in radiosensitivity.

10. Skin effects follow a _____ dose–response relationship.

   a. linear, nonthreshold
   b. linear, threshold
   c. nonlinear, nonthreshold
   d. nonlinear, threshold

## Exercises

1. What might be an appropriate way to communicate with a patient who expresses concern over "x-ray burns"?

2. Describe the relative radiosensitivity of the hematologic system.

3. What is the primary difference in radiosensitivity between the testes and ovaries?

4. What is the value of knowing information such as the acute radiation syndromes, when the technologist will probably never observe them in actual practice?

5. Describe the acute radiation syndromes. Is this consistent with information taught in the previous chapter (e.g., the law of Bergonie and Tribondeau)?

6. Discuss some of the problems with analyzing chromosomal defects in radiologic technologists.

## Answers

Questions

| | |
|---|---|
| 1. b | 6. c |
| 2. d | 7. b |
| 3. b | 8. b |
| 4. c | 9. c |
| 5. d | 10. d |

Exercises

1. The patient must be told that (1) the equipment used today is not capable of providing doses of radiation that will result in burns, and (2) the radiographer is a skilled professional who understands how to operate that equipment in the most efficient manner possible. This type of attitude and information giving applies to other disciplines, such as nuclear medicine technologists, who must comfort patients receiving "an injection of radiation," or radiation therapists, who must describe real effects of radiation while assuring the patient that this is in his or her best interest.

2. Hematologic cells are constantly being produced, with life spans that vary from a few days to about 4 months. Lymphocytes are considered to be one of the two most radiosensitive cells, whereas erythrocytes, with a relatively long life span and a fairly high degree of differentiation, are among the least radiosensitive cells. Their stem cells, erythroblasts, on the other hand, are more radiosensitive.

3. Oogonia multiply only in the fetus, whereas spermatogonia are continually renewing. Temporary sterility in the male will take 2 months to fully manifest because these cells require 3 to 5 weeks to mature. This eventual depletion of mature sperm is called maturation depletion.

4. As an informed professional, the radiologic technologist seeks to learn everything possible about radiation and the effects of radiation. In some cases, the technologist will be expected to teach others, such as patients, about radiation (see the first exercise question), and this requires knowledge of items that may not seem 100% relevant to daily clinical practice such as positioning.

5. Because of their degree of differentiation and reproductive activity, the dose–response relation of the acute syndromes (hematologic syndrome requires the lowest doses, central nervous system syndrome, the highest) follows material presented in the previous chapter. Also, the existence of a latent period, in which the cells in the system are either recovering or beginning to manifest lethal effects, is consistent. As Chapter 6 noted, cells can recover from the effects of radiation. This depends on the dose received and the relative radiosensitivity of the cell.

6. Some of the problems include:

   - There was a lack of knowledge of dose received.
   - The group was small.
   - There were possible confounding effects; for example, was the damage due to radiation or to exposure to various illnesses in the hospital setting?
   - A statistically significant increase does not mean that observable effects will be seen.

CHAPTER

**8**

# Late Effects of Radiation

### Steven B. Dowd • Elwin R. Tilson

## Chapter Objectives

At the end of this chapter, the student should be able to:

1. Synthesize a list of radiation studies to determine relative risks from radiation and discuss their applicability to diagnostic imaging and therapeutic uses of radiation.

2. Differentiate between the radiation incidents at Three Mile Island and Chernobyl.

3. Differentiate the three methods of stating cancer risk.

4. Describe the risks for various types of cancer.

5. Describe types of local tissue damage from irradiation.

6. List the results of genetic studies.

7. Define the doubling dose.

8. Explain the concept of genetically significant dose.

9. List the stages of fetal development.

10. Describe possible effects to the embryo and fetus from radiation.

**Important Terms**

absolute risk
additive
all or none effect
ankylosing spondylitis
cataractogenesis
causal relationship
certainty effect
dosimetry
doubling dose

epidemiology
excess risk
fetal (growth) stage
genetically significant dose (GSD)
hydrocephaly
hypertrophy
latent period
maturation depletion
microcephaly
neonatal death
organogenesis
osteosarcoma
radiation carcinogenesis
radiocarcinogenic
relative risk
postpartum mastitis
preimplantation
prenatal death
radiation carcinogenesis
synergistic
Thorotrast

## INTRODUCTION

In this chapter, we will be examining common late effects from radiation exposure. The term *late effects* refers to long-term effects such as malignant disease, local tissue damage, life-span shortening, genetic damage, and potential effects to the fetus. We will briefly review some of these here and discuss their implications to the health of the general population and the radiologic technologist.

## MODERN RADIATION INCIDENTS

Although it is very rare for any group of people to be exposed to high levels of radiation, such accidents do still occur, unfortunately. These accidents are important for two reasons—because they are public health problems and because they give researchers the opportunity to study the impacts of high levels of radiation does. Two radiation incidents that stand out in recent history are Three Mile Island, in the United States (1979), and Chernobyl, in what was then the USSR (1986). Many other less severe accidents and experiments in which small groups were exposed are detailed by the U.S. Department of Energy's Office of Human Radiation Experiments at http://www.ohre.doe.gov/.

### Three Mile Island

Radioactivity released from Three Mile Island was relatively low. About 10 MCi of xenon-133 and 15 Ci of iodine-131 were released. This translated into a radiation dose to the surrounding population of about 8 mrem (0.08 mSv) over a radius of 10 miles and about 2 mrem (0.02 mSv) over a radius of 50 miles.

Conservative estimates indicate that about 0.7 additional cancer deaths could be expected in the population of about 2 million people living within that 50-mile radius. The expected cancer mortality in that region is 330,000 over the lifetime of that population. Prudently, the governor of the state first recommended evacuation of pregnant women and children within a 5-mile radius; the Nuclear Regulatory Commission then recommended an evacuation within a 10-mile radius of the plant.

An interesting risk–benefit consideration to come out of the Three Mile Island incident was Titterington's contention that the antinuclear backlash that resulted from a fairly benign incident has resulted in an increased dependence on coal-generated electricity. He contends that this has resulted in an additional 100 deaths per year due to mining and transportation deaths, as many as 125,000 cases per year of chronic respiratory disease (from burning coal), and possibly 1 million person-days of aggravated heart and lung symptoms.

## Chernobyl

The incident at Chernobyl was of much greater impact. This explosion and fire at the nuclear power plant had serious consequences. Many tons of uranium dioxide were released into the atmosphere, along with cesium-137 and iodine-131, by-products of the reactor. Iodine-131 has a short half-life of 8 days and produces effects mostly to the thyroid, where it tends to concentrate. On the other hand, cesium-137 has a half-life of 30 years and concentrates mainly in muscle, spleen, and liver, although it could be found throughout the body.

Of the 444 workers on site, 203 suffered from acute radiation syndrome (discussed in Chapter 7). Most of the individuals were young, between the ages of 25 and 35. Of 105 individuals who received doses of 100 to 200 rem (1–2 Sv), there were no deaths. Of 53 workers who received from 200 to 400 rem (2–4 Sv), one died. Of the 23 people who received 400 to 600 rem (4–6 Sv), 7 died. Twenty-one of the 22 people who received 600 to 1600 rem (6–16 Sv) died.

The fact that so many individuals in the 400 to 600 rem group survived indicates that the $LD_{50/30}$ (the lethal dose that will kill 50% of the population in 30 days) may not be accurate, especially with newer methods of bone marrow transplantation. There was still a good survival rate in the group that did not receive bone marrow transplants. It has been theorized from this accident that bone marrow transplants are not needed until 800 rem (8 Sv) has been reached, although their limit of effectiveness appears to be about 1000 rem (10 Sv). In fact, rejection of transplants (because the patients were not immunosuppressed) was a major problem. Dr. Gale, leader of the transplantation team, considered giving some individuals more radiation to cause immunosuppression to a point where they would accept the transplant, but he decided not to because of the potential misunderstandings that could result.

Most deaths were due to skin burns and damage to the gastrointestinal tract and lungs. The potential long-term effects are the subject of much disagreement among scientists. Theoretically, it should take at least three generations before these are well defined.

One hundred thirty-five thousand people were evacuated from a 30-kilometer (about 20-mile) radius of the reactor. They were exposed to an average of 12 rem (12 cSv), with a high of 45 rem (45 cSv) and a low of 6 rem (6 cSv). There were mostly live births among the 2000 women who were pregnant. Abortion was fairly common in the USSR at that time, and the number of miscarriages and abortions is not known.

## GENERAL CONCEPTS OF EPIDEMIOLOGY

Population studies use an epidemiologic approach. Epidemiology is the study of the distribution and causes of disease in human populations. It is an observational, not experimental, science; that is, it collects information from a human population. For example, the cause of spina bifida (a birth defect affecting the closure of the spinal column) was not understood. One of the main causes of the condition was found through an early epidemiologic study. When the individual cases of spina bifida were plotted on a map of England, it was noted that there was a very high rate of this defect in one particular area of the country. Upon closer examination, the distribution of the defect appeared almost cone shaped, with the tip of the cone over one particular industrial city. Another interesting aspect noted was that the concentration of cases got greater as the cone got near the city in question. When the data were closely examined, the distribution of the disease was then found to very closely match the prevailing

---

### More Information:
### Chernobyl

Although there is little evidence of increased congenital abnormalities and adult cancers in the population around the Chernobyl accident, there has been a documented dramatic increase in childhood thyroid cancers in Belarus, the Ukraine, and the Bryansk region. A recent review found more than 100 articles on this single subject in a 3-year period in the medical literature. In areas that received heavy contamination, this increased incidence has been as high as 100 times what is found in the general population. A number of studies have compared the incidence of various thyroid conditions in children in the contaminated area with that in children from other regions and other countries, and with documented previous cases found in cancer registries. Evi-

dence exists that the p53 tumor suppressor gene has been affected in many of the individuals exposed to fallout. A possible confounding factor is the iodine deficiency already seen in the region, which some believe may have led to an overstatement of the actual number of cases.

Consider the following questions based on your readings:

1. Why has the incidence of adult cancer not yet perhaps shown an increase?
2. Why would children possibly be affected before adults? Why thyroid cancer?
3. Thyroid cancer is the third most common solid tumor in children. Will this make it easier or more difficult to study from an epidemiologic standpoint?

---

wind patterns as they passed over one particular industrial plant nearby. Based on the disease and environmental data, the final conclusion of this study was that one of the causes of spina bifida was a particular type of air pollution emitted from the plant. When that pollution was cleaned up, the rate of spina bifida in that area dramatically dropped.

Epidemiologic studies can be very powerful and are extremely useful in the study of many conditions or diseases because one should never purposefully hurt a human to study the disease (such as exposing people to a dose of radiation just to see what would happen). However, one of the problems with epidemiologic studies is that human populations do not separate themselves well into nice discrete groups, as can be done, for example, in experiments with fruit flies. This creates a problem because the researcher often ends up comparing not apples to apples but something like an apple to a different something that is also not quite an apple.

One of the basic question asked by any epi-

demiologic study of radiation effects is whether those exposed to radiation have a greater risk of developing a disease than those not exposed. Many of the epidemiologic studies of biologic effects of radiation have focused on cancer induction, also called *radiation carcinogenesis*. These consist of either animal experimentation or human population studies. There are four basic limitations on human population studies:

1. The observed incidence of cancer is compared with the expected incidence. This expected incidence comes from a control group of unexposed individuals. It is possible to select a group as a control that does not exactly match the exposed group in all other factors.
2. Even if an increase is seen, it may not be statistically significant.
3. It is not possible to isolate all factors involved. For example, uranium miners have a high incidence of lung cancer but are also usually heavy smokers. It is not

known if the effects of smoking and uranium mining on lung cancer are additive or synergistic. That is, the combined effects may be worse than simply adding the two together.

4. The dosimetry problem is probably the worst of all. We can only estimate doses, especially for the early studies. For example, the data for survivors of the atom bomb have been repeatedly revised based on dosimetry and radiation types, most recently in 1989. Another example is estimation of dose in relation to thyroid cancers in children treated for tinea capitis with therapeutic radiation. Dose was estimated in these studies based on a description of the treatment applied to a phantom. Such items as body size, shielding used, and beam quality are subject only to estimation.

Epidemiologic studies are used clinically to make value judgments about the use of radiation. As value judgments, rather than pure fact, there is some potential to make an incorrect decision.

Based on population studies, we describe the risk for cancer following irradiation three ways:

1. Absolute risk is a very common means of stating risk. It is expressed in terms of number of cases per 1 million people per rad (cGy) per year. This means that if the 1 million people were exposed to one rad (cGy) and the absolute risk was 5.5, we would expect to see 5.5 more cases of the disease among those million people than we would have normally expected. This of course assumes a linear dose–response relationship.

2. Excess risk describes the risk in terms of the number of excess cases observed over what would be expected spontaneously (naturally) in a population. If 52 cases of a disease are observed in a population exposed to 200 rad (2 Gy) and 47 were expected, the excess risk is 5.

3. Relative risk is used when the dose to which a population has been exposed is not precisely known. The number of people in the exposed population is compared with those not exposed as a control group. Relative risk rates tend to range from 1 to 10, with 1 representing no risk. Relative risk is expressed either as a number (e.g. 5) or as a ratio (e.g. 5 to 1).

Absolute risk and relative risk are the preferred models for expressing risk. Many texts list both values, because agreement does not exist as to which is the better means of expressing risk. The BEIR V Report used the relative risk model.

## LEUKEMIA

The first case of radiation-induced cancer was a skin cancer on the hand of a radiologist in 1902. Radiation was first noted in 1911 as a cause of leukemia, which has been implicated in more studies than any other disease. Only specific types are increased—acute and chronic myeloid leukemia in adults plus acute and chronic lymphocytic leukemia in children. From 1950 to 1956, 64 cases of leukemia were seen in survivors of Hiroshima and Nagasaki. Comparisons are often made between what would have been expected and what actually occurred. In Nagasaki, for example, where the dose received was primarily x-radiation of 20 to 50 rad (20–50 cGy), 7 cases of leukemia were expected and 20 occurred.

Patients were formerly treated for ankylosing spondylitis with fractionated radiation therapy of 100 to 2000 rad (20 Gy). A study in Great Britain focused on 15,000 patients treated from 1935 to 1944. The reported incidence of leukemia was 9.5 times what would have been expected. This group received an average dose of 370 rad (370 cGy) to the bone marrow, and 52 cases were observed, whereas 5.5 would have been expected.

Radiologists have been studied with conflicting results. Currently, no increased incidence of leukemia is observed in this group. Two earlier studies, one British and one American, had different results. The U.S. study found a threefold increase; the British study found no increased incidence of leukemia. Skin cancer is no longer a concern, but it was in the 1930s when the maximum permissible dose (MPD) was about 1 rad (cGy) per week.

## More Information:
## Epidemiology

*Epidemiology* means "the study of epidemics." Epidemiology's roots are in the study of infectious disease. John Snow's 1854 investigation of cholera, in which he was able to isolate the causative factor as contaminated water from one well (even though this was some years before the cholera bacillus was discovered), is often cited as the first epidemiologic study. Epidemiology has been used to determine the risk of disease from a variety of agents and was used to determine the correlation between smoking and lung cancer. More recently, epidemiology was used to discover the causative factor for AIDS. Epidemiologic data and findings are often used to decide where and how to direct health care dollars.

Epidemiology relies on a strong understanding of the scientific method, and epidemiologists have been called "disease detectives." Epidemiology and an understanding of the method are not confined to universities or large medical centers: many of the initial epidemiologic studies began with observant physicians who noted a disease entity that might overwise have been passed off as "occurring by chance" kept arising in a certain group (smokers, people living in a certain area of town, etc.). Since disease can be caused by agents that we cannot see (microbes or, closer to home for us, ionizing radiation), or that may take years after exposure to develop, observational techniques such as epidemiology will remain important for many years to come.

Therapeutic doses of iodine-131 have been implicated in leukemia incidence, but the results are not clear. Thorotrast (thorium dioxide), an alpha particle emitter, has been implicated in both liver cancer and leukemia.

Leukemia has the shortest latent period of any malignant disease—most sources list 5 to 7 years. The actual at-risk period is considered to be 20 years. Leukemia is considered to have an absolute risk, based on the atomic bomb data of 1.5 cases/$10^6$ people/rad (cGy)/yr. The ankylosing spondylitis study showed an absolute risk of 0.8 cases/$10^6$ people/rad (cGy)/yr. The relative risk at 600 rad (6 Gy) was 2.8 for the atomic bomb survivors and 9.5 for the ankylosing spondylitis patients.

Estimates of the risk of diagnostic x-ray in causing leukemia vary greatly. In 1986, Hall, a respected radiobiologist, estimated that less than 0.1% of all leukemias were caused by x-ray. In that same year, a *New England Journal of Medicine* article by Evans stated that about 1% of all leukemias were caused by x-ray. In 1992, Thomas and Preston-Martin, citing problems with the data used by the first two authors, estimated that 12% of leukemias were caused by diagnostic x-ray.

## OTHER MALIGNANT DISEASES

It is more difficult to "prove" that radiation causes forms of cancer besides leukemia. What we lack is hard data from human studies. However, ionizing radiation has definitely been implicated in cancers of bone, lung, skin, thyroid, and breast. When we describe the potential for radiation to induce cancer, we cannot predict this potential for any one individual. There are too many confounding factors, such as dosimetry, health status of the individual, organs exposed, and potential for repair. Table 8–1 demonstrates our range of knowledge about radiation and its effects from a high to a low level of knowledge. Our level of understanding correlates with the sequence of events from exposure to expressed effect; that is, we understand very well the initial events of radiation production, radiation dose, and atomic level interactions, but have a poor knowledge of effects on the cell, tissues, and organism.

Table 8–1  Continuum of Radiation Effects

| Level of Understanding | | | |
|---|---|---|---|
| **High** | **Good** | **Medium** | **Poor*** |
| Radiation production | Chemical effects | Single-cell effects | Cellular carcinogenesis |
| Dosimetry | | | Tissue-level effects |
| Atomic-level interactions | | | Host effects |
| | | | Clinical cancer induction |

*These are poorly understood as a result of confounding and synergistic effects that may not be due to radiation (e.g. combining smoking with radiation exposure).

## Bone Cancer

Osteosarcoma, or bone cancer, was observed in the radium dial painters, a group composed primarily of women who painted luminescent radium on watch hands and faces. Although the possible effects to the wearer were small (1 mrem/yr was estimated), the painters were taught to lick the tips of the brushes to a fine edge. Each brush still contained small

---

### Radiologic Technologists and Occupational Exposure

One study, still in the preliminary stages, has explored the relation between occupational exposure and risks such as cancer induction in radiologic technologists. Some 104,000 technologists participated in the study. These individuals were mostly female and white, and had an average of 12 years of work experience. Initial findings follow:

1. Cancer was found in 3.6% of respondents, with 1517 cases of skin cancer, 726 cases of cervical cancer, 665 cases of breast cancer, 242 cases of uterine cancer, 220 cases of thyroid cancer (9500 reported a "thyroid condition"), 76 cases of lung cancer, and 42 cases of leukemia.
2. Birthing experiences were similar in female technologists (9% observable defects) and spouses of male technologists (8%).
3. Ninety-eight percent indicated wearing a monitor of some kind; 95% wore lead aprons.
4. Fluoroscopy or other procedures were not shown to increase mean scores of exposure.
5. Ten percent indicated that their training had them take radiographs on other students.
6. Technologists were found to be more likely to use radiologic services than the general public, increasing their overall dose.
7. Average exposure in the 58% of technologists who could be traced through commercial dosimetry records was less than 1 rad (1 cGy).

This ongoing study should provide the profession with a better knowledge of the risks of low levels of radiation. By the time this text is in print, several new articles should have been published based on the original study and the follow-up study completed in 1998. These articles will look at specific types of cancers in technologists and should give a better understanding of what risks exist from occupational exposure.

amounts of radium. Radium goes to bone and has a half-life of 1620 years, which means that it basically remains in the human at full strength throughout the life span. These individuals exhibited an increased incidence of bone cancer. A 1978 study of 1474 women employed before 1930 in the industry found 61 cases of bone cancer, as well as 21 cases of carcinoma of the paranasal sinuses and mastoid.

Osteogenic sarcoma induced by radiation appears to follow the linear quadratic model, based on the studies of radium dial painters. The radium dial painters showed a relative risk of 122 to 1. The calculated absolute risk is 0.11 cases/$10^6$ people/rad (cGy)/yr.

It is, of course, difficult to compare radium dial painters to diagnostic radiation workers since radium salts emit alpha and beta particles. These high-LET radiations were harmful because they were ingested (eaten) and were deposited in bone in a manner similar to calcium. The bones most often affected were the femur, mandible, and pelvis. Some of these individuals received organ doses of up to 50,000 rad (500 Gy).

## Lung Cancer

An increased incidence of lung cancer was not observed in the chest fluoroscopy study mentioned earlier, but it has been noted in miners. Inhalation of radon gas was implicated as the carcinogen. As mentioned earlier, most of the miners were also smokers, which compounds the effect. Uranium miners were exposed to up to 3000 rad (30 Gy). The increased incidence of lung cancer was 6 to 8 times what would be expected in nonsmokers. It was 20 times higher in smokers.

About half of the miners died of lung cancer, an increased incidence thought to be due to radon exposure. Radon, which has also received media attention, is a gas that emanates through rock. Breathed radon is deposited in the lung spaces and emits alpha particles until it decays to a stable lead isotope. Increased lung cancer was also seen in atomic bomb survivors who were at least 35 years old at the time of the blast.

The dose–response relationship for radiation-induced lung cancer is thought to be linear and nonthreshold. An absolute risk of 1.3 cases/$10^6$ people/rad (cGy)/yr has been calculated based on observations of over 4000 uranium miners.

## Radon Exposure

Radon is associated with two exposure factors: (1) high indoor radon levels in houses, caused by natural deposits or uranium in the soil, and (2) active or passive exposure to cigarettes, which give off radon when burned. The U.S. Senate considers radon a serious enough health problem to have authorized several millions annually to fund programs established by the 1988 Indoor Radon Abatement Act. Certain areas in Great Britain have been found to have radioactive levels of radon higher than some areas in the path of the Chernobyl explosion.

The average indoor level for radon is 1 pCi/L; the Environmental Protection Agency (EPA) equates high levels (100 pCi/L) with 20,000 chest x-rays per year; 200 pCi/L is associated with smoking four packs of cigarettes a day. The EPA attributes 5000 to 20,000 lung cancer deaths per year to radon.

Others have questioned the value of spending this money when public health issues surrounding the diagnostic use of radiation are possibly of greater importance. Some have stated that credentialing of operators of x-ray equipment should take a stronger focus. Many individuals believe that exposure to radon is not probable (few homes, most in specific areas, have elevated levels of radon) and that the lives saved are not worth the financial investment. Certainly, this is another example of value judgments being made based on scientific information.

### Skin Cancer

Skin cancer induced by radiation follows a threshold dose–response relationship. It usually begins with the development of a radiodermatitis. At 500 to 2000 rad (5 to 20 Gy), there is a 4 to 1 relative risk of developing skin cancer; this rises to 27 to 1 when the dose reaches 6000 to 10,000 rad (60–100 Gy).

### Thyroid Cancer

A variety of studies have implicated radiation exposure in thyroid cancer. Children with enlarged thymus glands (thymus hypertrophy) were treated with radiotherapy, primarily in the 1930s and 1940s. Of 2872 children who received an average of 119 rad (119 cGy), 24 cases of thyroid cancer were observed, with 0.24 cases being the expected incidence. This is a 100-fold increase. In unexposed siblings used as the control group, no cases of thyroid cancer were seen in a group of 5055.

Children were also formerly treated for tinea capitis (ringworm) with radiation therapy. Of 10,842 children exposed to an average of 9 rad (9 cGy), 23 developed thyroid cancer whereas 5 cases would have been expected. Through studies on children exposed to nuclear fallout from atom bomb testing (the Marshall Islanders), the latent period (the time from exposure to incidence of the effect) of thyroid cancer has been established at 10 to 20 years. Children were also treated for various benign diseases such as tonsillitis and acne, in some cases until the 1960s. A fourfold increase in incidence of thyroid cancer has been observed in this group. Increased incidence of skin cancer was also noted in the acne and ringworm group. Incidence of thyroid cancer through radionuclides (iodine-131) applied diagnostically has not been shown.

Thyroid cancer follows a linear, nonthreshold dose–response relationship. Various studies have reported different levels of absolute risk. In a group of children irradiated for enlargement of the thymus, the absolute risk was reported as 2.5 for tinea capitis (ringworm) and was set at 8.3 cases/$10^6$ people/rad (cGy)/yr. An Israeli study of tinea capitis set the *radiocarcinogenic* thyroid dose at 9 rad (9 cGy). It is not clear that this is accurate, because other studies have indicated that Jewish individuals have an increased risk of thyroid cancer. Some have also indicated that it is not possible to set a radiocarcinogenic thyroid dose.

The radiocarcinogenic thyroid dose is important for radiation protection purposes. Many individuals have opted for thyroid shields (see Chapter 10) during fluoroscopy because of concern over the radiogenic dose. Radiation-induced thyroid tumors occur at a fourfold higher level in females over males. This is thought to be due to the fluctuating hormonal status of women. This may make the wearing of thyroid shields more acute for women.

The carcinogenic capability of internal sources of radiation due to radioactive $^{131}$I is not well known. Animal studies indicate that $^{131}$I is as effective as x-ray in producing cancer. In adults treated for hyperthyroidism with $^{131}$I, increased risk of cancer has not been observed. However, the latent period appears to be at least 10 years, with the peak incidence believed to be 15 to 25 years. The potential latent period is 40 years after irradiation. $^{131}$I imaging of the thyroid has largely been discontinued because of the high thyroid dose associated with the radionuclide.

### Breast Cancer

Breast cancer has been described in at least three studies of female survivors of Hiroshima and Nagasaki, radiation treatment of benign breast diseases such as postpartum mastitis, and fluoroscopy for tuberculosis. Of the 531 women studied in the postpartum mastitis group (mean dose of 247 rad [247 cGy]), breast cancer incidence doubled from 3.2% expected to 6.3% actual.

These studies indicate that radiation can induce breast cancer. This has been, and will continue to be, important because of the possible development of breast cancer from diagnostic mammography. Some studies have indicated a relative risk for breast cancer as high as 10 to 1. One study of pneumothorax fluoroscopy indicated that cancer induction from radiation fits the linear dose–response curve. This is not wholly clear, although the pneumothorax studies are the best so far in terms of dose and population size.

The postpartum mastitis group, in which breast cancer incidence approximately doubled, set the absolute risk at 8.3 cases/$10^6$

people/rad (cGy)/yr and the relative risk at about 2.5 to 1. The pneumothorax fluoroscopy studies set absolute risk at 6.2 cases/$10^6$ people/rad (cGy)/yr. This is much higher than estimates from atomic bomb survivors, which set the absolute risk at 1.5 cases/$10^6$ people/rad (cGy)/yr.

In that same group, no increased risk was seen in the 40- to 49-year-old age group. There were more young women in the first two groups. This seems to indicate that breast irradiation in later years is safer. From this, it could be concluded that the benefit of mammography appears to outweigh risk in women over age 40, although this cannot be determined from a few studies (see "Risk–Benefit Considerations for Mammography"). Table 8–2 summarizes absolute risk values of the cancers described here.

**Table 8–2** Cancer Risk Based on Absolute Risk

| Cancer Type | Absolute Risk (cases/$10^6$ people/rad [cGy]/yr) |
|---|---|
| Bone cancer | 0.11 (radium dial painters) |
| Leukemia | 0.8 (ankylosing spondylitis) |
| | 1.5 (atomic bomb) |
| Lung cancer | 1.3 (uranium miners) |
| Breast cancer | 1.5 (atomic bomb) |
| | 6.2 (pneumothorax fluoroscopy) |
| | 8.3 (postpartum mastitis) |
| Thyroid cancer | 2.5 (thymus) |
| | 8.3 (tinea capitis) |

## Risk–Benefit Considerations for Mammography

In 1976, Bailar suggested that the risk of radiation-induced breast cancer from mammography was greater than the benefit associated with the detection of breast cancer. His calculations showed that, with an average dose to the breast tissue of 2 rad (2 cGy) per examination, 370 breast cancers could be induced in a group of 1 million women aged 35 to 49. He also calculated 148 deaths from breast cancer in that group.

Also in 1976, however, what could be called the second generation of mammography screen/film was introduced. This film was 15 times faster than previous screen/film combinations. In 1978, a third generation of mammography film was introduced that reduced exposure by another 50%. The American College of Radiology (ACR) recommends that the average dose in mammography be no more than 0.3 rad (3 µGy) per view, and many facilities average 0.1 rad (1 µGy) per view. With a four-view examination (two views of each breast), the average dose then ranges from 0.4 to 1.2 rad (1.2 cGy) maximum.

The guidelines set forth by the American Cancer Society and the ACR for mammographic screening of asymptomatic women are as follows:

- a baseline mammogram between the ages of 35 and 40.
- mammograms at 1- to 2-year intervals from age 40 to 49.
- annual mammograms after age 50.

These are not universally accepted, although they are based on reasonable assumptions of risk versus benefit. Some screening programs have found that younger patients could benefit from mammographic screening by detecting rarer but more aggressive malignancies sometimes found in younger women. For example, women under the age of 40 account for 6.5% of breast cancers per year. A study conducted at Memorial Sloan-Kettering in New York found value for mammographic screening in women aged 35 to 39 years. Other authors have suggested that mammograms are of no value for women under age 50. These debates will continue, as will efforts to minimize mammographic dose.

Table 8–3   Studies Showing Evidence of Carcinogenesis in Humans

| Group | Strong Association | Weak Association (suggested) |
|---|---|---|
| Japanese atom bomb survivors* | Leukemia, thyroid and breast cancer | Stomach, esophagus, bladder, and salivary gland cancer |
| Marshall Islanders | | Thyroid cancer |
| Radium dial painters | Bone cancer | Colon cancer |
| Early radiologists | Leukemia, skin cancer | Lymphoma, brain cancer |
| Multiple chest fluoroscopy | Breast cancer | |
| Infants with enlarged thymus | Thyroid cancer | Leukemia, skin and salivary gland cancer |
| Thorotrast | Leukemia, liver cancer | Lung and kidney cancer |
| In utero exposures | Leukemia | |
| Thyroid cancer patients treated with I-131 therapy | | Leukemia |
| Uranium miners | Lung cancer | |

*Recent studies have shown that the incidence of solid tumors has increased over time among the atom bomb survivors whereas leukemia incidence has slowly declined.

## Conclusions about Radiation-Induced Cancers

Table 8–3 summarizes some of the studies of humans that show both strong and weak evidence of cancer in humans. Table 8–4 summarizes studies of patients exposed to internal radionuclides. Table 8–5 summarizes studies of patients exposed to diagnostic radiation. There are also nine generalizations that should be noted regarding radiation carcinogenesis:

1. A single exposure can be enough to elevate cancer incidence several years later.
2. There is no radiounique cancer.

3. Almost all cancers are increased with irradiation.
4. The breast, bone marrow, and thyroid are seen as especially radiosensitive.
5. The most prominent (most studied and implicated) radiogenic tumor is leukemia.
6. Solid tumors have a minimum latent period of 10 years. Leukemia's latent period is thought to be 5 to 7 years. Some texts cite shorter latent periods of 2 to 3 years for leukemia and 5 years for solid tumors.
7. The age of the irradiated individual is probably one of the most important factors. For example, the immature breast is more sensitive to radiation than the mature breast.

Table 8–4   Studies of Patients Exposed to Internal Radionuclides

| Group | Association |
|---|---|
| German patients (bone disease; Ra-224) | Bone cancer (strong); liver and breast cancer (weak) |
| Polycythemia vera patients (P-32) | Leukemia |
| Thorotrast patients (Th-232) | Liver cancer, leukemia (strong); bone cancer (weak) |
| Thyroid cancer patients (I-131) | Leukemia, bladder cancer |

Table 8–5   Studies of Patients Exposed to Diagnostic Radiation

| Group | Association |
|---|---|
| Tuberculosis patients | Breast cancer |
| Spinal x-rays for scoliosis | Breast cancer patients |
| Patients receiving prenatal x-rays | Leukemia, other childhood cancers |

8. The percentage increase in cancer incidence per rad (cGy) varies between organs and types of cancers.
9. To provide for safety, dose–effect curves are best assumed to be linear.

## LOCAL TISSUE DAMAGE

### Skin

The skin is a highly vascular, very large organ (about 1.8 m²) that consists of an outer layer (epidermis), connective tissue (dermis), and a subcutaneous layer of fat and connective tissue. The epidermis consists of mature, postmitotic cells and, at the basal or basement layer, precursor cells, which are radiosensitive. The function of the skin is to cover the body with a protective barrier against microbes and chemicals, help control body temperature, help regulate blood flow, and excrete wastes.

In addition to the changes discussed in Chapter 7, chronic, long-term irradiation of the skin can result in nonmalignant changes. The early radiologists also developed hands and forearms that were very weathered in appearance, similar to those of individuals with many years of exposure to the sun. Sometimes the skin became tight and brittle, leading to cracking and flaking (see the photos in Chapter 7 for an example of some of this cracking and flaking in addition to the amputations for skin cancer). Radiation induced changes in the skin occur in the basal layer.

Other late changes found in the skin are atrophy, fibrosis, change in pigmentation, ulceration, and necrosis. At radiation doses over 1000 rad (10 Gy), the skin may not regenerate and permanent depilation (loss of hair) will occur.

Today's practice of diagnostic imaging and therapy does not lead to such changes in the technologist. The highest hand doses are seen in nuclear medicine technologists, but even these doses are too low to lead to these changes. However, such changes are still a possibility for radiation therapy patients, and this is taken into account when treatment plans are developed. Unfortunately, radiation "skin burns" are again being seen in some patients who have very high-dose fluoroscopy studies such as cardiac catheterization. These often lead to fibrosis (scar tissue) and the degeneration of tissue (atrophy). Atrophy is the most common late change seen in the skin from radiation, and it is usually minimal. See Chapter 11 for more information on these high-dose examinations.

### Reproductive System

In males, the reproductive system consists of testicles, the penis, the semen transport ducts, the Cowper gland, which produces seminal fluids, and the prostate gland. In females, the reproductive system consists of the uterus, the ovaries, the fallopian tubes connecting the uterus and ovaries, and the vagina. The function of the reproductive systems, obviously, is procreation. The male gonads are filled with tubules in which precursor cells are continuously maturing into sperm. The female ovaries contain many thousands of oocytes (eggs), which, when fertilized, can develop into the fetus. All of the oocytes are present at birth, and normally only one matures each month.

Other than experimental studies and statistical extrapolation, we simply do not have good information on the effects to the gonads caused by small amounts of radiation. Cytogenetic damage, doubling dose, and genetically significant dose are concepts used to discuss potential damage from low-level doses. These will be discussed later in this chapter. We do have reasonably good information about the effects of higher doses to the reproductive system.

In the male, moderate doses (over 100 rad or 1 Gy) damage and depopulate the spermatogonia through a process called *maturation depletion*. In this process, the precursor cells, which are more radiosensitive, are destroyed and are not available when they would normally have become the mature sperm. This results in sterility. Temporary sterility has been seen with doses as low as 250 rad (2.5 Gy), and permanent sterility is usually seen at between 500 and 600 rad (5 to 6 Gy). Impotency in which the sex drive is diminished is related to suppression of testosterone production and is seen only at very high doses—over 3000 rad (30 Gy). Generally, the male reproductive system is considered radioresistant except for the testes, which are considered moderately radiosensitive. Even though the system is considered radioresistant, the potential for chromosomal damage (discussed in Chapter 6 and later in this chapter) is significant and must be of the utmost concern. Disruption of the male reproductive system (except for possible chromosomal damage) is not of concern in radiography or nuclear medicine. However, protection against chromosomal damage is very important. Both chromosomal damage and system disruption are of major concern in radiation therapy.

The female reproductive system is considered moderately radioresistant. The various types of follicles (egg sacs in the ovaries) have different radiosensitivities, ranging from radiosensitive to radioresistant. As with males, a moderate dose can cause temperate sterility. Permanent sterility in females is a function of age, with more radiation required in younger women and an average dose of about 600 rads (6 Gy) needed. As with the males, damage to the reproductive system is not of concern for radiography or nuclear medicine, although, again, chromosomal damage is a serious concern. Also, damage to the system and chromosomal damage is of great concern in radiation therapy, as it is with males.

### Eyes

Generally, the eye is considered radioresistant except for the lenses, which are moderately radiosensitive. The major outcome from exposure to the lens seems to be cataract formation. The process of *radiation cataractogenesis* (the formation of cataracts due to radiation exposure; Figure 8–1) remains somewhat controversial, although not as controversial as in the 1970s, when some believed that low doses to the eye (e.g. a few rad) might cause cataracts. Some of the problems with studies of cataractogenesis have been that they have been ex post facto (after the fact), the exact amount of radiation to the eyes of subjects is not known, and the latent period for cataract formation may be up to 30 years. There are well-documented cases of radiation cataractogenesis at high doses in radiation therapy patients and cyclotron physicists. The dose–response relationship is thought by most investigators to be a threshold, nonlinear response. At 1000 rad (10 Gy) to the eye, all of those irradiated will develop cataracts. The threshold may be about 200 rad (2 Gy) for a single dose, but this is not certain. For fractionated doses, it may be as high as 1000 rad (10 Gy).

Some technologists and physicians, especially those working in relatively high-dose areas such as angiography, wear protective lens shields. Although this may be unnecessary, each individual should practice personal radiation protection as he or she sees fit. For example, one study found that physicians in training (radiology residents) received a high enough dose to the lens of the eye to warrant wearing protective lens shields.

For radiography and nuclear medicine patients, radiation cataractogenesis is not usually a major concern. There are some high-dose examinations, such as conventional tomography of the head and neck, in which protective lens shields can be advocated for patient use. Usually in computed tomography (a relatively high-dose examination), and especially in pediatric studies, axial views of the brain are taken at a 20-degree angle to the canthomeatal line in order to minimize dose to the lens of the eye (see also Chapter 11). In radiation therapy, protection of the lenses of the eyes is a major concern in treatment planning.

### Hemopoietic System

The hemopoietic system consists of the blood-forming (marrow) organs, circulating blood, and the lymphoid system. Although all bones have marrow, the marrow responsible for supplying mature cells to the blood is primarily located in the ribs, the ends of long bones, vertebrae, the sternum, and the skull. The function of the bone marrow system is to produce the mature components of the circulating blood through the process of differentiating stem or precursor cells into the three major types of blood cells: erythrocytes (RBCs), leukocytes (WBCs), and thrombocytes, or platelets. (Refer back to Chapter 7 for a review of blood component formation.) Because the bone marrow is primarily made up of stem cells, it is radiosensitive. If marrow is exposed to doses above 1000 rad or 10 Gy, there are significant, potentially life-threatening outcomes. (See "Acute Radiation Syndromes" in Chapter 7.) The major long-term effect to the bone marrow comes from sublethal doses above 100 rad (1 Gy). In these situations, the ability of

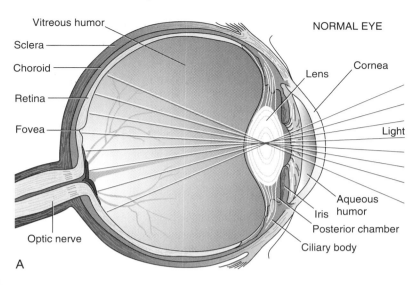

**Figure 8–1** Cataract formation.

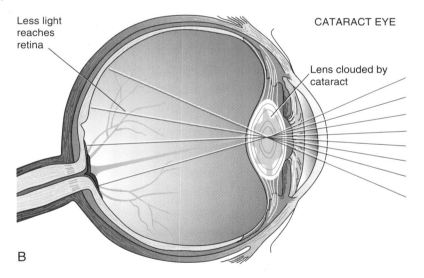

the marrow to produce blood cells may be permanently damaged and not enough cells would then be produced.

Slightly more than half of the volume of blood is made up of plasma (the liquid portion of the blood), proteins, and electrolytes (salts). Less than half of the volume of circulating blood is made from cells. The function of the circulation blood is to transport oxygen, carbon dioxide, hormones, antibodies, nutrients, and waste

products. The blood also serves as a fluid reservoir that helps balance the osmotic pressure and control body temperature. Because the red blood cells (erythrocytes) and the thrombocytes (platelets) are fixed, postmitotic cells, the circulating blood is considered radioresistant.

The lymphoid system consists of the lymph nodes, thymus, spleen, tonsils, and some bone marrow. The primary function of the lymphoid system is body defense through the formation of white blood cells (lymphocytes). White blood cells are moderately radiosensitive.

In radiography and nuclear medicine, there are no long-term effects except possible chromosomal changes in lymphocytes. In radiation therapy, long-term suppression of blood formation is of concern and must be taken into account when developing a treatment plan. In some rare cases, radiation therapy is actually used to suppress the lymphoid system for certain types of medical procedures.

## Cardiovascular System

The cardiovascular system consists of the blood vessels (vasculature) and the heart. Overall, the system is considered radioresistant. The vasculature is considered moderately radioresistant, as blood vessels are mostly made up of highly differentiated, nonmitotic cells. The major exception to this are the endothelial cells, which are responsive to radiation doses. Specifically, if exposed to a moderate radiation dose, endothelial cells may be stimulated to divide excessively, leading to an occlusion (blockage) of the blood vessel or lose of elasticity. When elasticity is lost, pinpoint hemorrhaging may occur. If exposed to high doses, the endothelial cells are killed off and a blood clot may form and either occlude the vessel or break off and occlude another vessel. In either case, the loss of the blood supply will lead to tissue death (necrosis) or the formation of fibrotic (scar) tissue.

Small vessels are more radiosensitive than are large ones simply because it takes a much smaller occlusion or clot to block a small blood vessel than a large one. Consequently, most of the damage seen related to blood vessels occurs in organs with a large blood supply and an extensive network of small vessels such as the liver or kidneys.

The heart is radioresistant because it is a muscle with fixed, postmitotic cells. We do not see any damage to the heart itself until the dose reaches about 4000 rad (40 Gy). At that level, pericarditis (inflammation of the cardiac sac) or pancarditis (inflammation of the heart) may result and lead to permanent tissue damage and even death.

Based on the amount of radiation necessary to cause a long-term effect in the cardiovascular system, radiation therapy treatment planning is the only area in which this must be taken into account.

## Respiratory System

The respiratory system consists of the nose, pharynx, trachea, and lungs. The function of the respiratory system is the exchange of gases inside the pulmonary region of the lungs. Specifically, air travels through the nose and/or mouth, the pharynx, and the trachea to the main bronchi of the lungs. From there the air travels through more and more branching of the bronchi until it reaches the alveoli, or air sacs. The alveoli are made up of small air-filled sacs surrounded by blood-carrying capillaries. Because of the close proximity of the air and the blood, oxygen can diffuse into the blood and carbon dioxide can diffuse into the air sac in a process called *respiration*. The respiratory system is considered moderately radioresistant. The only major long-term radiation effect seen in the respiratory system is fibrosis (scar tissue) development in the lungs from acute radiation pneumonitis. Fibrosis and pneumonitis are not areas of concern for radiography or nuclear medicine, as they are usually seen only in doses over 2500 rad (25 Gy). These are of importance in radiation therapy, though, and must be taken into consideration.

## Digestive System

The digestive system is also referred to as the GI system and consists of the mouth, esophagus, stomach, small bowel, and large bowel, as well as auxiliary organs such as the salivary glands, the pancreas, the liver (discussed below), and the gallbladder—in other words, the track through the body starting with the mouth and ending with the anus. The functions of the digestive system are to break food down into macromolecules simple enough to be absorbed as nutrients in the small bowel, to transport fluids to the large bowel, where they are absorbed by the blood, and to transport waste material out of the body. The radiosensitivity of the digestive system is determined by the portion of the system we are referring to.

The system has areas that are lined with mucous membrane, which contains highly mitotic and undifferentiated cells. Other areas are primarily made up of differentiated cells that seldom divide. Overall, the digestive system is considered moderately radiosensitive, with the small bowel section being radiosensitive. Doses over 500 rad (5 Gy) can cause atrophy, strictures, fibrosis, and ulceration in the GI tract. Doses over 1000 rad (10 Gy) have been shown to permanently destroy the villi of the small intestines. This leads to ulceration, fibrosis, and necrosis (tissue death).

Because the doses necessary to cause long-term effects in the GI tract are higher than those usually found in nuclear medicine and radiography, they are not normally a consideration. In radiation therapy, however, GI impacts are one of the major considerations when planning a treatment protocol.

### Liver

The liver is the largest single organ inside the body. It is made up of hepatic cells whose function it is to manufacture, store, and excrete digestive enzymes and chemicals such as bile. Because the hepatic cells are highly differentiated and do not normally divide, the liver would appear to be moderately radioresistant. However, it is actually considered to be moderately radiosensitive, in part because it has a very large blood supply. As noted above, vascularity is moderately radiosensitive because of potential damage to the endothelial cells. Damage to the liver such as radiation hepatatis usually results from damage to the blood supply to the liver.

There are no known dangers to the liver from radiography or nuclear medicine doses. In therapy, care must be taken if the dose to the liver is above 35 Gy (3500 rad), as vascular damage can occur.

### Urinary System

The kidneys, ureters, bladder, and urethra make up the urinary system. The function of the urinary system is the elimination of waste products from the blood and the maintenance of water, electrolyte, and acid/base balances.

The ureters and urethra are transport systems, the bladder is a storage system, and the kidneys do the actual cleansing of the blood. This is accomplished by selectively filtering water, waste products, salts, and toxins out of the blood and into the urine. Inside the kidneys is a large network of blood vessels and nephrons, which carry out the filtration and excretion process. The urinary system is considered relatively radioresistant, as the only long-term effect of note is atrophy and renal failure from chronic radiation nephritis. As 2500 rad (25 Gy) to both kidneys can lead to renal failure and death, protection of the kidneys is important in radiation therapy planning. No long-term effects are known from radiography or nuclear medicine studies.

### Growing Bone and Cartilage

The function the skeletal system is to act as a framework to support all of the organs of the body, protect vital organs, and to grow mature blood components (discussed above). Mature bone and cartilage are radioresistant, as their cells are fixed and postmitotic. However, as osteoblasts and chondroblasts are stem cells found in growing bone and cartilage respectively, they are moderately radiosensitive. Doses of over 100 rad (1 Gy) to children have been shown to cause a temporary halt in the mitosis of the osteoblasts and/or chordroblasts. This can lead to reduced height by the time they are adults. Doses above 1000 rad (10 Gy) can lead to a permanent suppression of mitosis and can have a severe impact on both the size and shape of a child's bones in adulthood.

Long-term bone and cartilage damage are not seen with radiography. The potential does exist for bone damage in children who receive certain types of nuclear medicine studies that concentrate the radiopharmaceuticals in the growth areas. Stunted growth and some learning difficulties can occur in children under 2 years of age with radiation therapy doses over 2000 rad (20 Gy).

### Central Nervous System

The central nervous system consists of the brain and the spinal cord. As both consist of fixed, postmitotic nerve cells, they are radioresistant.

There are no known effects to either the brain or the spinal cord at doses below 1000 rad (10 Gy). At about 2000 rad (20 Gy), necrosis and fibrosis can occur. As in other organs that are mostly made up of radioresistant cells, much of the damage to the central nervous system comes from damage to blood vessels. At the level of dose needed to cause CNS damage, there are no known dangers from radiography or nuclear medicine studies. As a 2000 rad (20 Gy) dose is possible in radiation therapy, care must be taken to avoid exposing the CNS any more than necessary.

## LIFE-SPAN SHORTENING

No data indicate that radiation causes a specific life-span shortening in humans. That is, the life-span-shortening effects of radiation are due to other radiation-induced effects such as leukemia. In the 1930s, radiologists were reported to have a life span of about 5 years less than a control group of other physicians. Because of socioeconomic background, physicians in general would be expected to have similar life spans, so radiation was implicated as the specific cause. However, a repeat of this study in the 1960s indicated that such a difference no longer existed. The lack of a current difference is attributed to improved radiation protection practices.

No life-span shortening has been observed in the atomic bomb survivors, radium dial painters, or diagnostic imaging patients. A study of radiographers who trained as field operators in World War II also found no such effects. These individuals were exposed to large amounts of radiation as a result of the poor design and shielding of the equipment, as well as the fact that their training involved producing at least one full set of diagnostic radiographs on another trainee. Seven thousand of these individuals have been observed, with no effects noted.

## GENETIC DAMAGE

The weakest area of understanding in radiation bioeffects is that of genetics. Most data come from experiments on fruit flies and mice at high doses and are extrapolated to low doses to humans. The human data that we have has provided no positive observations of genetic effects, and the only study that has provided us with the requisite three generations of data is the follow-up of atomic bomb survivors.

Two researchers have produced the bulk of research on genetic effects. First, H.J. Müller's experiments with fruit flies (*Drosophila melanogaster;* Figure 8–2) led to a variety of conclusions:

1. There was no increase in the quality of mutations or the types of observed mutations. Instead, radiation was found to increase those types of mutations found spontaneously in nature.
2. Most mutations observed were recessive. Thus, both parents had to carry the gene for the effect to be observed in the offspring.
3. No threshold was observed. Lethal mutations increased equally with equal increases in dose; thus, the effects observed were linear, nonthreshold.
4. It did not matter whether one large dose or many small doses (fractions) were given, so long as the total amount of radiation was the same. This suggests that mutations were single-hit phenomena and were cumulative in nature.

A husband and wife team (Russell) experimented with millions of mice over many years (the "megamouse" experiment). Their data differed from Müller's in that a dose administered over a long period showed less genetic effect than one large dose.

Technologists should not make too much or too little of these studies. It is easy to assert that humans are not fruit flies or mice, or that "everything causes cancer." These studies have shown that radiation has genetic effects. This is a risk. It can also be assumed that some effects are cumulative and some are not; the best assumption to make is that all effects are cumulative until we have evidence to the contrary. In 1932, the National Council on Radiation Protection (NCRP) lowered the maximal permissible dose (MPD; now referred to as dose limits) based on Müller's work and his description of genetic effects as linear. That basic philosophy holds today: there must be a reason for the exposure that outweighs the potential risk.

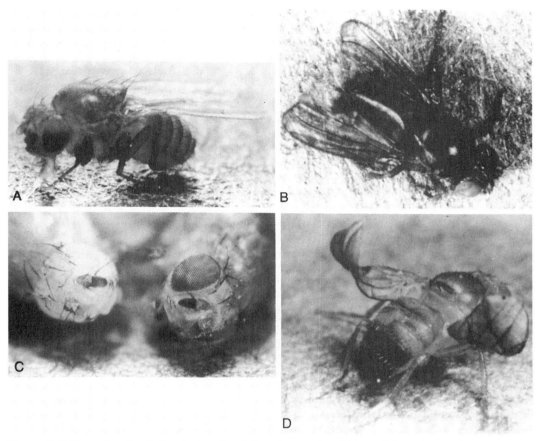

**Figure 8–2** Normal and radiation-induced mutational examples of *Drosophila melanogaster.* The mutations were induced by doses of 20 to 40 Gy (2000 to 4000 rad) delivered to male ancestors. (Insects are far more resistant to high doses of radiation than are mammals.) The mutations were observed in insects many generations removed from the irradiated insects. *(A)* Normal body, eye color, and wing form of a female fruit fly. *(B)* Radiation induced recessive mutation of ebony body color. *(C)* Sex-linked mutation of eye color. The fly on the left is a white-eyed mutation. The eyes of the fly on the right demonstrate the normal color. *(D)* Male fruit fly demonstrating a dominant curly wing mutation associated with inversion. (Courtesy of Seymour Abramson, Ph.D., University of Wisconsin, Madison; reprinted with permission from Wagner LK: Radiation Bioeffects and Management Test and Syllabus. Reston, VA, American College of Radiology, 1991, pp 232–233.)

## Cytogenetic Damage

It has been said that mutations currently alter the reproductive fitness or life span of 10% of the population. From human follow-up studies and animal experiments, data suggests that radiation can cause the following:

- leukemia and other forms of neoplasm
- altered sex ratios (changing the ratio of males to females in a population)
- increased spontaneous abortion or stillbirth
- increased infant mortality

- increased congenital effects
- decreased life expectancy
- dominant inheritable diseases:

    achrondroplastic dwarfism
    polydactyly
    Huntington's chorea

- recessive inheritable diseases:

    cystic fibrosis
    Tay-Sachs
    hemophilia
    albinism

The causal relationship is better established for some of these conditions than it is for others. One of the roles of the technologist is to improve the health of the population. Because these are long-term effects, we do not normally see them. They occur many years later in the exposed children of patients. The responsibility we hold as informed professionals is that we know what the potential genetic effects of radiation are and work to minimize them.

### Doubling Dose

From experiments, the concept of a doubling dose has resulted. This is the dose of radiation that produces twice the frequency of genetic mutations as would have been observed without radiation. Mutations exist in nature with a certain frequency. The current accepted estimate for spontaneous mutation is 6%, which corresponds well with the number of observed congenital abnormalities (4% to 6%). Of course, not all mutations can be detected, and some congenital abnormalities are not genetic in nature.

Müller's fruit fly studies and early reports on the atomic bomb survivors indicated that the doubling dose in humans was 20 to 200 rad (0.2 to 2 Gy). Recently, figures of 50 to 250 rad (0.5 to 2.5 Gy) have been cited as the doubling dose in humans, based primarily on the mega-mouse experiments. It has also been estimated that the doubling dose in females is 40% or more above the value for males. Whalen and Balter note that "Mother Nature thus seems to be protecting her own since ovarian shielding during abdominal x-ray examinations is not usually feasible." Based on the Russell experiments, it appears that mutation rates are lower in females (compared with males) at low dose rates but higher than males at higher dose rates.

### Genetically Significant Dose

The genetically significant dose (GSD) is an average calculated from actual gonadal doses received by the whole population. It takes into account the expected contribution of these individuals to exposed children. It is assumed that this dose, if received by every member of the population, would have the same genetic effect as doses received by those individuals actually exposed to ionizing radiation.

The GSD concept assumes that the long-term effects of radiation can be averaged over a population. It is calculated by a complex statistical formula that looks at the average gonadal dose per examination, the number of persons receiving x-ray examinations, the total number of persons in the population, and the expected number of future children per person.

Although this *would not be an accurate calculation of the GSD,* the concept can be simplified as follows: if two individuals receive radiation of 100 and 50 mrad, and a third receives none, the average to that small "population" of three people is 50 mrad (100 + 50 = 150; 150 ÷ 3 = 50). Of course, it takes many more people than that to make a population, and this is a much simpler averaging than the GSD. The future genetic effects to that population are based on a 50-mrad exposure, even though one person received twice that amount and one individual received nothing.

### FETAL IRRADIATION

The fetus passes through three basic stages of development (Figure 8–3). The first is preimplantation, which in humans is the period from conception to 10 days following conception. In this stage, the fertilized ovum is dividing, forming a ball of undifferentiated cells.

Stage two is organogenesis, in which the cells are implanted in the uterine wall. This stage occurs through the sixth week after conception. In this stage, cells begin differentiating into organs. For example, neuroblasts typi-

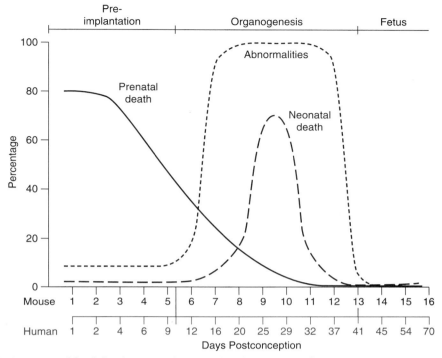

**Figure 8–3** Stages of fetal development. (Reprinted with permission from Thompson MA: Principles of Radiation Protection for Nurses and Other Medical Facility Personnel. Birmingham, AL, University of Alabama at Birmingham, 1986.)

cally form on the 18th day of gestation, and the eyes on the 20th day of gestation.

Stage three is the fetal or growth stage. This is the period following the sixth week after conception. It is, as the name implies, primarily a period of growth rather than new development. The main exception is the central nervous system (CNS), which is still highly undifferentiated in the fetus. Complete development of the CNS does not typically occur until the 12th year of life in humans.

Radiation is a known teratogen. A teratogen is an agent that causes birth defects. Other teratogens include rubella, alcohol, lithium, and mercury. The effects of radiation on the embryo and fetus depend on two factors: the stage of development and the radiation dose. The principal effects of radiation on an embryo or fetus are:

- embryonic, fetal, or neonatal death.
- malformations.
- growth retardation.
- congenital defects.
- cancer induction.

In the earliest stages of development, for example, radiation exposure may destroy enough of the cells to terminate the pregnancy. However, since the cells are still undifferentiated (not specialized) at this point, if enough cells survive to continue to reproduce, the only effect is a delay in development. This is known as the "all or none effect" (see p. 161).

In the middle stages of development, when parts are not fully formed, radiation exposure may cause damage to a part or stunt its development. Late effects of radiation are the most common in later stages, when the fetus is growing rather than developing. Since the CNS remains highly undifferentiated, large doses of radiation (e.g. 25 rad [25 cGy]) can have a variety of effects on it. Radiosensitivity begins to decrease at 20 weeks, but the fetus then becomes more susceptible to late effects and CNS effects.

Dekaban performed the most complete study of embryonic and fetal effects due to large amounts of (therapeutic) radiation. His conclusions, based on a dose of 250 rad (25 cGy) or more, were these:

1. Delivered before the second or third week of gestation, this dosage will most likely result in prenatal death, but few abnormalities will be seen in children carried to term.
2. Irradiation between weeks 4 and 11 of gestation can result in severe abnormalities of multiple organs, especially the skeletal system and the CNS.
3. Mental retardation and microcephaly are frequent if the radiation is delivered between weeks 11 and 16 of gestation.
4. Functional defects can result after week 20, although the fetus is in general less radiosensitive after this time.

Table 8–6 describes some anomalies in relation to human gestational days and radiation exposure. These are extrapolated from mouse data compiled by Rugh. Tables 8–7 and 8–8 illustrate the doses to the embryo from some representative examinations to lend clarity to the material presented here. Developmental defects are considered to have a nonstochastic risk; radiogenic carcinoma is considered to be a stochastic risk.

## Prenatal Death

Exposures of 5 to 15 rad (5 to 15 cGy) in the preimplantation stage can result in prenatal death, or death before birth. An in utero exposure of 10 rad (10 cGy) in the first 2 weeks can result in a spontaneous abortion. However, the natural occurrence of spontaneous abortion is 25% to 50%, and 10 rad (10 cGy) would raise this response by only 0.1%. All these doses are

**Table 8–6  Radiation Damage in Terms of When Irradiated**

| Anomaly | Gestational Days |
|---|---|
| Cataracts | 0–6 |
| Exencephaly (herniation of the brain) | 0–37 |
| Embryonic death | 4–11 |
| Anencephaly or microcephaly | 9–90 |
| Anophthalmia | 16–32 |
| Cleft palate | 20–37 |
| Skeletal disorders | 25–85 |
| Growth disorders | 54+ |

**Table 8–7  Doses to Embryo From Selected Radiographic Procedures***

| Examination | Dose (mrad) |
|---|---|
| Barium enema† | 800 |
| Cholecystogram | 10 |
| Intravenous pyelogram | 800 |
| Pelvis | 200 |
| Upper gastrointestinal series† | 50 |

*Based on an average number of films per examination.

†Refers to overhead films *only.* Fluoroscopic exposure is not included.

**Table 8–8  Whole-Body Dose to Embryo from Selected Radiopharmaceuticals***

| Radiopharmaceutical | Dose (mrad/mCi) |
|---|---|
| I-123 sodium iodide | 32 |
| Tc-99m pertechnetate | 27–39 |
| Tc-99m DTPA | 35 |

*Assumes conceptive age of 1.5 to 6 weeks.

From: Wagner, LK, Mettler FA: Diagnostic x-ray and radionuclide studies during pregnancy. *In* Wagner LK: Radiation Bioeffects and Management Test and Syllabus. Reston, VA, American College of Radiology, 1991.

to the embryo, not the external dosage received by the mother.

In the preimplantation stage, there is typically an "all or none" response in that either a radiation-induced spontaneous abortion occurs or no effects are seen. This type of all or none response usually requires high doses of radiation. At day 1 of preimplantation, 200 rad (2 Gy) leads to death in 80% of humans; at day 9, this same dosage has a 30% fatality rate. Embryonic resorption may occur, and the mother may never know she was pregnant.

### Neonatal Death

Neonatal death is death at birth. It is considered to be a rare form of radiation response. According to the mouse data, it appears to occur primarily as a result of irradiation in the later stages of development of organogenesis and the

fetal stage, as well as at high doses. In the fetal stage, the $LD_{50}$ approaches that of adults.

### Congenital Malformation

Congenital abnormalities such as microcephaly (abnormally small head) or hydrocephaly (commonly called "water on the brain," an expansion of the head due to an increased amount of fluid in the ventricles) can result from radiation exposure in the organogenesis stage. This risk lessens somewhat in the fetal stage but remains high. It is not observed if irradiation occurs during preimplantation. It has been said that 10 rad (10 cGy) of exposure in this stage increases the number of abnormalities by 1%. A parallel can be drawn with exposure to rubella (German measles) and the drug thalidomide, which are thought to cause similar effects in the organogenesis stage.

## The 10–25 Rule

Dr. Stewart Bushong, in his lectures around the country, expounds his "10–25 rule" regarding radiation exposure and pregnancy. Bushong developed this rule after he noted in a national woman's magazine an article about a woman who had a two-view lumbar spine examination because of lower back pain. She later found that she was pregnant, and her physician informed her that he had consulted with a number of "experts" and recommended that she terminate the pregnancy because of the severe effects that could occur.

Bushong notes that this examination probably resulted in a dose of about 100 mrad to the fetus. His 10–25 rule uses both common sense and a knowledge of radiobiology. It states that:

- Doses of less than 10 rad (10 cGy) should never be an indication to terminate a pregnancy.

- Doses of between 10 and 25 rad (10 and 25 cGy) are a gray area in which the determination to terminate a pregnancy depends on the time of exposure.

- At doses of over 25 rad (25 cGy), termination of a pregnancy should be considered.

Additionally, Bushong states that the safest time to be irradiated in pregnancy is during the first 2 weeks, contrary to what many people believe. Because of the all or none effect (see text), there will either be a spontaneous abortion or the child will be carried to term with no ill effects. This is, of course, a value decision based on a knowledge of radiobiology; other individuals might consider the possibility of a spontaneous abortion unacceptable.

In 1930, Murphy and Goldstein observed the children of women who had therapeutic radiation while pregnant. Twenty-eight of 75 children had abnormalities, primarily CNS and skeletal defects. A large degree of microcephalic idiocy (16 of the 28) and of hydrocephaly was observed.

## Childhood Malignancy

In the fetal stage, few abnormalities are noted with radiation exposure. Instead, late effects of radiation such as cancer (especially leukemia) are more likely. It has also been stated, however, that 50 rad (50 cGy) to the fetus probably is necessary to bring about an increase in late effects.

## Diminished Growth and Development

Diminished growth and development is theoretically possible at all stages but occurs primarily during the latter part of gestation and possibly during the very early stages of gestation. Hall stated that growth retardation will not be seen with irradiation in the preimplantation stage, will be temporary with irradiation in the organogenesis stage, and will be permanent if the fetus is irradiated during the fetal stage. During the later stages, this is thought to be due to cell depletion, with a consequent reduction in size. No congenital abnormalities are observed, but the individual will have a somewhat reduced physical size. The children born at Hiroshima were noted later in adolescence to be about 7 lb lighter, 1 inch shorter, and about 50% smaller in head circumference than nonirradiated children.

## SUMMARY

Radiation effects in terms of carcinogenesis have been studied for many years. Although there are a variety of problems with these studies because of dosimetry, extrapolation, and other factors, it has been shown that radiation increases the incidence of leukemia, as well as thyroid, breast, bone, skin, liver, and lung cancer. Radiation has also been implicated in can-

cer of the stomach, esophagus, bladder, salivary glands, colon, lymphoma, and brain.

The radiation incidents that stand out in recent history are Three Mile Island in 1979 and Chernobyl in 1986. Radioactivity released from Three Mile Island was relatively low, but the explosion at Chernobyl resulted in both high and low doses that had immediate and as yet undetermined long-term effects.

Based on population studies, there are three ways to express risk of cancer from radiation: absolute, excess, and relative risks. Leukemia has been implicated more than any other form of cancer and has the shortest latent period of any malignant disease (5 to 7 years), with an at risk period of 20 years. Bone, lung, skin, thyroid, and breast cancer have also been strongly implicated as being caused by radiation.

At today's dose levels, radiation poses no risk to skin. Other than experimental studies and statistical extrapolation, little information is available on the effects to the gonads from small amounts of radiation. Radiation cataractogenesis remains somewhat controversial. The dose–response relationship is a threshold, nonlinear response.

Life-span shortening as observed in humans is nonspecific. No life-span shortening was observed in a group of military radiologic technologists who received relatively high doses as a result of being required to perform full sets of radiographs on fellow trainees.

Genetic effects are the weakest area of understanding in radiation bioeffects. Most data are extrapolated from animal studies at high doses to low doses in humans. Radiation increases mutations found spontaneously in nature, and most radiation-induced mutations are recessive. Effects are linear and nonthreshold, and it is not clear whether mutations are cumulative.

Radiation causes a variety of types of cytogenetic damage. The doubling dose is the dose of radiation that produces twice the frequency of genetic mutations as would have been observed without radiation. The genetically significant dose is an average calculated from actual gonadal doses received by the whole population; the concept assumes that the long-term effects of radiation can be averaged over a population.

For radiation effects, three basic stages of development are used. The first is preimplantation, which in humans is the period from conception to 10 days following conception. Stage two is organogenesis, in which the cells are implanted in the uterine wall. Stage three is the fetal or growth stage. This is the period following the sixth week after conception.

The effects of radiation on the embryo and fetus depend on the stage of development and the radiation dose. The principal effects of radiation on an embryo or fetus are embryonic, fetal, or neonatal death; malformations; growth retardation; congenital defects; and cancer induction.

## Questions

1. The preferred methods of expressing the risk of cancer induction from radiation exposure are:

   I. absolute risk.
   II. excess risk.
   III. relative risk.

   a. I and II only      b. I and III only
   c. II and III only    d. I, II, and III

2. The malignancy with the shortest latent period is:

   a. bone cancer.       b. breast cancer.
   c. leukemia.          d. thyroid cancer.

3. Which of the following are radiation effects that are well understood?

   I. cellular carcinogenesis
   II. dosimetry
   III. radiation production

   a. I and II only      b. I and III only
   c. II and III only    d. I, II, and III

4. Which of the following types of cancer induced by radiation appears to have a threshold?

   a. leukemia           b. lung cancer
   c. skin cancer        d. thyroid cancer

5. The threshold for cataractogenesis (fractionated doses) appears to be:

   a. 25 rad (cGy).      b. 100 rad (cGy).
   c. 200 rad (cGy).     d. 1000 rad (cGy).

6. Which of the following were findings of H.J. Müller's experiments on fruit flies?

   I. There was an increase in the quality of mutations.
   II. Most mutations observed were recessive.
   III. No threshold was observed.

   a. I and II only      b. I and III only
   c. II and III only    d. I, II, and III

7. Which of the following is the correct order of development?

   I. fetal stage
   II. preimplantation
   III. organogenesis

   a. II, III, I         b. III, II, I
   c. I, II, III         d. III, I, II

8. The $LD_{50}$ is similar to that of an adult:

   a. in the preimplantation stage.
   b. in organogenesis.
   c. in the fetal stage.
   d. only after birth.

9. In utero exposure to 10 rad (10 cGy) will raise the percentage of spontaneous abortions by:

   a. 0.01%.             b. 0.1%.
   c. 1%.                d. 10%.

10. Growth disorders would most likely occur from exposure following which conceptual days?

    a. 24                b. 34
    c. 44                d. 54

11. Which of the following are thought to follow a linear dose–response curve?

    I. leukemia
    II. cataractogenesis
    III. genetic damage

    a. I and II only     b. I and III only
    c. II and III only   d. I, II, and III

12. Solid tumors have a minimum latent period of:

    a. 1 year.          b. 5 years.
    c. 10 years.        d. 20 years.

13. The primary long-term effect of radiation observed in the radium dial painters was:

    a. lung cancer.     b. bone cancer.
    c. thyroid cancer.  d. leukemia.

14. In terms of cancer induction, which of the following are seen as especially radiosensitive?

    I. brain
    II. bone marrow
    III. thyroid

    a. I and II only    b. I and III only
    c. II and III only  d. I, II, and III

## Exercises

1. Determine and name (e.g. relative) each of the following risk factors:

   a. Five cases are expected in a population; ten are observed after exposure to 100 rad (1 Gy).
   b. 10 cases/$10^6$ people/rad (cGy)/yr means what?
   c. Compared with controls, the risk was 2.

2. Why do we have a poor knowledge of some radiation effects?

3. What is the evidence of life-span shortening in humans?

4. What were the findings in Müller's fruit fly experiments and the megamouse experiments? What was the main conflicting finding?

5. What elements must be calculated in the genetically significant dose?

6. What are the principal effects of radiation on an embryo or fetus?

7. Describe the all or none response.

8. What is the significance of central nervous system development in radiation effects to the fetus?

9. When will diminished growth and development most likely occur?

10. What did two studies of the effects of therapeutic radiation on the fetus discover?

11. Radiation has been shown to increase the incidence of what cancers?

12. Describe limitations on human population studies for radiation carcinogenesis. How does this limit our knowledge of the effects of radiation on personnel in diagnostic imaging?

13. What are some of the unclear issues of the accident at Chernobyl?

## Answers

Questions

| | |
|---|---|
| 1. b | 8. c |
| 2. c | 9. a |
| 3. c | 10. d |
| 4. c | 11. b |
| 5. d | 12. c |
| 6. c | 13. b |
| 7. a | 14. c |

Exercises

1. a. This is excess risk and would be assigned a value of 5 (10 − 5 = 5).

   b. This is absolute risk, and it means that in a group of 1 million people exposed to 1 rad (cGy), 10 will develop cancer as a result.

   c. This is relative risk, and it means that cancer induction has doubled (2×) as a result of radiation exposure.

2. Effects such as cellular carcinogenesis, tissue-level effects, host effects, and clinical cancer induction are poorly understood because of confounding and synergistic effects that may not be due to radiation. They could be due to exposure to other

diseases or risk agents such as chemicals or smoking.

3. The only evidence of specific human life-span shortening comes from a study of radiologists. Some animal studies have suggested that specific life-span shortening could occur, but life-span shortening in humans appears to be nonspecific (i.e. caused by cancer or effects other than the radiation itself).

4. Müller's studies indicated that (1) there was no increase in the quality of mutations or the types of observed mutations; (2) most mutations observed were recessive; (3) no threshold was observed; and (4) mutations were single-hit phenomena and were cumulative in nature.

   The megamouse experiments differed mainly in that a dose rate effect was seen: a given dose extended over a long period of time showed fewer effects genetically than one large dose.

5. The GSD assumes that the long-term effects of radiation can be averaged over a population. It is calculated by a formula that looks at the average gonadal dose per examination, the number of persons receiving x-ray examinations, the total number of persons in the population, and the expected number of future children per person. It is an average calculated from actual gonadal doses received by the whole population.

6. The principal effects are embryonic, fetal, or neonatal death; malformations; retardation of growth; congenital defects; and cancer induction. Whether these effects occur and their severity depend on the stage of development and the radiation dose.

7. An all or none response often occurs in the preimplantation stage. There is either a radiation-induced spontaneous abortion or no effects are seen. This type of all or none response usually requires high doses of radiation.

8. The CNS remains highly undifferentiated in the fetus and is not usually fully devel-oped until age 12 years. Large doses of radiation can have a variety of effects on the CNS, such as microcephaly or hydro-cephaly. Overall radiosensitivity begins to decrease at 20 weeks of gestation, but the fetus then becomes more susceptible to late effects and CNS effects.

9. Diminished growth and development occurs primarily during the latter part of gestation and possibly during the very early stages of gestation after irradiation. With irradiation, growth retardation will not be seen in the preimplantation stage, will be temporary in the organogenesis stage, and will be permanent in the fetal stage.

10. Murphy and Goldstein found that 28 of the 75 children in their study had abnormalities, primarily CNS and skeletal defects; 16 of these had microcephalic idiocy. Dekaban found, with 250 rad (2.5 Gy) or more, that (1) if delivered before week 2 or 3 of gestation, prenatal death is most likely, but few abnormalities will be seen in full-term children; (2) severe abnormalities of multiple organs, especially the skeletal system and the CNS, will result from radiation in weeks 4 to 11; (3) mental retardation and microcephaly are frequent if the radiation was delivered from week 11 to 16; and (4) functional defects can result after the 20th week, although the fetus is less radiosensitive in general.

11. Radiation has been shown to increase the incidence of leukemia and thyroid, breast, bone, skin, liver, and lung cancer.

12. The four basic limitations are (1) selection of a control group; (2) need to prove statistical significance; (3) difficulty in isolating factors; and (4) dosimetry. These limit our ability to properly study the effects of radiation on personnel. A control group must be chosen that exactly matches the group studied. Also, personnel exposed to ionizing radiation engage in the same risks as the rest of the population. Finally, we do not always know the dose that personnel were exposed to, especially in past situations, where dose was not always monitored.

13. Two issues are unclear:

    - The presence of cesium-137, which has a half-life of 30 years, raises questions of long-term effects. Theoretically, it should take at least three generations before these are well defined.

    - The widespread use of abortion in the USSR at that time clouds the issue of fetal effects. Also, the fact that so many individuals lived in the 400 to 600 rem group indicates that the $LD_{50/30}$ may not be accurate, especially with newer methods of bone marrow transplantation.

# CHAPTER 9

# Radiation Safety/Protection and Health Physics

Siamak Shahabi

## Chapter Outline

## Chapter Goals and Objectives

At the end of this chapter, the reader should be able to:

1. Describe the risk-versus-benefit decisions made by health and medical physicists.

2. List the agencies involved in making recommendations and setting regulatory guidelines for radiologic/diagnostic equipment.

3. Describe the role of the radiation safety officer.

4. Describe a typical radiation safety program.

5. List representative regulations for radiologic/diagnostic equipment.

6. Describe the role of the radiologic/diagnostic technologist in conforming to standards and regulations for radiation protection.

## Important Terms and Definitions

agreement state
American Registry of Radiologic Technologists (ARRT)
as low as reasonably achievable (ALARA)
beam quality
Code of Federal Regulations (CFR)
Conference of Radiation Control Program Directors (CRCPD)
dose equivalent limit
external exposure
half-value layer
health physicist
internal exposure
International Atomic Energy Agency (IAEA)
International Commission on Radiation Protection (ICRP)
International Commission on Radiological Units and Measurements (ICRU)
International Labour Organization (ILO)
Joint Commission of Accreditation of Healthcare Institutions (JCAHO)
linearity
maximum permissible dose (MPD)
medical physicist
National Evaluation of X-Ray Trends (NEXT)
National Research Council Committee on the Biological Effects of Ionizing Radiation (BEIR)
negligible individual risk level (NIRL)
planned special exposure (PSE)
primary barrier
prospective limit
radiation area
radiation safety officer (RSO)
rem bank
reproducibility
retrospective limit
secondary barrier

| | |
|---|---|
| shielding | U.S. Food and Drug Administration (FDA) |
| tolerance dose | U.S. Nuclear Regulatory Commission (NRC) |
| U.N. Scientific Commission on Effects of Atomic Radiation (UNSCEAR) | U.S. Occupational Safety and Health Administration (OSHA) |
| U.S. Environmental Protection Agency (EPA) | whole-body cumulative exposure |
| | x-ray compliance program |

## INTRODUCTION

This chapter discusses and reviews the fundamentals of radiation protection/safety, health physics, and the role of the health or medical physicist (who also is often the radiation safety officer for an institution that provides radiation therapy, a diagnostic radiology department, or both) in preparing radiation protection programs for compliance with federal and state rules and regulations/guidelines. The terms *health physicist, medical physicist,* and *radiation safety officer* are used interchangeably throughout the text because these professionals are concerned with the same basic common goal of providing radiation protection/safety. This is done for the sake of convenience but is not a wholly accurate means of referring to these individuals. As an example, the radiation safety officer at an institution may not be a physicist by training, but might be a radiologist, radiation oncologist, radiation therapist, or diagnostic technologist with advanced training and education.

In diagnostic imaging and radiation therapy, clinical medical physicists as well as health physicists and radiation safety officers are all concerned with the provision of radiation protection to occupationally exposed personnel, patients, and the general public.

Health physicists and clinical medical physicists are certified in a process similar to the certification of radiologic technologists and are designated certified health physicists or certified medical physicists in either radiation therapy or diagnostic radiology or both.

Although some of the topics here are discussed elsewhere in this textbook, the intent is to present them here from the standpoint of the individual who sets standards for institutional radiation protection programs, the

health or medical physicist or radiation safety officer.

No one standard set of regulations can cover comprehensively all facilities in the United States. Therefore, for safe practice the physicist or radiation safety officer at a facility must weigh risks versus benefits having knowledge of the federal and state rules and regulations and also the recommendations of national and international organizations.

A hospital, for example, will typically meet certain guidelines for accreditation by the Joint Commission on Healthcare Organizations (JCAHO) that relate to radiation exposure. However, accreditation is a voluntary process. In most cases, the institution will also meet state laws regarding radiation exposure. Also, laws at the federal level often are an outgrowth of recommendations of national organizations such as the National Council of Radiation Protection and Measurement (NCRP). For example, licensees of the Nuclear Regulatory Commission (the NRC is the U.S. agency that has control over the use of all reactor-produced radioactive materials) must meet standards for protection from radiation in Title 10, Part 20 of the Code of Federal Regulations. This is an outgrowth of recommendations found in NCRP Report No. 91.

One may summarize the roles of the different agencies stated above as follows: (1) The International Commission on Radiological Protection (ICRP) set the first radiation protection standards; (2) the National Council on Radiation Protection was established in the United States and has functioned as a primary standard setter in radiation protection; (3) The Nuclear Regulatory Commission (NRC) is a U.S. agency that regulates the safe use of reactor-produced radioactive materials in medical and nonmedical practices. Finally, the individual states regulate x-ray machines and naturally occuring radioactive materials such as radium and radon.

All of this will be discussed in more detail in this chapter. The reader should realize that the process of federal and state rule making in radiation protection is a complex one that may reflect many varying viewpoints of scientists and policymakers.

## RISK VERSUS BENEFIT

The exposure of the public, patient, and employee to ionizing radiation has, for the most part, been evaluated on a risk-versus-benefit basis. For the general public, any unnecessary exposure to ionizing radiation is an unacceptable risk with no benefit. As for patients, the risks of exposure are outweighed by the greater benefit of an accurate diagnosis or the successful treatment of a disease. The risks for employees who receive occupational exposures are controllable, and the benefits include better structural evaluations of building components (in industrial radiography), an accurate medical diagnosis or therapy, cleaner sources of energy, and breakthroughs in medical research. The list of possible benefits is virtually endless, but it should be remembered that, for every benefit resulting from medical and occupational exposure to radiation, there are risks.

Within a few weeks of Roentgen's discovery of x-rays in 1895, the value of x-rays as a diagnostic tool was realized. Early work with ionizing radiation soon revealed that there were risks involved. Physicians and other operators working with early fluoroscopic devices exhibited a higher than normal incidence of skin cancers, cataracts, and lesions of the distal digits of the hand. It soon became evident that the risks, when left uncontrolled, far outweighed the benefits. Controls needed to be established to make the risks manageable.

As understanding of the biologic effects of radiation exposure has evolved, so have radiation protection standards. For example, only short-term effects were recognized in the early days of radiology. It was usually thought that doses needed to be limited only in the short term and that a *tolerance dose* existed, below which no effects would be seen. In what was often called the "Golden Age of Radiology," a time during which standards for imaging were developed

(until the 1930s or 1940s), 1 roentgen per day was often considered acceptable. This exposure is about twice what the average technologist receives in *1 year* of exposure at today's levels.

As the long-term potential risks of radiation have become known, radiation protection standards have focused on minimizing the potential long- and short-term effects. This logical evolution in standards is shown in Table 9–1. Today, radiation protection programs are based on a simple philosophy—to keep exposures of patients, the general public, and personnel as low as reasonably achievable (ALARA). This is also referred to in some documents as *optimization*. ALARA assumes that the relationship between dose and risk is strictly linear and without a threshold. Although this may be an overly conservative model, it is desirable to overestimate rather than underestimate risk.

## ORGANIZATIONS THAT DERIVE STANDARDS

Many organizations contribute to radiation protection standards. Some report on scientific research into radiation and its effects, some make recommendations for standards, and others make and enforce regulations at the state and federal levels. The relationship between the "major players" is as follows (adapted from Hendee, (1992):

| UNSCEAR and BEIR reports | → | ICRP, NCRP, and CRCPD recommendations (also called reports in some cases) | → | State and federal (NRC, FDA, EPA) regulations |
|---|---|---|---|---|

Thus, reports lead to recommendations that become part of law. This section will discuss organizations that conduct reports or make recommendations that lead to standards for practice or laws regulating the use of equipment.

### International Commission on Radiological Units and Measurements (ICRU)

The International Commission on Radiological Units and Measurements (ICRU) was established in 1925 by the International Congress of Radiology. The goal of the ICRU is the devel-

Table 9–1  Evolution of Occupational Exposure Limits

| Time Period | Limit | Authority |
| --- | --- | --- |
| 1896 to early 1900s | Erythema dose | Generally accepted guideline |
| 1902 | Fogging of a photographic plate (dental film later used as a rudimentary film badge) | Rollins |
| 1920s–1940s | Tolerance dose | Generally accepted guideline |
| 1925 | 1/100 erythema dose (about 40 rem/yr) | Mutscheller |
| | 1/10 erythema dose | Sievert |
| 1931 | 0.2 R/day (about 40 rem/yr) | Advisory Committee on X-Ray and Radium Protection |
| 1936 | 0.1 R/day (about 20 rem/yr) | Advisory Committee on X-Ray and Radium Protection |
| 1959 | 5 rem/yr | NCRP |
| | Cumulative dose 5(N − 18) | |
| 1987 | 5 rem/yr | NCRP |
| | Cumulative dose = age in rem | |
| 1991 | 2 rem/yr | ICRP (not enforced yet in U.S.) |

opment of a common framework of scientific concepts based on an international consensus on matters relevant to the assessment of radiation for its safe and effective use.

## International Commission on Radiological Protection (ICRP)/National Council on Radiation Protection and Measurement (NCRP)

In 1928 the International Commission on Radiological Protection (ICRP) was formed, and in 1929 the National Committee on Radiation Protection and Measurement, which was later chartered by Congress in 1964 as the National Council on Radiation Protection and Measurements (NCRP), a not-for-profit corporation, was established. The ICRP and the NCRP exist as separate but cooperative entities today, with the following common objectives:

1. Collect, analyze, develop, and disseminate in the public interest information and recommendations about
   a. protection against radiation
   b. radiation measurements, quantities, and units, particularly those concerned with radiation protection
2. Provide a means by which organizations concerned with scientific and related aspects of radiation protection and of radiation quantities, units, and measurements may cooperate for effective utilization of their combined resources; stimulate the work of such organizations
3. Develop basic concepts about radiation quantities, units, and measurements; about the applications of these concepts; and about radiation protection, the ICRU, and other national and international organizations, governmental and private, concerned with radiation quantities, units, and measurements and with radiation protection.

The Council is made up of the members and the participants who serve on the 34 Scientific Committees of the Council. The Scientific Committees, composed of experts having detailed knowledge and competence in the particular area of the committees' interest, draft proposed recommendations. These are then submitted to the full membership of the Council for careful review and approval before being published. In 1987, the NCRP made new recommendations for limits on exposure to ionizing radiation in its Report No. 91. These were the first changes recommended since 1971 by this organization, and they had far-reaching effects on the radiation protection community. These are summarized later in this chapter. In 1991, the ICRP recommended a further reduction in exposure limits, recommending 2 rem (20 mSv) per year for occupational exposure.

## International Atomic Energy Agency

The International Atomic Energy Agency (IAEA) was established in 1957 by the General Assembly of the United Nations. It is an autonomous organization that fosters, encourages, and advises the development of peaceful uses of atomic energy throughout the world. It promotes the wider use of radioisotopes and radiation sources, primarily in industry. The IAEA publishes the *IAEA Bulletin* and *Meetings on Atomic Energy,* and is currently performing an evaluation of the radiologic consequences of Chernobyl at the request of the former USSR.

## International Labour Organization

The International Labour Organization (ILO) was established in 1919 and became associated with the United Nations in 1946. Panels of consultants work on special problems such as occupational health and safety in various industries, including radiation work.

## United Nations Scientific Committee on Effects of Atomic Radiation

The United Nations Scientific Committee on Effects of Atomic Radiation (UNSCEAR) was established in 1955 by resolution 913 of the General Assembly of the United Nations. Its aims are to assess and report on exposures of humans and the environment to ionizing radiation from natural sources, man-made practices, and accidental releases of radiation. They evaluate the risks of radiation exposure from epidemiologic and research findings.

## Conference of Radiation Control Program Directors

The Conference of Radiation Control Program Directors (CRCPD), established in 1968, is a not-for-profit professional organization made up of individuals in state and local government who regulate and control the use of radiation sources, and of individuals, regardless of employer affiliation, who have expressed an interest in radiation protection.

The CRCPD developed the Suggested State Regulations for Control of Radiation. This document provides the regulatory foundation for most state and local programs. The CRCPD also has developed other programs in the healing arts and the fields of environmental nuclear and general radiation protection to promote the safe and effective use of radiation. In the healing arts, the conference, in conjunction with the U.S. Food and Drug Administration, developed a quality assurance program for mammography and diagnostic procedures and helped establish the Nationwide Evaluation of X-Ray Trends (NEXT) program.

## National Research Council Committee on the Biological Effects of Ionizing Radiation

The National Research Council (NRC), not to be confused with the Nuclear Regulatory Commission (also NRC), is administered by the National Academy of Sciences, the National Academy of Engineering, and the Institute of Medicine. Five reports have been issued by the Committee on the Biological Effects of Ionizing Radiation (also called the BEIR Committee) since it was convened in 1955. The most recent report, BEIR V: *Health Effects of Exposure to Low Levels of Ionizing Radiation* (1990), is an update of studies of biologic effects of radiation and risk estimates estimated in the earlier BEIR reports. It is a controversial report that has been interpreted many ways by readers, some believing that it validated current practice as "safe," others thinking that it indicated that radiation risks are still not appropriately quantified.

## REGULATORY AGENCIES RESPONSIBLE FOR PROTECTING THE PUBLIC AND OCCUPATIONALLY EXPOSED PERSONNEL FROM UNNECESSARY EXPOSURE TO IONIZING RADIATION

### U.S. Nuclear Regulatory Commission (NRC)

Originally established as the U.S. Atomic Energy Commission (AEC) in the 1940s, the U.S. Nuclear Regulatory Commission (NRC) established regulations and standards for protection against radiation hazards arising out of the activities under licenses issued by the NRC. Prior to 1954, the atomic energy activities were restricted to the federal government. In 1954, Congress enacted the Atomic Energy Act of 1954 and made it possible for private commercial firms to enter the field. Because of the hazards, Congress determined these activities should be regulated under a system of licensing to protect the health and safety of radiation workers and the public.

For the interested student, specific regulatory information related to the NRC may be found in Title 10 of the Code of Federal Regulations (CFR) Chapter 1. Of particular interest are the requirements of 10 CFR 20, which outline basic radiation protection standards.

### Agreement States

Protection of the public health and safety had traditionally been a responsibility of the states, but the 1954 Act did not provide a specific role for the states. In 1959, Section 274 of the Atomic Energy Act was enacted to spell out a state role and to provide a statutory basis under which the federal government could relinquish to the states portions of its regulatory authority. The 1959 amendments made it possible for the states to license and regulate by-products, source materials, and small quantities of special nuclear materials.

The mechanism for the transfer of the NRC's authority to a state is an agreement between the governor of the state and the commission. Before transferring this authority, the NRC must determine that the state's radiation safety program is compatible with the commission's and that it is adequate to protect the public health and safety. It is also necessary that the state establish its authority by enacting enabling legislation.

Originally, primarily the southern states, New York, and California were members of NRC agreements transferring authority to a state. Twenty-nine states have entered into such agreements with the NRC. These states now regulate 55% of by-product, source, and special nuclear material licensees in the United States. These programs are routinely reviewed by the NRC to ensure that they are effective in protecting the public health and safety. The current agreement states are:

| | |
|---|---|
| Alabama | Nebraska |
| Arizona | Nevada |
| Arkansas | New Hampshire |
| California | New Mexico |
| Colorado | New York |
| Florida | North Carolina |
| Georgia | North Dakota |
| Idaho | Oregon |
| Iowa | Rhode Island |
| Kansas | South Carolina |
| Kentucky | Tennessee |
| Louisiana | Texas |
| Maine | Utah |
| Maryland | Washington |
| Mississippi | |

### U.S. Environmental Protection Agency (EPA)

The U.S. Environmental Protection Agency (EPA) was established in the executive branch as an independent effective December 2, 1970, as a result of the Reorganization Plan 3 of 1970. The Office of Radiation Programs coordinates with the NRC and state and local radiation programs in the development and enforcement of regulations related to the control of radiation in the environment.

### U.S. Food and Drug Administration (FDA)

The U.S. Food and Drug Administration (FDA) regulates the design and manufacture of electronic products by authority of the Radiation Control for Health and Safety Act of 1968. Medical x-ray equipment is designated an electronic product that may emit x-rays and other ionizing electromagnetic radiation.

The FDA established operational standards for x-ray equipment manufactured for sale in the United States. Specific standards for the beam quality, reproducibility of the beam and timer mechanisms, linearity of milliampere (mA) stations, beam collimation and alignment, and light field intensity, as well as special requirements for fluoroscopic equipment, were established to protect patients and occupationally exposed individuals from unnecessary exposure due to faulty manufacturing. These are listed later. The FDA conducts spot compliance inspections on equipment installed in x-ray facilities to determine the level of compliance with the standards.

For the interested student, further specific regulatory information related to the FDA may be found in Title 21 of CFR Subchapter J. Specifically, pages 477 to 488 of the April 1, 1992, edition contain most of the regulations relevant to radiographic and fluoroscopic equipment. According to the *Conventions Specific to the Radiography Examination* (ARRT, May 1993), sections of 21 CFR 1992 are covered on the radiography registry. A note about terminology used in regulations is in order. If a regulation uses the term *shall,* that means that this is a requirement and everyone must abide by this regulation. If the term *should* is used, this means that the regualtion is a suggestion and it is not mandatory for people to meet the suggestion. Some of the regulations are summarized next.

### Beam Quality

The half-value layer (HVL) of the useful beam for a given x-ray tube potential shall not be less than the appropriate level shown in Table 9–2. When multiple filters can be selected on a tube, an interlock system must be in place that will prevent x-ray emission if the minimum required filtration is not in place.

### Reproducibility of the Beam and Timer Mechanisms

Timers must terminate the exposure at a preset time interval, a preset product of current and time (mAs), a preset number of pulses, or

**Table 9–2   Half-Value Layers from 21 CFR***

| X-Ray Tube Voltage (kVp) | | Minimum HVL (mm of Aluminum) | |
|---|---|---|---|
| Designed Operating Range | Measured Operating Potential | Specified Dental Systems | Other X-Ray Systems |
| Below 50 | 30 | 1.5 | 0.3 |
| | 40 | 1.5 | 0.4 |
| | 49 | 1.5 | 0.5 |
| 50–70 | 50 | 1.5 | 1.2 |
| | 60 | 1.5 | 1.3 |
| | 70 | 1.5 | 1.5 |
| Above 70 | 71 | 2.1 | 2.1 |
| | 80 | 2.3 | 2.3 |
| | 90 | 2.5 | 2.5 |
| | 100 | 2.7 | 2.7 |
| | 110 | 3.0 | 3.0 |
| | 120 | 3.2 | 3.2 |
| | 130 | 3.5 | 3.5 |
| | 140 | 3.8 | 3.8 |
| | 150 | 4.1 | 4.1 |

*From this comes the often-repeated mandate that for tubes operating at or below 50 kVp, at least 0.5 mm of Al eq filtration is required; for tubes operating at from 50 to 70 kVp, at least 1.5 mm of Al eq filtration is required; and for tubes operating above 70 kVp, at least 2.5 mm of Al eq filtration is required.

a preset radiation exposure to the image receptor. For automatic exposure controls, the product of current and exposure time is limited to 600 mAs per exposure above 50 kVp.

### Linearity of mA Stations

The average ratio of exposure to the indicated mAs product in mR/mAs obtained at two consecutive tube current settings shall not differ by more than 0.1 times their sum, or:

$$X_1 - X_2 < 0.1(X_1 + X_2)$$

where $X_1$ and $X_2$ = the average mR/mAs values obtained at each of two consecutive tube current settings. Compliance is measured by making 10 exposures at each of two consecutive x-ray tube current settings made within 1 hour.

## Beam Collimation and Alignment

The minimum field size at a source-to-image receptor distance (SID) of 100 cm must be equal to or less than 5 × 5 cm. The x-ray field must be aligned to the center of the image receptor to within 2% of the SID. For positive beam limitation (PBL; automatic collimation), an exposure should not be possible when the length or width of the x-ray field exceeds the length or width of the image receptor by more than 3% of the SID. The operator must be able to undersize the field size as needed.

## Light Field Intensity

A light localizer used to define the x-ray field must provide an illumination of at least 160 lux (15 foot-candles) at 100 cm or the maximum SID, whichever is less. At that same distance, the edge of the light field must exhibit a contrast ratio of not less than 4.

## Special Requirements for Fluoroscopic Equipment

Requirements for fluoroscopic equipment include:

1. A protective barrier that must be in place for x-ray exposure to occur and that limits exposure that is not directed to the image receptor to less than 2 mR/hr at 10 cm.
2. A maximum exposure rate of 5 R/min at the point where the center of the useful beam enters the patient unless the high-level control (also called the fluoroboost) is activated. The fluoroboost must have a continuous audible signal when activated.
3. The source-to-skin distance shall be limited to not less than 38 cm on stationary fluoroscopes and not less than 30 cm on mobile fluoroscopes. Shorter source-to-skin operation is possible on some surgical equipment (e.g. mobile C-arms), but in no case can operation occur at less than 20 cm.
4. A timer device must be available that will signal the fluoroscopist when any preset

time (not to exceed 5 minutes) has been reached.

## U.S. Occupational Safety and Health Administration

The U.S. Occupational Safety and Health Administration (OSHA) is responsible for monitoring workplaces, especially in commercial industry. OSHA regulates the occupational exposure to radiation through 29 CFR 1910.

## State and Local Governments

All states, even those not part of the NRC agreement, have some form of regulation covering ionizing radiation equipment. Most state and local regulatory agencies operate under regulations patterned after the Suggested State Regulations for the Control of Radiation. These suggested regulations are prepared by the CRCPD, U.S. NRC, U.S. EPA, U.S. Department of Health and Human Services Public Health Service, and FDA.

## State Licensure of Radiologic Technologists

Certification of radiologic technologists through organizations such as the American Registry of Radiologic Technologists (ARRT) is a voluntary process designed to ensure safe operation of radiologic equipment. Although numbers vary, statistics indicate that as many as half the operators of radiologic equipment in the United States are not certified in the operation of equipment. Since studies such as NEXT have shown that certified operators provide better radiation protection to patients, many states have instituted licensure. Most states use the ARRT or similar criteria for licensure.

The goal of state licensure is to ensure that operators meet minimum standards. This ensures, to a degree, safe operation of equipment. In states with licensure, it often is the responsibility of the radiation safety officer to maintain records of certification of staff technologists.

## TYPICAL DUTIES OF A MEDICAL PHYSICIST OR RADIATION SAFETY OFFICER

A medical physicist evaluates the risk involved in being exposed to ionizing radiation to determine if there is a way to reduce the risk to the point that such an exposure will result in a benefit. The physicist does this by studying the information and regulations provided by such organizations and governmental agencies as those listed above, and then utilizes and interprets that material to protect individuals and population groups against the harmful effects of ionizing and nonionizing radiation.

### Radiation Safety Program

In medical, educational, or industrial radiation facilities, the radiation safety program should be under the direction of a formally designated radiation safety officer (RSO). Institutions handling radioisotopes must designate an RSO by the standards of rules and regulations of qualified agencies (e.g. nuclear regulatory commission). In addition to the RSO, a radiation safety committee should be formed and should include as members individuals from each department in which ionizing radiation is used. Ideally, this would include departments, such as surgery, radiation oncology, diagnostic radiology, nuclear medicine, and gynecology, in which radiation is used but non–radiation workers are not always aware of the proper uses and methods for radiation protection.

An operational and effective radiation safety program for a diagnostic radiology facility should include but not be limited to the following:

1. Introduction
   a. Objectives of radiation protection
   b. Tissues at risk: bone marrow, breast, thyroid, other organs, gonads, lens of the eye, and the fetus
   c. Risk assessment
   d. Maximum permissible dose equivalent
2. General concepts of exposure reduction
   a. Training of personnel
   b. Means of minimizing radiation exposure from examinations
   c. Reducing repeats
   d. Pregnant patients
3. Protection of personnel and patients
   a. Immobilization of patients
   b. Shielding
   c. Fluoroscopic examinations and exposure to personnel
   d. Eye protection
   e. Personnel monitoring
   f. Pregnant personnel
4. Emergency response

The RSO in most settings should be a qualified medical physicist who is responsible for the development of a comprehensive radiation safety program that oversees activities that include but may not be limited to the receipt, use, and disposal of radioactive material, radiation surveys, personnel and area monitoring, leak testing, shielding design, emergency response, and decontamination of radioactive spills. Thus, the RSO works not only in the departments of radiology, nuclear medicine, and radiation therapy, but also in areas, such as the operating room, where either radiation (intraoperative radiation therapy) or radioactive material is used. These activities are just a few of the duties performed by a physicist or RSO.

### Radiation-Shielding Design

Shielding design includes an evaluation of the use of ionizing radiation with respect to the environment within which it is used. In an x-ray facility, there may be several x-ray rooms, each with its own unique components and workloads, and adjoining rooms or areas. Occupationally and nonoccupationally exposed individuals in such a facility may be exposed to primary and scatter radiation resulting from the use of this equipment.

A medical physicist evaluates a set of plans prior to the construction of an x-ray facility to determine the need for lead or concrete equivalent shielding required to protect both occupationally and nonoccupationally exposed individuals from unnecessary exposure to ionizing radiation. The plans should indicate the normal location of the x-ray-producing equipment's collimator, the general orientations of the radiation beam, the locations of any windows and doors, and the location of the control booth, the surrounding adjacent area, and the control console. In addition, the structural composition and thickness of all walls, doors, floors, and ceilings should be determined, along with the floor-to-ceiling height for each room. Then, the occupancy of all adjacent areas is evaluated and a model of the x-ray-producing equipment is developed from information about the equipment's maximum energy (kVp) and maximum mA.

From the information collected, combined with information about the types of examinations or treatments that will be performed, an anticipated workload in mA-minutes per week can be derived and used in calculations to determine the thickness of lead or lead equivalent shielding necessary to protect the adjacent areas from primary and scatter radiation. The workload is derived by listing the types and quantities of examinations performed and the associated technique factors for each examination.

The two barrier types considered in shielding an x-ray room are the primary and secondary protective barriers. The primary barrier is designed to attenuate radiation resulting from the primary x-ray beam. Primary barriers are generally installed on walls where vertical cassette holders are used in chest examinations or when the primary x-ray beam is directed at specific walls while performing cross-table examinations. The secondary barrier is designed to attenuate radiation resulting from leakage from the protective housing and radiation scattered from an irradiated object, usually the patient. Typically, the greater of the two secondary barrier thicknesses is selected as the value for the barrier, and one HVL of the lead or lead equivalent shielding is added to this value to provide added protection from stray radiation.

The dose rate in any unrestricted area cannot exceed 2 mrem in any 1 hour, and the total effective dose equivalent cannot exceed 100 mrem annually. This is only 20% of previous guidelines and has caused many physicists to recalculate and redesign protective barriers.

For the interested student, the entire shielding evaluation procedure is outlined in detail in NCRP Report No. 49, *Structural Shielding Design and Evaluation for Medical Use of X-Rays and Gamma Rays of Energies up to 10 MeV* (1976). Additional reading on this subject may be found in the 1989 text *Introduction to Health Physics,* by Herman Cember. The special insert also works one example for the interested student.

## Advanced Information:
## Sample Barrier Calculation: Shielding Evaluation of a Cardiac Cath Lab

### General Construction

*Floor:* Concrete slab on grade

*Ceiling:* Four-inch concrete slab. Second-floor interface. The primary beam will not be aimed in this direction.

*Walls:* The exterior wall, labeled F, is composed of 8 inches of poured reinforced concrete with a brick veneer. All interior walls are constructed with 4-inch metal studs covered on each side with 5/8-inch gypsum board. All walls will be considered secondary barriers with the exception of the control booth, which will be considered a primary barrier to provide added protection to the operator.

*Anticipated workload:* 1000 mA-min/wk at 125 kVp (approximately 24 patients/day)

*Beam orientation:* The primary beam is directed toward the floor in most procedures. On occasion, the imaging gantry may be turned approximately 35 to 45 degrees off the vertical axis, but not to the extent that any wall may be considered a primary barrier.

### Primary Barrier Calculation

$$K_{ux} = \frac{P(d_{pri})^2}{WUT}$$

## Sample Barrier Calculation: Shielding Evaluation of a Cardiac Cath Lab *(Continued)*

Where:

$P$ = weekly design exposure rate in roentgens

$d_{pri}$ = distance from the source of radiation to the person being protected

$W$ = anticipated workload in mA-min/wk

$U$ = use factor assigned for the wall being evaluated

$T$ = occupancy factor of the area being evaluated

### Wall A

$W$ = 1000 mA-min/wk

$P$ = 0.1 R for occupationally exposed personnel

$U = 1$

$T = 1$

$d_{pri}$ = 5.64 m

$K_{ux} = \dfrac{0.1(5.64)^2}{1000(1)(1)} = 0.0032$

The amount of lead shielding necessary to provide an adequate primary barrier is determined by interpreting the value $K_{ux}$ = 0.0032 on the graph depicted in Figure 1 of Appendix D to NCRP Report No. 49, page 91 (Figure 9–1). This value is approximately 1.2 mm of lead. There is a commercially available thickness of lead, 1.19 mm, which is inadequate. The next commercially available thickness is 1.5 mm. This shall be the required thickness:

### Leakage Barrier Calculation

$B_{ix}5 = \dfrac{P(d_{sec})2\ (600)I}{WT}$

Where:

$d_{sec}$ = distance from the source of radiation to the person being protected

$I$ = maximum continuous rated tube current

All other symbols have the same meaning as previously indicated.

### Wall A

$W$ = 1000 mA-min/wk

$P$ = 0.1 R for occupationally exposed personnel

$T = 1$

dsec = 5.64 m

$I$ = 4 mA

$B_{lx} = \dfrac{0.1(5.64)^2(600)5}{1000(1)} = 9.5429$

The amount of lead shielding necessary to provide an adequate barrier against leakage radiation is determined by interpreting the value $B_{lx}$ = 9.5429 on the graph depicted in Figure B-3 of NCRP Report No. 49, page 57. Since this value exceeds 1, there is no need for additional shielding against leakage radiation.

### Scatter Barrier Calculation

$K_{ux} = \dfrac{P(d_{sca})^2(d_{sec})2(400)}{aWTF}$

Where:

$d_{sca}$ = distance from the source of radiation to the person being protected

$a$ = ratio of scattered to incident exposure

$F$ = field area of the scatterer in cm$^2$

All other symbols have the same meaning as previously indicated.

Values for a, F, I, and $d_{sca}$ are taken from Table B-3, NCRP Report No. 49, page 61.

### Wall A

$W$ = 1000 mA-min/wk

$P$ = 0.1 R for occupationally exposed personnel

## Sample Barrier Calculation: Shielding Evaluation of a Cardiac Cath Lab *(Continued)*

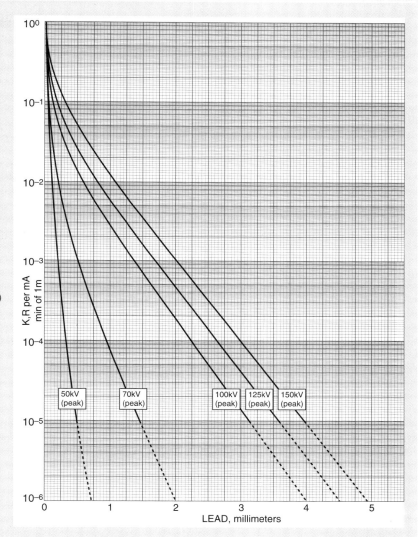

**Figure 9–1** Graph to determine lead shielding for a primary barrier. (Adapted with permission from NCRP Report No. 49.)

$$T = 1$$
$$d_{sca} = 0.45 \text{ m}$$
$$d_{sec} = 5.64 \text{ m}$$
$$I = 4 \text{ mA}$$
$$K_{ux} = \frac{0.1(0.45)^2(5.64)^2(400)}{0.0015(1000)(1)(400)} = 0.4294$$

The amount of lead shielding necessary to provide an adequate barrier against leakage radiation is determined by interpreting the value $K_{ux} = 0.4294$ on the graph depicted in Figure 1 of Appendix D to NCRP Report No. 49, page 91. This value is approximately 0.3 mm of lead. Since five-eighths-inch gypsum board provides

## Sample Barrier Calculation: Shielding Evaluation of a Cardiac Cath Lab *(Continued)*

lead equivalent shielding of approximately 0.15 mm of lead, the existing gypsum shall be adequate for the purposes intended.

Figure 9–2 is a diagram depicting the elements of shielding of a cardiac cath laboratory discussed here.

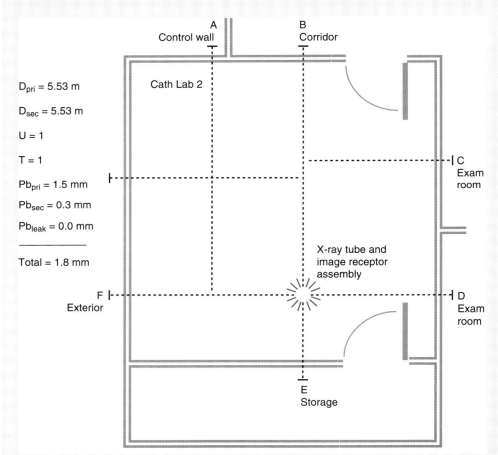

$D_{pri} = 5.53$ m

$D_{sec} = 5.53$ m

$U = 1$

$T = 1$

$Pb_{pri} = 1.5$ mm

$Pb_{sec} = 0.3$ mm

$Pb_{leak} = 0.0$ mm

___

Total = 1.8 mm

A  Control wall

B  Corridor

Cath Lab 2

C  Exam room

X-ray tube and image receptor assembly

F  Exterior

D  Exam room

E  Storage

**Figure 9–2** Shielding of a cardiac cath laboratory. All areas are considered to be occupationally exposed since access is controlled. The weekly design exposure is P = 0.1 R.

### Work Area Definitions

An unrestricted area is one where radiation levels are essentially the same as background radiation. These areas require no monitoring, posting, or control requirements. A restricted area limits access to protect individuals from undue risk to exposure to radiation or radioactive materials. There are three categories of restricted areas:

1. *Radiation area*—where the radiation level could result in an individual's receiving more than 5 mrem but less than 100 mrem in 1 hour. To determine these levels, measurements must be taken 30 cm from the source or from the surface where the radiation emanates.

   *Requirements:*
   a. Controlled access.
   b. A sign of purple, magenta, or black on a yellow background reading "Caution–Radiation Area" with the three-blade radiation symbol (Figure 9–3).

2. *High-radiation area*—where the radiation level could result in an individual receiving more than 100 mrem in 1 hour.

   *Requirements:* Entrances must have an access control feature such as door interlocks to prevent unauthorized entry and inadvertent radiation exposure.

3. *Very high-radiation area*—where the radiation could result in an individual receiving in excess of an absorbed dose of 500 cGy in 1 hour. These are not commonly found in diagnostic imaging departments.

## X-Ray Compliance Program

A typical x-ray compliance program inspects the x-ray equipment and reviews the records of facilities using x-ray equipment to determine compliance with federal, state, and local regulations governing the production and use of ionizing radiation. Most compliance programs will inspect each facility under their jurisdiction at least once every 2 years.

The primary method used to test x-ray equipment is known as the BRH Test Method. The FDA's Bureau of Radiological Health (BRH; now called the Center for Devices and Radiological Health [CDRH]) developed a testing method to determine whether manufacturers were in compliance with the standards specified in FDA regulations (20 CFR, Subchapter J).

This test method evaluates x-ray equipment for compliance with standards for beam quality, reproducibility, linearity, beam alignment, and collimation. These are typically part of a departmental quality assurance program. These tests

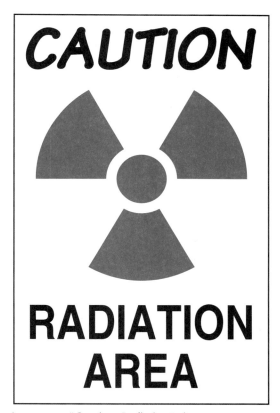

**Figure 9–3** "Caution: Radiation" sign.

are often conducted by a medical physicist trained in quality assurance methodology.

Records reviewed during inspections include radiation safety manuals, equipment registrations, tests, and surveys, personnel-monitoring program records, patient holding logs, and the posting of notices and instructions to workers.

## Personnel-Monitoring Program

The two most commonly used methods of personnel monitoring are the film badge and the thermoluminescent dosimeter (TLD), which are used to measure whole-body radiation exposure. These were discussed in earlier chapters.

Film was first used as a monitoring device by radiation workers, who carried small pieces of dental film in their pockets. Exposure was determined by the amount of fogging of the film, or simply the gross density on the film. This method was later refined through the development of film badges that allow a more accurate estimation of exposure.

The film badge consists of two pieces of photographic film wrapped in light, tight paper that is then inserted into a film badge holder. The film badge holder is usually a plastic casing that has a filter array designed to differentiate between the energies of the exposure received. As the film is exposed to radiation, the silver halide in the photographic emulsion darkens. If the film badge has been exposed to a wide range of energies, a filter pattern will be evident. The optical density of the exposure in each filter area is measured and compared to a known standard optical density to determine the exposure received. Film badges are adequate for measuring exposures from 10 to 1800 mR of radium gamma rays.

TLDs are crystals made of calcium fluoride with manganese as an impurity (or, more commonly, lithium fluoride) that emit light (thermoluminescence) when heated after being exposed to radiation. TLDs are commonly used as ring badges. The RSO for a facility will determine which monitors are most appropriate based on an assessment of the advantages and disadvantages of the monitor and the types of exposures that can be expected. An RSO also determines, based on probability of exposure and cost of the monitoring program, which individuals should be badged. Although in some cases it may seem best to badge all employees, even secretaries and patient transporters, the added cost and low risk of exposure (based on surveys of the areas using radiation-detection devices) may not indicate that badging is advisable.

In both clinical and private office x-ray facilities, the personnel-monitoring program is the front-line defense against potential overexposure to ionizing radiation. It is important that the employer and the employee understand that the personnel-monitoring program is in place to make each aware of the hazards of working with ionizing radiation. By observing trends in monthly exposure readings, the potential of a future overexposure can be prevented, thus reducing the possibility of future adverse conditions.

*Overexposure* is, of course, a relative term unless state or national guidelines have been exceeded. The nature of an overexposure should be defined in the facility's radiation safety program. The RSO will counsel the employee, and this counseling session is often documented in case further problems arise. The RSO is also responsible for setting guidelines for the institutional monitoring program (such as where to wear a film badge) and should be consulted if questions arise about the program.

A personnel-monitoring program is mandatory if any individual working with ionizing radiation receives or is likely to receive a whole-body dose in excess of 25 mR in any 1 week, can be expected to receive 10% of the maximum permissible dose (MPD), enters a high-radiation area, operates mobile x-ray equipment, operates photofluoroscopic equipment, or services an operable x-ray machine. It is important to understand that the exposure value of 25 mR in any 1 week is not meant to represent an exposure rate. This simply means any whole-body dose in any 7-day period.

## Maximum Permissible Dose/Dose Equivalent Limits

The maximum permissible dose (MPD) limit was the limit placed on all exposures resulting from internal and external sources of radiation. ICRP Publication 26 (1977) limits the annual occupational exposure to 50 mSv (5 rem) per year and the dose limit for members of the public to 10% of the occupational limit (500 mrem). Effective January 1, 1994, the NRC is setting new MPD limits based on NCRP Report No. 91, which limits the annual occupational exposure to 50 mSv (5 rem) per year and the dose limit for members of the public to 1 mSv (0.1 rem) per year.

The term *maximum permissible dose* should not be used any more, since it implies that there is an acceptable dose of radiation. The term *dose equivalent limits* is now preferred (see the text box for the calculation of effective dose equivalents). Of course, in clinical practice, many individuals will continue to use the term *MPD*. The ARRT uses the terminology *dose equivalent limits* (formerly MPD) on the radiography registry.

Another new area in regulations is occupational dose limits for minors (workers under the age of 18). Their limit is 10% of the annual dose limits specified for adults.

**Table 9–3** Summary of Recommendations[a] from NCRP Report No. 116: *Limitation of Exposure to Ionizing Radiation*

|  | SI Units | British Units |
|---|---|---|
| A. Occupational exposures[b] | | |
|   1. Effective dose limits | | |
|     a. Annual | 50 mSv | 5 rem |
|     b. Cumulative | 10 mSv × age | 1 rem × age |
|   2. Equivalent dose annual limits for tissues and organs | | |
|     a. Lens of eye | 150 mSv | 15 rem |
|     b. Skin, hands and feet | 500 mSv | 50 rem |
| B. Guidance for emergency occupational exposure[b] | Section 14, NCRP Report No. 116 | |
| C. Public exposures (annual) | | |
|   1. Effective dose limit, continuous or frequent exposure[b] | 1 mSv | 100 mrem |
|   2. Effective dose limit, infrequent exposure[b] | 5 mSv | 500 mrem |
|   3. Equivalent dose limits for tissues and organs[b] | | |
|     a. Lens of eye | 15 mSv | 1500 mrem |
|     b. Skin, hands and feet | 50 mSv | 5 rem |
|   4. Remedial action for natural sources: | | |
|     a. Effective dose (excluding radon) | > 5 mSv | >500 mrem |
|     b. Exposure to radon decay products | $> 7 \times 10^{-3}$ Jh m$^{-3}$ | $> 7 \times 10^{-3}$ Jh m$^{-3}$ |
| D. Education and training exposures (annual)[b] | | |
|   1. Effective dose limit | 1 mSv | 100 mrem |
|   2. Equivalent dose limit for tissues and organs | | |
|     a. Lens of eye | 15 mSv | 1500 mrem |
|     b. Skin, hands and feet | 50 mSv | 5 rem |
| E. Embryo–fetus exposures[b] (monthly) | | |
|   1. Equivalent dose limit | 0.5 mSv | 50 mrem |
| F. Negligible individual dose (annual)[b] | 0.01 mSv | 1 mrem |

[a]Excluding medical exposures.

[b]Sum of external and internal exposures but excluding doses from natural sources.

From National Council on Radiation Protection and Measurements (NCRP) Report No. 116: *Limitation of Exposure to Ionizing Radiation*, Bethesda, MD, 1993.

The summarized recommendations of NCRP Report No. 91 can be found in Table 9–3.

## Calculating Dose Equivalent Limits

Although radiation workers are allowed 5 rem (50 mSv) per year (the *prospective* limit for whole-body exposure), they cannot simply accumulate this amount each year for an indefinite period. Prior to the release of NCRP Report No. 91, this was allowed through the formula:

$$H = 5 \times (N - 18) \text{ rem}$$

where H = dose equivalent limit (also called the rem bank or *retrospective* limit for cumulative whole-body exposure) and N = age in years. Thus, a 35-year-old worker, assuming no prior exposure, could have 80 rem in the rem bank, and could exceed the 5 rem/yr

limit (by small amounts of 10 to 15 rem) until that "bank account" was depleted. The new recommendations of NCRP Report No. 91 indicate that the rem bank cannot exceed the individual's age in rem. Our example worker's rem bank is now 35 rem. In SI units, the rem bank is calculated by multiplying the age times 10 mSv. A 35-year-old worker's limit is 350 mSv. The ARRT now considers the formula 5(N − 18) obsolete.

Initial cumulative whole-body exposures are higher than those previously used (from 10 to 20 rem for our 20-year-old worker) for younger workers but are lower over the life span (a 60-year-old radiation worker's cumulative whole-body exposure would have been 210 rem; now it is 60 rem).

Also, special exposures are now treated under the concepts of planned special exposures

---

**EXAMPLE 1**

Based on ICRP Publication No. 26 (the "old" standard), a 20-year-old radiation worker's cumulative whole-body exposure is:

$$H = 5 (20 - 18)$$

$$H = 5 \times 2$$

$$H = 10 \text{ rem}$$

---

**EXAMPLE 2**

Based on NCRP Report No. 91 (the "new" standard), the same radiation worker's cumulative whole-body exposure is:

$$H = \text{age in rem}$$

$$H = 20$$

*or*

$$H = N \times 10 \text{ mSv}$$

$$H = 20 \times 10 \text{ mSv}$$

$$H = 200 \text{ mSv}$$

---

(PSEs) and emergency situations. PSEs are for adult workers who are likely to receive more than the occupational limits when alternatives to avoid high exposures are unavailable or impractical. These must be planned in advance and are not likely to occur in diagnostic imaging or therapeutic uses of radiation. Doses of greater than 10 rem (single dose) are justified only in lifesaving situations.

### Negligible Individual Risk Level

NCRP Report No. 91 defines the negligible individual risk level (NIRL) as "a level of average annual excess risk of fatal health effects attributable to irradiation, below which further effort to reduce radiation exposure to the individual is unwarranted." It considers the risks as *trivial* in comparison with the risk of fatality associated with normal activities (recall the risk comparisons made in Chapter 1) and believes that the risk can thus be dismissed from consideration.

The NIRL is an outgrowth of the legal concept *de minimis non curat lex,* which means "the law is not concerned with trifles." If a practice results in a dose or risk that is so low that trying to regulate it would be a waste of resources best directed elsewhere, it is not the concern of regulatory agencies.

The NIRL can be seen as a type of threshold (although it does not strictly meet the criteria for a threshold given in previous chapters) and

---

## Effective Dose Equivalent and Dose Equivalent

*1. Effective dose equivalent*

Since whole-body doses are rarely uniform in occupational exposure, a method is needed to weigh partial-body doses into effective dose limits (formerly called *maximum permissible doses*). The method used by the NCRP in its Report No. 91 is the effective dose equivalent. The effective dose equivalent is the sum of the products of the dose equivalent to the organ or tissue and

the weighting factor applicable to each of the body organs or tissues that are irradiated. The effective dose equivalent equation is given as:

$$H_E = \Sigma \, W_T \, H_T$$

Essentially, this equation states that the probability of a stochastic effect, $H_E$, in any tissue is proportional to the dose equivalent, $H_T$, to that tissue. $H_T$ is the mean dose equiv-

## Effective Dose Equivalent and Dose Equivalent *(Continued)*

alent received by the organ or tissue, and $W_T$ is the weighting factor of tissue T. The values of $W_T$ for various types of organs and tissues are given in the table below. The weighting factor represents the proportionate risk of tissue or organ when the whole body is irradiated uniformly, and the values are derived from risk coefficients (i.e. risk per unit dose equivalent). Since the sensitivities of various tissues to exposure from ionizing radiation differ, the probability of a stochastic effect due to an exposure is also different for various tissues. Please remember that we are concerned primarily with the stochastic or long-term effects from low doses of radiation in occupational exposure.

### Organ Dose Weighting Factor $W_T$*

| Organ or Tissue (T) | $W_T$ |
| --- | --- |
| Gonads | 0.25 |
| Breast | 0.15 |
| Red bone marrow | 0.12 |
| Lung | 0.12 |
| Thyroid | 0.03 |
| Bone surface | 0.03 |
| Remainder† | 0.30 |
| Whole Body‡ | 1.00 |

*The $W_T$ values are taken from ICRP Report No. 26: Recommendations of the International Commission on Radiological Protection. New York: Pergamon Press, 1977.

†*0.30 results from 0.06 for each of five "remainder" organs (excluding the skin and the lens of the eye) that receive the highest dose.

‡For the purpose of weighting the external whole-body dose (for adding it to the internal dose), a single weighting factor, $W_T$ = 1.00, has been specified. The use of other weighting factors for external exposure will be approved on a case-by-case basis until such time as specific guidance is issued.

### EXAMPLE

The data just given can be used as follows to calculate effective dose in the example following.

An individual receives the following doses:

100 cGy to the lung
50 cGy to the thyroid
100 cGy to the bone marrow

Using the effective dose equation, one can obtain:

$$(100 \times 0.12) + (50 \times 0.03) + (100 \times 0.12) = 12 + 1.5 + 12 = 25.5 \text{ cGy}$$

The effective dose equivalent is 25.5 cGy, which indicates that the combined doses received will have the same potential effect to the individual as if he or she had received 25.5 cGy of whole-body exposure.

*2. Dose equivalent*

The dose equivalent is defined as the dose, D, times a quality factor, Q. The quality factor takes into account the biologic effectiveness of the radiation type or simply represents the relative degree of biologic damage each type of radiation causes. Q has a value of unity (1.0) for x- and gamma rays (photons) and electrons and has higher values for other types of radiation such as neutrons, protons, and alpha particles. The old unit for equivalent dose is the rem, which in the case of x-rays is equivalent to rad or cGy. In the SI system if the dose is given in grays (Gy), then the unit of equivalent dose is sieverts (Sv), which equal 100 rem. It is defined as:

Equivalent dose (H) = Dose $\cdot$ Q

is used as a lower limit for ALARA. That is, below that level, it is not useful to try to limit exposure anymore. The exposure level currently considered appropriate for the NIRL is 1 mrem. Thus, activities that result in an exposure of 1 mrem do not warrant further efforts to reduce dose. This 1 mrem is not a yearly exposure to an individual but is exposure from an activity or a source of radiation.

## Internal and External Exposure

In the clinical environment it is possible that occupationally exposed personnel may be exposed to more than one source of ionizing radiation. Under new requirements specified in 10 CFR 20, the RSO is required to monitor both internal and external occupational exposures to ionizing radiation and to report such exposures to the individual exposed. If internal exposure exceeds 10% of the applicable limit, both internal and external exposure must be considered in determining an employee's annual dose limit. X-ray departments (radiation therapy and diagnostic radiology) will typically not have to be concerned with internal exposure; but other departments may, such as nuclear medicine.

## Exposure Control

Occupational exposure is defined as the exposure of an individual to ionizing radiation in a restricted area in the course of employment in which the individual's duties involve exposure to ionizing radiation, provided that the term *occupational dose* does not include any exposure of an individual to radiation for the purposes of medical diagnosis or medical therapy.

An individual's occupational exposure is relatively easy to control if it is remembered that the three most effective means of controlling exposure to ionizing radiation are time, distance, and shielding. Individuals working in a radiology department should always be aware of their position relative to the primary x-ray beam and the amount of time spent working around the radiation beam.

In addition to time, distance, and shielding, the individual working in a radiology department should be aware of the term *as low as reasonably achievable (ALARA)*, described earlier in this chapter. ALARA means making every rea-

sonable effort to maintain exposure to radiation as far below the dose limit as is practical and consistent with the purposes intended.

## The Control Booth

Adequate shielding design and operational procedures will aid the technologist in maintaining ALARA. The shielding in and design of the control booth are important in providing protection to the technologist and staff. The minimum design requirements for an x-ray control booth are as follows:

1. The floor area of the booth shall not have less than 7.5 square feet of unobstructed floor space with no dimension less than 2 feet. This area shall be free of any encumbrance or obstruction.
2. The wall shall be at least 7 feet high and shall be permanently fixed to the floor or other structure as necessary.
3. If a door or movable panel is used as an integral part of the control booth, it shall be interlocked with the control panel such that an x-ray cannot be initiated with the door open.
4. The switch shall be fixed within the booth at a position at least 30 inches from any open edge of the booth wall closest to the examining table and shall allow the operator to use most of the viewing window.
5. The viewing method may be a window, a mirror, or an electronic device. Regardless of the viewing method, the operator must have full view of any occupant of the room and view of any entry into the room. If any entrance cannot be seen by the operator, that entrance shall be equipped with an interlock device that prevents the operation of the x-ray equipment when the entrance is open. If the viewing method is a window, the window shall have a viewing area of at least 1 square foot and be positioned so that some portion of the window is at least 5 feet above the floor; the distance between the opening edge of the control booth and the edge of the window shall not be less than 18 inches, and the glass in the window shall have the same lead equivalency as the shielding required for the control booth wall.

In most cases, an x-ray room will be arranged such that the operator will be in a shielded position while taking x-rays. This shielded position is generally in the control booth or behind a movable shield. On rare occasions, it might be necessary to assist the patient in maintaining the proper position or to hold the film during a radiographic procedure. It is on these occasions that the x-ray technologist, acting as a human holder, receives the highest exposure as a result of the proximity of the human holder to the primary beam and the soft scatter off the patient.

If possible, all other methods of obtaining proper positioning should be exhausted before assisting the patient, assuming the medical needs of the patient are not critical. If there is no other alternative, the individual assisting the patient is required to wear proper protective clothing. In most states, the proper clothing consists of a leaded apron or whole-body protective barrier of not less than 0.25 mm of lead equivalent shielding and if exposed to the primary beam, not less than 0.5 mm of lead equivalent shielding.

## Other Occupational Areas

There are a variety of areas in which the medical physicist and RSO must constantly work to minimize occupational exposure. These are angiography, cardiac catheterization, and C-arm fluoroscopy. Although technologists and radiologists are educated in radiation safety and thus know how to limit their exposure, a variety of other individuals such as cardiologists and nurses who also work in these areas must be educated to minimize their exposures. For example, Connett (1987) found that nurses had over 10 times the eye dose of radiographers in cardiac catheterization. Cardiologists received over 3 times the eye dose of radiologists in the same setting. It is the radiographer's responsibility to reinforce instructions given by the RSO to nurses and other health professionals, and always to function as an educator to reduce exposure to patients and other health workers.

## Patient Exposure

The relationship between exposure and technique factors can be best seen by understanding the method of x-ray production described in earlier chapters.

Most states do not limit the exposure received by a patient during a diagnostic radiographic procedure, but the operator should be aware that it is best to use technique factors that will produce the desired diagnostic quality while keeping the patient's exposure ALARA. Proper selection of techniques also reduces the number of retakes necessary as a result of underexposing or overexposing the film. The proper selection of the technique may be achieved by utilizing manual technique charts or by selecting the proper tube voltage (kVp) and current (mA) while using the phototimer.

In the case of manual techniques, a chart of applicable technique factors for all commonly performed procedures with a specific x-ray machine is required by most state and local regulatory agencies. This chart should show the patient's anatomic size versus the technique factor to be used, the type and size of film or film/screen combination to be used, the type and focal distance of the grid to be used, if any, the SID, and the type and location of gonadal shielding to be used. With experience and careful attention to the patient's anatomic size, this can prove to be a most effective method of determining the correct technique.

Most modern x-ray equipment uses a phototiming system (automatic exposure controls) that measures the amount of radiation exiting the patient to determine whether adequate exposure is present to produce a film of diagnostic quality. The use of phototiming can decrease the amount of exposure a patient receives because the number of retakes due to poor technique selection have been reduced. However, phototimers have been known to fail, and there is still the possibility that the operator will select an inadequate kVp or mA relative to the patient's anatomic size. In such cases, the technique chart can prove to be a valuable backup. Also, Smith and colleagues (1989) and Plaut (1993) indicate that phototimers are valuable primarily for less-experienced radiographers. No difference in exposure is noted with experienced radiographers using phototimers.

## ROLE OF THE RADIOLOGIC TECHNOLOGIST IN MEETING REGULATORY REQUIREMENTS

### Administrative and Operational Controls

Each facility is responsible for the development of administrative and operational controls to provide for the protection of both the occupationally exposed personnel and members of the public. This may be accomplished by putting policies and procedures in a written radiation safety manual. The responsibility of an employee working with ionizing radiation is to be familiar with the provisions of any regulatory requirements and the administrative and operating procedures that apply to the work being performed. The observance of these responsibilities will ensure the protection of the individual, co-workers, and patients.

One example is overexposure of patients due to machine malfunction. The machine may continue exposing after an exposure (the mA meter should always be checked to be sure that exposure has terminated), or a fluoroscopic switch might become caught under the wheel of a gurney used to transport the patient. A variety of information must be recorded if such an incident occurs, including the patient's name, build, and position during the exposure; personnel in the room; and whether the machine was set manually or was on automatic factors.

### Protective Aprons, Gloves, and Gonadal Shielding

A question that arises often is, "When should protective aprons, gloves, and gonadal shielding be used while performing a radiographic procedure?" This question is answered in most states by a regulatory requirement generally adopted from the CRCPD *Suggested State Regulations:*

> Except for patients who cannot be moved out of the room, only the staff and ancillary personnel required for the medical procedure or training shall be in the room during the radiographic exposure. Other than the patient being examined:
>
> (a) All individuals shall be positioned such that no part of the body will be struck by the useful beam unless protected by 0.5 millimeters lead equivalent.
>
> (b) Staff and ancillary personnel shall be protected from the direct scatter radiation by protective aprons or whole body protective barriers of not less than 0.25 millimeters lead equivalent.
>
> (c) Patients who cannot be removed from the room shall be protected from direct scatter radiation by whole body protective barriers of 0.25 millimeters equivalent or shall be positioned so that the nearest portion of the body is at least 2 meters from both the tube head and the nearest edge of the image receptor.

As to gonadal shielding, a shield of not less than 0.25 mm of lead equivalent is required to be used on all patients who have not passed the reproductive age, except for cases in which the gonads are of diagnostic interest or the shield would interfere with the diagnostic procedure.

### Holding Patients or Film

When a patient or film must be provided with auxiliary support during a procedure, the operator should use the following guidelines to determine the best method of support to achieve the desired diagnostic quality.

The primary choice for auxiliary support should always be a mechanical holding device if the technique factors allow it. Such devices can include the use of Pigg-o-stats and swaddling for infants and small children, sandbags or straps to isolate and steady the area of interest, support sponges and pillows to position the patient properly, and portable film stands. In the event that none of these devices provides adequate support for the patient or film, a human holder is to be considered the last choice.

If it is necessary for the patient or film to be held by a human holder, (1) written safety procedures are required to determine the method of selecting the human holder, (2) the human holder is required to wear the appropriate leaded apron and gloves as required by the state or local regulatory agency, (3) no one individual shall be used routinely as a human holder, and (4) in any case in which the patient is required to hold the film, except during intraoral examinations, any portion of the body other than the area of clinical interest struck by the primary beam must be covered by not less than 0.5 mm of lead equivalent material.

## X-Ray Log

Most facilities keep a record of procedures performed daily in a logbook, which lists the patient's name, the type of examination, the technique factors, the number of films taken, the initials of the technologist performing the procedure, and the date the procedure was performed. In addition to this information, if it is necessary to use a human holder during the procedure, the name of the human holder should also be noted, as well as the number of exposures for which the human holder was used.

A logbook helps track the frequency of examinations requiring a human holder and reduces the possibility of one individual's being used on a regular basis to be the human holder. If there are a great number of examinations requiring assistance, there will be an associated increase in the risk involved. Along with the increased risks come increased liability. If proper records are maintained, both the risk and the liability are reduced. Another use for the log is to follow up on pregnant patients who were exposed to radiation before their pregnancy status was known. In the future, such logs may form evidence in radiation protection lawsuits. It can reasonably be assumed that as patients become more assertive about their quality of care, they will begin to question their radiation exposure as well.

In addition to the department log, another publication that can have a great effect on dose reduction is an up-to-date departmental procedure manual. Ideally, this manual should be revised on a regular basis, should reflect current practice in radiology, and should be developed through input from all concerned parties. One example of how an up-to-date manual can minimize patient exposure can be seen in the following scenario. A new radiographer consults the manual and finds that four overhead films are to be taken following an upper GI. However, the department routine has changed to three views, two that are the same as the old routine and one new view. The patient will receive two additional films, which will approximately double the dose. This is not an unusual experience and relates to proper inservice education of new staff as well as to keeping publications current.

## The Pregnant Patient

The simplest method of determining whether a patient might be pregnant is to ask the time since the last menstrual period. All female patients who have not passed the reproductive years can be asked this question prior to any examination in which the abdomen is exposed to ionizing radiation. However, this question can be seen as embarrassing, especially if the question is asked of a young female patient by a male technologist. It is also not foolproof; however, there are no foolproof methods of determining the pregnancy status of a patient.

Other methods of avoiding exposure to the fetus include the 10-day rule, pregnancy testing, and signs that indicate that patients should inform technologists if they might be pregnant. Plaut (1993), based on ICRP recommendations, suggests an extension of the 10-day rule called the *28-day rule*. This rule holds that exposure can be made in the 28-day period following menstruation rather than in 10 days. Under the all-or-none effect, this rule certainly makes sense (review Chapter 8 for the all-or-none effect).

Direct irradiation of the abdomen (elective procedures) of the pregnant patient should be avoided during the first and second trimesters. If possible, the examination should be delayed until after delivery or at least the third trimester. This is often a multifaceted decision. It is usually assumed that the patient's primary physician, in cases of known pregnancy, has weighed a risk-versus-benefit decision and has concluded that the examination is necessary. This may not always be an accurate assumption. In some cases, the primary physician may assume that the radiologist will make this decision.

The physicist may be responsible for calculating the dose received by a pregnant patient. The radiographer will often be responsible for providing information about the exposure, such as technical factors used, positions, and so on. A sample calculation is given in the text box on page 190.

## The Pregnant Employee

The dose to an embryo or fetus of a pregnant employee due to occupational exposure is limited to 0.5 rem for the duration of the pregnancy. This dose is determined to be the sum of the deep-dose equivalent of the declared pregnant woman and the dose to the embryo or fetus from radionuclides in the embryo or fetus and in the declared pregnant woman. If the dose to the embryo or fetus is found to have exceeded 0.5 rem or is within 0.05 rem of this dose by the time the woman declares the pregnancy to the employer, the employer is deemed to be in compliance with the 0.5-rem limit if the additional dose to the embryo or fetus does not exceed 0.05 rem for the duration of the pregnancy. A total of 500 mrem to the mother is equivalent to less than 10 mrem to the embryo or fetus.

Regulations use the term *declared pregnant woman*. This term implies that a pregnant worker must advise her employer *voluntarily* and *in writing* of her pregnancy and estimated date of conception. Formal, voluntary notification is the only means by which the employer can ensure that dose to the fetus can be limited during the pregnancy.

The employer is required to make an effort to avoid substantial variation above a uniform monthly exposure rate to a declared pregnant woman to ensure that the exposure to the embryo or fetus does not exceed the limits specified. This does not mean that the declared pregnant woman should be removed from duty. It means that upon examination of the employee's previous exposure history, an evaluation of the work environment should be performed to determine the potential of receiving exposures that would exceed the 0.5-rem limit, and then the employee's work habits should be adjusted to reduce risks.

Diagnostic exposures of pregnant workers are not included in these limits. Thus, each worker must personally decide if she needs an examination in consultation with her physician.

## Posting of Notices to Employees

In states that regulate the production and use of ionizing radiation, the employer is required

---

## Calculating Dose to the Fetus

There are a variety of procedures for calculating fetal dose. The following is based on one method described by Hendee and Ritenour (1993).

A patient receives 4 minutes of fluoroscopy at 100 kVp and 2 mA, and three spot films at 80 kVp and 30 mAs over an 18-cm-thick abdomen. The tube-to-tabletop distance was 0.5 m. Later, it is determined that the patient was pregnant during the examination.

A rule of thumb holds that exposure will not exceed 1 R/mA-min at 1 m. At 0.5 m, according to the inverse square law, exposure will be 4 R/mA-min (the inverse square law is covered in greater depth in Chapter 10). Skin dose to the patient during fluoroscopy is determined as follows:

$$\text{Exposure} = 4 \ (\text{R}/(\text{mA-min})) \times (2 \ \text{mA}) \times (4 \ \text{min}) = 32 \ \text{R}$$

Spot-film skin exposure will be determined as follows:

$$\text{Exposure} = (4 \ \text{R}/\text{mA-min}) \times \left[ \frac{(30 \ \text{mAs/film})(3 \ \text{films})}{60 \ \text{sec/min}} \right] = 6 \ \text{R}$$

Total skin exposure is 32 + 6, or 38 R. The most conservative assumption (which will give the *highest* estimate) is that beam transmission through the abdomen is 0.5% of incident exposure. It is assumed that the fetus sits midpoint in the abdomen. Transmitted fetal dose will be the square root of total transmitted exposure (the square root of 0.5% = 57%). The maximum exposure to the fetus will be:

$$\text{Exposure} = (38 \ \text{R})(0.07) = 2.66 \ \text{R}$$

If overhead films were taken, a similar procedure would be used to calculate exposure from overhead films. This example shows the need to keep accurate exposure records on all patients in case questions arise in the future.

to post a copy of documents titled "Notice to Employees." These documents provide the employee with information concerning the agency responsible for enforcing regulations, explain the employer's reponsibility to apply these regulations to work involving sources of ionizing radiation, and explain the employee's responsibility to become familiar with the regulations and any operating procedures developed by the employer. A sample notice is included in Figure 9–4.

## Working with the Health Physicist, Medical Physicist, or Radiation Safety Officer

Radiologic technologists should be familiar with the individual at their facility who is responsible for developing and implementing radiation protection practices. Since both radiologic technologists and RSOs are professionals with an interest in the same goal (quality patient care coupled with radiation protection), they should seek means to work as partners in patient care. Technologists should feel free to make sugges-

---

## Review of Radiation Quantities and Units

**Exposure:** This represents the amount of ionization or charge (either positive or negative) produced in a confined mass of air. Its unit is the roentgen (R). The new SI unit is coulomb per kilogram (C/kg), where

$$1 \text{ roentgen} = 1 \text{ R} = 2.58 \ 10^{-4}$$
coulomb/(kg of dry air)

**Absorbed dose:** This is defined as the energy of x- or gamma-ray radiation absorbed per unit mass. This quantity is usually measured in water to simulate human soft tissue. It basically represents the energy deposited in water or tissue. The old unit for absorbed radiation is the rad and the new unit is the gray (Gy), which is equivalent to 100 rad or 100 cGy. Therefore, 1 cGy is equal to 1 rad.

**Equivalent dose:** This is defined as the dose, D, times a quality factor, Q. The quality factor takes into account the biologic effectiveness of the radiation type. The Q has a value of unity (1.0) for x- and gamma rays (photons) and also electrons. The old unit for equivalent dose is the rem, which in the case of x-rays is equivalent to rad or centigray (cGy). In the SI system if the dose is given in grays (Gy), then the unit of effective dose equivalent is sieverts (Sv), which is equal to 100 rem.

Equivalent dose (H) = Dose × Q

**Effective equivalent dose:** In most cases the whole body will not be radiated uniformly. For example, the dose to the lungs as a result of inhalation of radon gas, which emits alpha particles, is much greater than the dose to the rest of the body from natural background radiation. Another concern may raise the question, "How much of this dose should be accounted in annual whole body dose?" To take account of this non-uniformity, the effective equivalent dose concept is introduced. Therefore, the effective dose equivalent is the amount of radiation dose that would result in the same radiation risk if the same dose is given to the whole body.

*Conversion factors:*
1 rad ≈ 1 rem (H = D × Q)
1 Roentgen = 1 R ≈ 1 rad (1 rad is the absorbed dose from an exposure of 1 R)
1 cGy = 1 rad
1 Gy = 100 cGy = 100 rad
1 Sv = 100 rem
1 Sv = 1000 mSv
1 rem = 10 mSv
1 mSv = 0.1 rem
1 mSv = 100 mrem
1 mSv = 1000 mSv
1 mSv = (1/1000) mSv

ALABAMA DEPARTMENT OF PUBLIC HEALTH

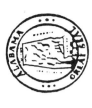

# NOTICE TO EMPLOYEES

## STANDARDS FOR PROTECTION AGAINST RADIATION

IN ALABAMA REGULATIONS FOR CONTROL OF RADIATION, THE ALABAMA DEPARTMENT OF PUBLIC HEALTH HAS ESTABLISHED STANDARDS FOR YOUR PROTECTION AGAINST RADIATION HAZARDS

### Your Employer's Responsibility

Your employer is required to—

1. Apply these regulations to work involving sources of radiation;
2. Post or otherwise make available to you a copy of the Alabama Department of Public Health regulations, licenses, and operating procedures which apply to work you are engaged in and explain their provisions to you; and
3. Post any Notice of Violation involving radiological working conditions.

### Your Responsibility as a Worker

You should familiarize yourself with those provisions of the Alabama Department of Public Health regulations and the operating procedures which apply to the work you are engaged in. You should observe their provisions for your own protection and protection of your co-workers.

### What is Covered by These Regulations

1. Limits on exposure to radiation and radioactive material in restricted and unrestricted areas.
2. Measures to be taken after accidental exposure.
3. Personnel monitoring surveys and equipment.
4. Caution signs, labels, and safety interlock equipment.
5. Exposure records and reports.
6. Options for workers regarding Alabama Department of Public Health inspections.
7. Related matters.

### Reports on Your Radiation Exposure History

1. The Alabama Department of Public Health regulations require that your employer give you a written report if you receive an exposure in excess of any applicable limit as set forth in the regulations

or in the license. The basic limits for exposure to employees are set forth in Sections 6-3.101, 6-3.103, and 6-3.104 of the regulations. These sections specify limits on exposure to radiation and exposure to concentrations of radioactive material in air and water.

2. If you work where personnel monitoring is required and if you request information on your radiation exposures,

(a) Your employer must give you a written report, upon termination of your employment, of your radiation exposures, and

(b) Your employer must advise you annually of your exposure to radiation.

### Inspections

All licensed or registered activities are subject to inspection by representatives of the Alabama Department of Public Health. In addition, any worker or representative of workers who believes that there is a violation of Act No. 582, Regular Session, 1963, the regulations issued thereunder, or the terms of the employer's license or registration with regard to radiological working conditions in which the worker is engaged, may request an inspection by sending a notice of alleged violation to the address given below. The request must set forth the specific grounds for the notice and must be signed by the worker or by the representative of the workers. During inspections, agency inspectors may confer privately with workers, and any worker may bring to the attention of the inspectors any past or present condition which he or she believes contributed to or caused any violation as described above.

### Inquiries

Inquiries dealing with the matters outlined above can be sent to the Alabama Department of Public Health, Environmental Health Administration, State Office Building, Montgomery, Alabama 36130. Telephone—(205)832-5992.

## POSTING REQUIREMENTS

COPIES OF THIS NOTICE MUST BE POSTED IN A SUFFICIENT NUMBER OF PLACES IN EVERY ESTABLISHMENT WHERE EMPLOYEES ARE EMPLOYED IN ACTIVITIES LICENSED OR REGISTERED, PURSUANT TO PARTS 6-2, 6-5, OR 6-8, BY THE ALABAMA DEPARTMENT OF PUBLIC HEALTH, TO PERMIT EMPLOYEES WORKING IN OR FREQUENTING ANY PORTION OF A RESTRICTED AREA TO OBSERVE A COPY ON THE WAY TO OR FROM THEIR PLACE OF EMPLOYMENT.

Prepared by Division of Primary Prevention for Division of Radiological Health

**Figure 9–4** Sample notice to employees.

## Basic Principles of Radiation Protection

The three basics principles of radiation protection are time, distance, and shielding

*Time:* decreasing exposure time will decreases the amount of radiation to the personnel.

*Distance:* the amount of radiation level decreases by the square of the distance from the radiation source.

*Shielding:* introducing shielding between personnel being exposed and the source will reduce the radiation levels. The fluoroscopy aprons provide safe protection against radiation from CT scanners if necessary.

Limits outside CT room: the radiation dose limit in public areas (e.g. an adjacent secretary's office), the continuous dose limit to the public, is set at 100 mrem/year or 2 mrem/week.

## ALARA

The acronym ALARA stands for "as low as reasonably achievable." The basic principle behind ALARA is that personnel working with or around radiation-producing sources should try to keep their exposure to radiation as low as reasonably possible while performing their tasks. In performing these tasks it is assumed and understood that the radiation workers will receive some radiation. To maintain minimum (low) levels of exposure of the personnel, proper techniques should be employed. The implementation of the ALARA principle is the responsibility of the employer, but the responsibility for ALARA practices falls on both the radiation workers and the employer. The maximum permissible dose a radiation worker is allowed to receive is 5 rem per year (5000 mrem per year or 1250 mrem per quarter). In establishing an ALARA program the exposure level is set at lower value, normally 1/10 of the maximum permissible dose, allowing 125 mrem in a calendar quarter. The exposure level above 125 mrem triggers an investigation to study the situation and see if it is possible to reduce the radiation exposure received by the personnel. (It is important to note that the factor 1/10 is an arbitrary factor that may differ from program to program and is not an NRCP recommendation.)

tions to the RSO in matters of radiation safety, and RSOs should consult with staff technologists on means of reducing exposure. A technologist with an interest in career advancement in the areas of health physics or quality assurance should consider volunteering for service on the institutional radiation safety committee. Technologists have worked with health/medical physicists in developing articles for publication in technologist journals such as *Radiologic Technology*. This helps other technologists implement safer practices at their own institutions.

### SUMMARY

The role of the individual assigned as a physicist or RSO to radiology facilities is to ensure that facilities comply with regulations and recommendations regarding the use of ionizing radiation. These regulations and recommendations are based on the feeling that all exposures must be kept as low as reasonably achievable, the ALARA concept.

A variety of organizations make reports and recommendations for the use of ionizing radiation. These include the International Commission on Radiological Units and Measurements (ICRU), International Commission on Radiological Protection (ICRP), National Council on Radiation Protection and Measurement (NCRP), International Atomic Energy Agency (IAEA), International Labour Organization (ILO), U.N. Scientific Commission on Effects of Atomic Radiation (UNSCEAR), Conference of Radiation Control Program Directors (CRCPD), and National Research Council Committee on the Biological Effects of Ionizing Radiation (BEIR). The major players in this arena are the ICRP, NCRP, CRCPD, and BEIR.

Regulatory agencies responsible for protecting the public and occupationally exposed personnel from unnecessary exposure to ionizing radiation include the U.S. Nuclear Regulatory Commission (NRC), the U.S. Environmental Protection Agency (EPA), the U.S. Food and Drug Administration (FDA), and the U.S. Occupational Safety and Health Administration (OSHA), as well as and state and local governments.

Typical duties of the physicist or RSO include administration of a radiation safety program, performing radiation-shielding design, determining compliance with work area definitions, and administering an x-ray compliance program and personnel-monitoring program to include compliance with maximum permissible doses and dose equivalent limits.

The radiologic/diagnostic technologist also has a role in meeting regulatory requirements, including the following:

a. complying with administrative operations and controls;
b. wearing protective aprons and gloves, and providing gonadal shielding to patients;
c. knowing in what situations to hold patients or films;
d. proper use of the x-ray log;
e. knowing how to work with the pregnant patient and potentially pregnant patient; and

f. knowing departmental guidelines for the pregnant employee.

The technologist should also work as a professional with the RSO in setting departmental guidelines.

## Questions

1. Which of the following organizations provide reports and recommendations?

   I. UNSCEAR
  II. ICRP
 III. NRC

a. I and II only      b. I and III only
c. II and III only     d. I, II, and III

2. The organization that regulates the design and manufacture of x-ray equipment is:

a. ICRP.          b. NRC.
c. FDA.           d. OSHA.

3. The minimum field size at 100 cm must not be less than or equal to:

a. 131 cm.       b. 232 cm.
c. 535 cm.       d. 10,310 cm.

4. Exposure from a fluoroscopic unit that is not directed to the image receptor must be less than _____ mR/hr at 10 cm.

a. 1             b. 2
c. 5             d. 10

5. In *no* case may a mobile C-arm be operated at less than _____ cm source-to-skin distance.

a. 10          b. 20
c. 30          d. 40

6. An area where the radiation level could reach 60 mrem/hr would be classified as a:

a. radiation area.
b. high-radiation area.
c. very high-radiation area.
d. dangerous radiation area.

7. What term is preferred over MPD (maximum permissible dose)?

a. maximum limited dose
b. maximum dose limits

c. dose equivalent limits

d. minimum dose

8. A 30-year-old radiation worker would be allowed, under newer standards (NCRP Report No. 91), _____ rem whole-body cumulative exposure.

   a. 5                   b. 10
   c. 20                  d. 30

9. If holding a patient, any area of the body struck by the beam must be covered with _____ mm of lead equivalent.

   a. 0.25                b. 0.5
   c. 2.5                 d. 5.0

10. A total of 500 mrem to the mother (occupational exposure) would be equivalent to about _____ mrem to the fetus.

    a. 500                b. 50
    c. 10                 d. less than 1

11. Which of the following statement(s) is (are) true?

    a. The annual radiation dose limits are the same for occupational/radiation workers and the general public.
    b. The annual radiation dose limit for the general public is set not to exceed 1 mSV (100 mrem) for continuous or frequent exposure.
    c. The annual radiation dose limit for radiation workers is set not to exceed 2 mSv (200 mrem).
    d. The annual radiation dose limit for the general public is set not to exceed 5 mSv (500 mrem) for infrequent exposure.
    e. Both b and d

12. The radiation dose to an embryo or fetus of a pregnant radiation worker is restricted to radiation exposure of no more than:

    a. 1000 mrem and 0.5 mrem per month.
    b. 500 mrem and 0.1 mrem per month.
    c. 500 mrem and 50 mrem per month.
    d. 1000 mrem and 0.1 mrem per month.

13. The principle behind ALARA states that:

    a. Exposure of personnel to a radiation source should be kept to zero.
    b. Exposure of personnel to any radiation source should be kept as low as reasonably achievable considering the economic and social aspects.
    c. Personnel are allowed to receive radiation doses up to 5 cGy biannually.
    d. Personnel are allowed to receive radiation doses up to 500 cGy per year.
    e. Both c and d

14. Which of these statement(s) is (are) true?

    a. The annual maximum permissible dose to the whole body (general public) is 50 rem.
    b. The annual maximum permissible dose to the lens of the eye (general public) is 5 rem.
    c. The level of dose limit for minors (under age 18) is lower than that for grown adults.
    d. The maximum dose allowed to a fetus/embryo of a radiation worker is set at 0.5 rem and 0.05 rem/month.
    e. The annual maximum permissible dose to the whole body (radiation worker) is 5 rem.

15. The three basic principles that guide radiation protection are:

    a. time, distance, and the tube voltage kVp.
    b. distance, shielding, and tube current mAs.
    c. time, tube voltage kVp, and tube current mAs.
    d. time, distance, and shielding.
    e. none of the above

16. Which one of the following is correct for a pregnant radiation worker?

    a. Personnel monitoring radiation badges are to be worn only 3 hours a day.
    b. Personnel monitoring radiation badges are to be worn only once a week.
    c. Personnel monitoring radiation badges are to be worn at all times during the pregnancy while performing any radiation-related duties.
    d. Personnel monitoring radiation badges are to be worn only for the first month of the pregnancy.

17. Which one of the following is true?

    a. Personnel monitoring radiation badges for pregnant women should be worn on the finger only.

    b. Personnel monitoring radiation badges for pregnant women should be worn on the chest only.

    c. Personnel monitoring radiation badges for nonpregnant women should be worn either on the collar or the abdomen or both.

    d. None of the above

## Exercises

1. Define the term *declared pregnant woman.*

2. What information must be known following an overexposure?

3. Describe the negligible individual risk level (NIRL).

4. What was the tolerance dose?

5. What is the primary purpose of the BEIR Committee?

## Answers

Questions

| | |
|---|---|
| 1. a | 10. c |
| 2. c | 11. e |
| 3. c | 12. c |
| 4. b | 13. b |
| 5. b | 14. b, c, d, and e |
| 6. a | 15. d |
| 7. c | 16. c |
| 8. d | 17. c |
| 9. b | |

Exercises

1. This means that a worker must notify her employer of a pregnancy voluntarily and in writing of both the pregnancy and estimated date of conception. This will help the employer keep the dose to the fetus as low as possible.

2. Although various facilities may require a variety of information to be kept, in general, the patient's name, build, positions during the exposure; personnel in the room; and factors (manual or automatic) must be reported following an overexposure.

3. The NIRL is an outgrowth of *de minimis non curat lex,* meaning "the law is not concerned with trifles." Risks from such an exposure are considered "trivial" and thus not worth the concern of regulatory agencies. Currently, 1 mrem is considered the level of the NIRL per exposure or activity.

4. The tolerance dose was considered to be a "safe dose" of radiation. During the 1930s and 1940s, it was thought that about 1 R/day was considered an acceptable dose below which no effects would be seen. This is about what the average technologist receives today in 2 years.

5. The Committee on the Biological Effects of Ionizing Radiation (BEIR) is a part of the National Research Council. They have issued five reports since 1955 on the biologic effects of radiation. The most recent report (BEIR V) has updated previous studies and risk estimates, and has been interpreted by some as calling current standards "safe," by others as calling for more research into radiation risks.

## CHAPTER 10

# Protecting the Radiographer and Other Workers

Steven B. Dowd • Elwin R. Tilson

## Chapter Objectives

At the end of this chapter, the student should be able to:

1. Describe the relationship between time and radiation exposure.
2. Describe how distance can be used to reduce personal exposure.
3. Solve problems related to the inverse square law.
4. List types of shields.
5. Develop means for personal protection of the pregnant radiographer.
6. State the first rule of mobile radiography.
7. List means by which the patient and operator can be protected during mobile radiography.
8. Give means by which the teachable moment can be used to educate individuals about radiation protection.
9. List means of reducing patient dose in fluoroscopy.
10. Describe the best means of reducing patient and operator dose in fluoroscopy.

---

<u>**Important Terms**</u>

Bucky slot shielding device
cataractogenesis
distance
lead aprons
lead gloves

oncogenic
primary barriers
secondary barriers
shielding
teachable moment
thyroid shields
time

---

## INTRODUCTION

Although the patient should be the only individual exposed to the primary beam, personnel may be exposed to secondary scatter radiation or leakage radiation from the tube. Examinations with a possibility of high exposure to the worker include interventional procedures, fluoroscopy, and mobile radiography.

This chapter will describe means through which the radiographer can practice personal radiation protection. Because some of these methods relate to patient radiation protection, this subject will also be discussed here. However, patient radiation protection will be discussed in greater detail in Chapter 11. Remember that, in general, methods used to reduce patient dose also reduce the dose of the radiographer. Patient advocates lobby for the role of the patient as an equal partner in the patient–professional relationship. Personal radiation protection and radiation protection of the patient should be seen as simultaneous goals of the professional practice of radiography.

Radiographers should not routinely hold patients unable to cooperate during a procedure. If immobilization devices are unavailable or cannot be used, assistance should be secured from non–radiation workers, preferably a family member or friend. No one should ever routinely hold patients. If a patient must be held, the individual holding the patient should remain at right angles to the primary beam and should also wear a lead apron and, if possible, lead gloves. See the section on immobilization for additional guidelines on using human immobilizers.

The three most important principles of radiation protection will be discussed in greater detail below. As professionals, radiographers should always be asking how they can improve their radiation protection practices. Time, distance, and shielding are the factors most modifiable for radiation protection.

## TIME

The radiographer must reduce the amount of time spent in the area of the radiation source. Time and radiation exposure are directly proportional. If the amount of time spent in the area of the source doubles, radiation exposure also doubles.

In technical factor selection, we know that doubling the time of exposure doubles the intensity of radiation and patient dose. A technique of 400 mA and 0.1 second (40 mAs) provides half the exposure of 400 mA and 0.2 second (80 mAs; these assume manual timed techniques rather than phototiming). Similarly, halving the time the radiographer spends in the vicinity of a source of radiation halves personal exposure.

This relationship may be calculated as follows:

$$\frac{t_1}{t_2} = \frac{I_1}{I_2}$$

$t_1$ = first time of exposure

$t_2$ = second time of exposure

$I_1$ = first intensity

$I_2$ = second intensity

This assumes that mA and other exposure factors are held constant, and is similar to the formula for mAs and exposure:

$$\frac{mAs_1}{mAs_2} = \frac{I_1}{I_2}$$

For example, if the radiographer's initial intensity is 10 mrem based on 10 minutes of exposure, what will this exposure be if the time of exposure is reduced to 5 minutes?

$$\frac{10}{5} = \frac{10}{x}$$

It is fairly easy to see that x will equal 5 on the right-hand side.

Here's a second example: If the radiographer receives 50 mrem during 15 minutes of exposure, what will exposure be if the time is cut to 5 minutes?

$$\frac{15}{5} = \frac{50}{x}$$

Cross-multiplying gives 15x = 250, or x = 16.67. Thus, exposure has been reduced by a factor of 3, which is consistent with the time change.

## DISTANCE

Distance is the most effective means of reducing radiation exposure. At a distance of 1 meter from the scattering object (the patient), the intensity of radiation in fluoroscopy decreases to 0.1% (one thousandth) of the original value.

The inverse square law, which states that radiation intensity varies to the inverse of the square of the distance, holds true for the primary beam (Figure 10–1), which is considered a point source of radiation, and after about 1 m for secondary scatter radiation. A point source of radiation is the original source of radiation such as the primary x-ray beam or a radionuclide source. Extended sources are objects that give off scatter, such as the patient or other objects in the area. For example, an intensity from a point source of 100 mrad (1 mGy) at 20 inches diminishes to 25 mrad (0.25 mGy) at 40 inches. This does not hold true for secondary scatter radiation because the patient is an extended source of radiation. However, the basic concept is the same: remain as far from the source (patient) as possible. The exposure switch on fixed radiographic equipment is attached to keep the operator behind the control booth.

## Applications of the Inverse Square Law

Although it is important that radiographers be able to calculate inverse square law problems, students should first seek to learn basic applications of the inverse square law. As will be discussed later, just learning a formula is contrary to professional practice and to really understanding how the inverse square law works. Memorizing formulas and their paper-and-pencil applications will only limit your understanding of the inverse square law to just that, paper-and-pencil applications.

Radiographers should know the following applications of the inverse square law:

- If distance is cut in half, intensity will increase by a factor of four (4 times original intensity).
- If distance is doubled, intensity will decrease by a factor of four (one fourth of original intensity).

There are two components to the inverse square law:

- The inverse refers to the fact that an opposite occurs; that is:
  1. As distance increases intensity decreases.
  2. As distance decreases intensity increases.
- The square refers to the fact that the numerical change is squared. The square of 2 is 4; thus, as above, if distance is doubled, intensity is cut by one fourth (the inverse square of 2 is 1/4). If distance is halved, intensity increases by 4 (the inverse square of 1/2 is 4/1, or 4).

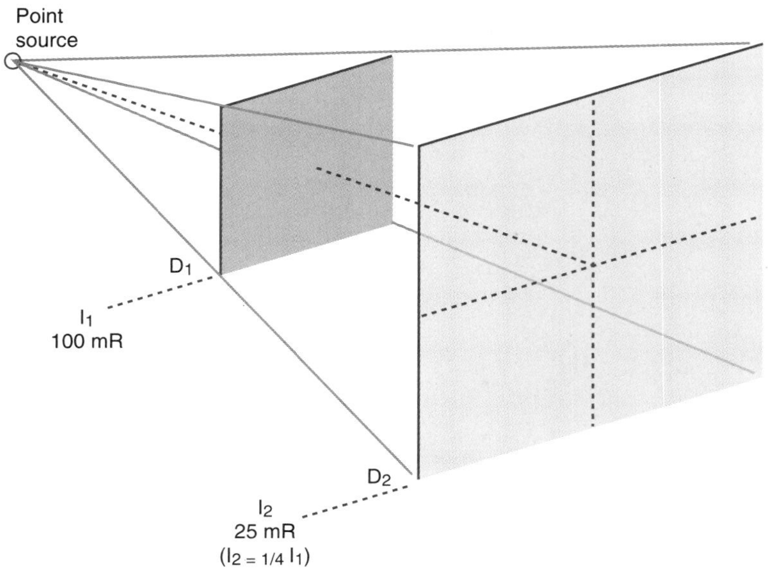

**Figure 10–1** Illustration of the inverse square law.

## Calculating Inverse Square Law Formulas

The formula for the inverse square law is as follows:

$$\frac{I_1}{I_2} = \left(\frac{d_2}{d_1}\right)^2 \quad \text{or} \quad \frac{I_1}{I_2} = \frac{D_2{}^2}{D_1{}^2}$$

$I_1$ = first intensity    $I_2$ = second intensity

$d_1$ = first distance    $d_2$ = second distance

Students usually learn best to solve inverse square law problems by breaking down the solution of the problem into multiple steps. Substituting the numbers from the above example:

Step 1:

$$\frac{100}{25} = \left(\frac{40}{20}\right)^2 \quad \text{set-up}$$

Step 2:

$$\frac{40^2}{20^2} = \frac{1600}{400} \quad \text{square distance values}$$

Step 3:

$$\frac{100}{25} = \frac{1600}{400} \quad \text{substitute values}$$

Step 4: We can verify the correctness of the numbers by cross-multiplying:

$$100 \times 400 = 40,000$$
$$25 \times 1600 = 40,000 \quad \text{check answer}$$

### EXAMPLE

A radiographer receives 10 mrem of exposure at 1 foot. What will this individual's exposure be at 2 feet?

$I_1$ = 10 mrem      $d_1$ = 1 foot

$I_2$ = x      $d_2$ = 2 feet

Step 1:

$$\frac{10}{x} = \left(\frac{2}{1}\right)^2 \quad \text{set-up}$$

Step 2:

$$\frac{10}{x} = \frac{4}{1} \qquad \text{square distance values}$$

Step 3:

$$4x = 10 \qquad \text{cross multiply}$$
$$x = 2.5 \qquad \text{divide}$$

Exposure will be quartered, to 2.5 mrem

---

**EXAMPLE**

A radiographer receives 10 mrem of exposure at 1 foot. How far back would this individual have to step to reduce exposure to 5 mrem?

$$I_1 = 10 \text{ mrem} \qquad d_1 = 1 \text{ foot}$$
$$I_2 = \phantom{0}5 \text{ mrem} \qquad d_2 = x$$

---

Step 1:

$$\frac{10}{5} = \left(\frac{x}{1}\right)^2 \qquad \text{set-up}$$

Step 2:

$$\frac{10}{5} = \frac{x^2}{1^2} \quad \text{or} \quad \frac{10}{5} = \frac{x^2}{1}$$

Step 3:

$$5x^2 = 10 \qquad \text{cross multipy}$$

$$x^2 = 2 \qquad \text{divide}$$

$$x = 1.41 \qquad \text{square root}$$

Exposure will be reduced to 5 mrem at 1.41 feet.

### Understanding the Inverse Square Law

As discussed earlier, understanding the inverse square formula and its uses in clinical practice is more important than working problems. When solving problems using the inverse square law, an important first step is presolving. Presolving involves collecting all data relevant to the problem and then formulating a "best guess" as to the solution. At first, until the student is able to better understand the application of the formula, this involves a guess as to whether intensity will increase or decrease. As distance increases, intensity will decrease. This knowledge alone can be helpful in clinical practice, or in multiple choice certification examination questions, for example:

Increasing distance from 1 to 3 meters will change the original intensity of 100 mR to:

    a. 900 mR      c. 33 mR
    b. 300 mR      d. 11 mR

Understanding that (1) radiation exposure will decrease limits the possible choices to c or d. Understanding that (2) if distance is tripled, radiation exposure decreases by one ninth (inverse square of 3) limits the possible choices to d only. Students who know only the formula make two common mistakes: (1) they invert one of the values, or (2) they forget to square. Making mistake 1 would have led to answer a. Making mistake 2 would have led to answer b. If this is unclear, the student should read the first section of this chapter related to the inverse square law.

Students should work to understand the inverse square law before memorizing the formula. Memorizing a formula does not signify understanding of a principle. Understanding principles, rather than merely applying them, is one of the hallmarks of a professional.

Also, memorizing formulas will not be helpful in clinical practice. In clinical practice, there is rarely time to calculate a formula. The practicing radiographer must rely on using intuition and estimates that are based on an understanding of principles.

Finally, understanding is helpful when problems do not meet the strict criteria of a memorized formula. For example, increasing distance from 20 to 30 inches will have what effect on radiation exposure?

This problem confuses some students who have memorized the formula. They expect to see three numbers and solve for a fourth. This problem can be solved as follows:

$$\left(\frac{D_1}{D_2}\right)^2 = \text{change in exposure due to distance}$$

$$\left(\frac{D_1}{D_2}\right)^2 = \left(\frac{20}{30}\right)^2$$

400/900 reduces to 4/9. 4/9th of the original intensity of 40 gives the new intensity of 17.6.

A student with an understanding of the formula and who is able to presolve will be better able to exercise the logic needed for these problems and apply the inverse square law to clinical settings. Appendix A contains more problems with answers using the inverse square law.

## SHIELDING

The third method of reducing exposure to the radiographer is shielding. Shielding consists of either fixed structural barriers (made of lead or concrete) or devices such as mobile shields and lead aprons. Lead is the material preferred for shielding. Its high atomic number (82) ensures that a majority of the scatter photons are absorbed. Shielding is measured in terms of half-value layers (HVLs; the amount of material needed to reduce radiation exposure in half) and tenth-value layers (TVLs; the amount of material needed to reduce radiation exposure to one tenth of the original amount). Refer back to Chapters 2 and 9 for a complete description of barriers; they will be reviewed briefly here.

Fixed barriers are classified as either primary or secondary barriers. A primary barrier is any wall (such as one supporting an upright film holder) or other barrier that can be struck by the primary beam. It must be at least 7 feet high. The beam cannot be directed toward secondary barriers, which can be struck only by secondary/scatter radiation. The control booth is usually considered a secondary barrier; the ceiling always is. When a control booth is considered a secondary barrier, x-rays will have scattered at least twice before reaching the radiographer. This reduces the intensity of the

beam to one millionth (one thousandth times one thousandth; see above) of the original value.

Shielding is conceptually easy to understand (something that attenuates x-rays), but it is just as often misunderstood. Lead and other materials don't magically absorb x-rays and make them disappear; materials such as lead, due to factors such as atomic weight, have an increased attenuation. However, lead can also allow some radiation to pass through (and it often does, especially at high energy levels such as the primary beam); and even materials such as lead generate some secondary/scatter radiation, which exits the back of the shield.

There are no absolutes. A lead shield that provides 97% attenuation at 50 kVp might only provide 50% attenuation at 100 kVp. Like other devices, lead aprons and other forms of shielding are just one piece of the puzzle in providing adequate radiation protection.

### Lead Aprons

For lead aprons to be effective, the lead must not be cracked; thus, aprons should not be handled carelessly or folded. Lead aprons are made of powdered lead incorporated in a flexible binder of rubber or vinyl (Figure 10–2). They provide an attenuation of radiation equivalent to that of 0.25 mm (if used only as a secondary barrier to absorb scatter radiation), 0.5 mm (in 1989, NCRP Report No. 102 stated that attenuation for lead aprons shall be 0.5 mm of lead equivalent for fluoroscopy, as they are primary barriers), or 1 mm of lead. [A reminder: when used in regulations, the term *shall* means "must" and the term *should* means "recommended."] A 0.5-mm lead equivalency should attenuate 90% of the radiation at 75 kVp (Bushong, 1997). Greater lead equivalencies translate into greater weight (up to 20 lb), which can lead to back strain and slowed movement.

Some manufacturers have begun making aprons using composite materials—a combination of barium, tungsten, and lead. This material can provide a better attenuation of radiation (lead has a diminished ability to absorb radiation between the energies of 50 and 88 keV) and has a reduced weight of 30%. Some indi-

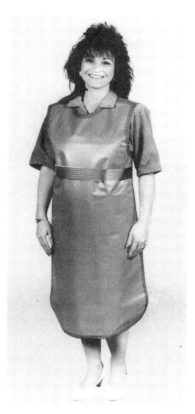

**Figure 10–2** Lead apron. (Courtesy of Nuclear Associates, 100 Voice Road, Carle Place, NY 11514.)

viduals have developed back pain from lead aprons, which has also resulted in the development of specially designed aprons (Figure 10–3).

A regular lead apron covers about 75% to 80% of the active bone marrow in the body. The bone marrow outside the apron is contained primarily in the skull, the arms, and the clavicles, assuming that the operator is facing the beam.

Maternity aprons are also available. For example, Picker markets a Sentry-Lite Maternity Apron (Figure 10–4). This apron provides 0.5 mm of lead equivalent protection throughout and 1 mm of lead equivalent protection of the fetus through an extra band of lead. This extends the full width of the apron from the xiphoid process to about 8 cm below the symphysis pubis.

### Lead Gloves

In addition to regular lead gloves (Figure 10–5), which provide 0.25 mm or more of lead equivalent protection (0.25 mm is the minimum for fluoroscopy, according to NCRP Report No. 102), radiation-resistant sterile gloves are also available (Figure 10–6). Made of lead-loaded rubber, these gloves are very thin to permit flexibility and dexterity. They lack the attenuation of regular lead gloves.

## Tales from the Internet Listservs . . . Radioactive Aprons?

In 1997, one issue that arose on both the AHRA and RadSci Internet discussion sites was the fact that several manufacturers had unknowingly used radioactive lead in the development of their aprons, exposing wearers to a small—but over time, perhaps not so small—amount of radiation. Although these aprons have since been recalled, in the future apron buyers might wish to consider adding an additional test to their QC measures—using a GM counter or other means of detecting radioactivity along with radiographing or fluoroscoping aprons to ensure that they are not cracked, as the "regular" checks will not detect low-level radioactivity.

## Common Mistakes in the Use of Lead Aprons

1. A new radiology nurse is very sure to put on her apron but also tries to stand with her back to the patient during fluoroscopy to minimize her gonadal exposure. Of course, due to backscatter, this can be seen as worse than no protection at all.
2. Tony, the portable technologist, always slings his apron, folded over twice, over his portable machine. By now the lead is so cracked that a radiograph of it would resemble a map of the California freeway system.
3. Sheila doesn't realize that lead aprons are designed to eliminate scatter rather than the primary beam and figures she can stand in the primary beam while holding a patient so long as she is wearing her lead apron.

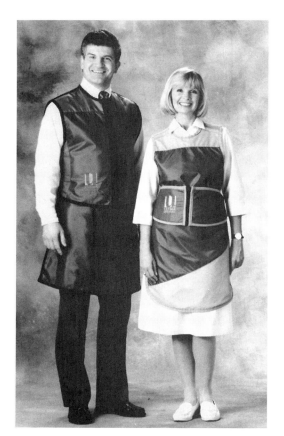

**Figure 10–3** Specially designed aprons for the relief of back pain. (Reprinted with permission from Buyer's Guide, vol 4. Mayfield Village, OH, Picker International, Inc.)

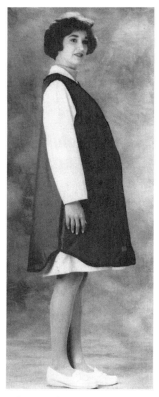

**Figure 10–4** Sentry-Lite maternity apron. (Reprinted with permission from Buyer's Guide, vol 4. Mayfield Village, OH, Picker International, Inc.)

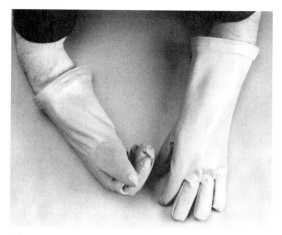

**Figure 10–5** Lead gloves. (Reprinted with permission from Buyer's Guide, vol 4. Mayfield Village, OH, Picker International, Inc.)

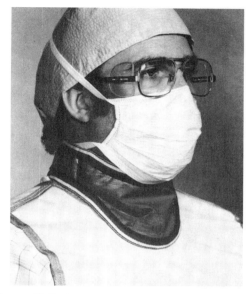

**Figure 10–7** Thyroid shield. (Courtesy of Nuclear Associates, 100 Voice Road, Carle Place, NY 11514.)

## Thyroid Shields

The second highest dosage to the fluoroscopist (radiologist) is to the thyroid. The average dose can be as high as 6 mrad per examination; this could provide a yearly occupational exposure to the thyroid of many rems in a year. This does not mean that all machines and examinations provide this dose; machines vary, and physicians vary greatly in how they perform fluoroscopy. A recent study by Nicklason et al. (1993) found exposures to the head and neck of about 261 mrem per year without a thyroid shield and 40 mrem with a thyroid shield. Use of a thyroid shield (Figure 10–7), depending on placement and lead equivalency (as well as the intensity of scatter), can reduce dose by a factor of up to 10.

As discussed in Chapter 8, some individuals have opted for the use of thyroid shields during fluoroscopy because of concern over the radiogenic dose for thyroid cancer. Because radiation-induced thyroid tumors are four times more likely to occur in females than in males as a result of the fluctuating hormonal status of women, women may feel a greater need to wear thyroid shields. In any case, this is an individual choice. Since thyroid shields are relatively inexpensive (less than $50), individuals who feel they need one, but work in an institution that does not provide thyroid shields, should consider buying one for personal use.

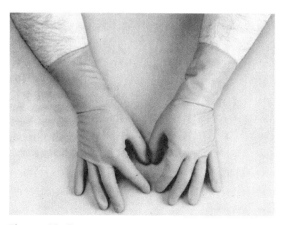

**Figure 10–6** Sterile lead gloves. (Reprinted with permission from Buyer's Guide, vol 4. Mayfield Village, OH, Picker International, Inc.)

## Mobile Shields

Mobile shields, unlike fixed barriers, are devices that can be moved around the room. They are sometimes used in angiography so

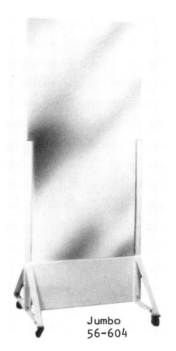

Jumbo
56-604

**Figure 10–8** Mobile shield. (Courtesy of Nuclear Associates, 100 Voice Road, Carle Place, NY 11514.)

that the physician has a barrier to step behind during rapid filming (Figure 10–8).

## Protective Facewear and Eyewear

Eyeglass lens materials have been recommended for the protection of eyes from the cataractogenic (causing the formation of cataracts) effect of radiation, primarily during fluoroscopic procedures. The need for these has never been proved; cataractogenesis is based on data from cyclotron physicists and radiotherapy patients. The radiation therapy patients developed cataracts 20 years after a therapeutic exposure of 200 rads from a radium source. Fluoroscopists in training (e.g. radiology residents), as opposed to other workers who receive smaller amounts of radiation during fluoroscopy, may need these devices.

These lenses, available commercially, contain a variety of materials of high atomic number such as lead or barium. Cousin and colleagues found that lead-containing glass was superior, reducing dose by up to 98%, and that large lenses were superior to small lenses. They also recommend using a face mask of leaded glass or a freely supported and properly positioned leaded barrier in addition to the lenses. Figure 10–9 shows one type of radiation protection glasses. This provides 0.75 mm of lead equivalent protection. Regular glasses of photochrome or crown glass reduce the dose by about 50%.

## THE PREGNANT RADIOGRAPHER

The future working habits of pregnant radiographers should be based on previous radiation exposure history as well as the current work setting. It is usually best for the radiographer to rotate out of areas such as fluoroscopy and mobile radiography. An additional monitor may also be provided to be worn at waist level to determine fetal dose. Pregnant radiographers and workers should never hold patients, according to NCRP Report No. 102 (1989).

Only when pregnant workers inform their employers of their pregnancy status do they become what is known as *declared pregnant workers*. Obviously, an employer cannot provide protection until the pregnancy status of the worker is

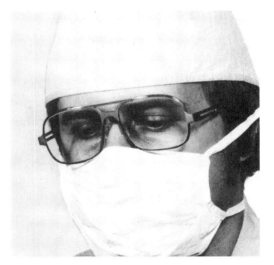

**Figure 10–9** Radiation-shielding glasses. (Courtesy of Nuclear Associates, 100 Voice Road, Carle Place, NY 11514.)

known. Rotation changes are best made in conjunction with the radiographer, the radiographer's personal physician, and the radiation safety officer, although the final decision rests with the radiographer. The most important factor is the relationship between the employer and employee. The employer is responsible for providing a safe work setting; however, the employee must also observe rules of safe practice.

In no case can a radiographer's employment be terminated because of pregnancy. The NCRP, in its Report No. 116, has recommended a monthly dose equivalent of 50 mrem (0.5 mSv) to the embryo/fetus (excluding medical and natural background radiation) once the pregnancy is known. This is different from previous recommendations that allowed an overall dose limit of 0.5 rem (5 mSv) during the entire gestational period based on the philosophy that a monthly limit would better control exposure during sensitive periods of gestation.

There is no such thing as a radiounique effect; that is, a variety of other factors such as air pollution, food additives, tobacco, and stress can lead to the same effect to the fetus as radiation exposure. It is as difficult to mandate a "safe" dose for the fetus as for the adult, even though we know that developing cells are more sensitive to radiation. This is, of course, consistent with the law of Bergonie and Tribondeau. The National Academy of Science has stated, however, that it is uncertain that a dose of less than 1 rad would have any effect at all on the fetus.

Wagner and Hayman (1982) studied women radiologists and concluded that the possibility of malformation of the fetus would increase from the normal level of 4 in 100 cases to 4.02 in 100 cases with an exposure of 1 rem (this exposure, of course, far exceeds acceptable limits). With that same exposure, they calculated that the probability of cancer would increase from the normal incidence of 4.07 per 100 cases to 4.17 per 100. Many authorities think that even at 5 rad, there is a virtual lack of risk of congenital anomalies and malformations. They also believe that the risk of carcinogenesis is much lower than other risks associated with pregnancy. Figure 10–10

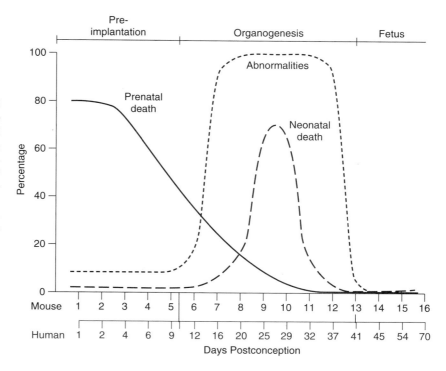

**Figure 10–10** Potential effects of radiation of the fetus, by gestational weeks. (Reprinted with permission from Thompson MA: Principles of Radiation Protection for Nurses and Other Medical Facility Personnel. Birmingham, AL, University of Alabama at Birmingham, 1986.)

**Table 10–1** Overview of Potential Effects of Occupational Radiation on the Fetus

| Time | Principal Response | Natural Incidence | Dose-Related Incidence |
|------|-------------------|-------------------|------------------------|
| 0–2 weeks | Spontaneous abortion | 25–50% of all conceptions | 1% increase per 10 rad |
| 2–8 weeks | Congenital anomalies | 5–10% of all live births | 1% increase per 10 rad |
| 0–9 months | Childhood malignancy (leukemia) | 4/100,000 live births | 2/100,000 per rad |

Data from Bushong SC: Policies for managing the pregnant employee. Radiology Manage 6(3):2–7, 1984.

summarizes the potential effects following radiation of the fetus by gestational weeks; Table 10–1 summarizes these in general terms along with natural incidence and dose-related incidence of the effect.

Bushong's (1984) estimate of childhood malignancy in Table 10–1 is lower than that cited in Chapter 8, where it was stated that probably 50 rad was needed to induce late effects, especially later in a pregnancy. Bushong himself notes in the article that this is "detectable only by exceedingly large-scale epidemiologic studies." It must also be noted again that a variety of factors influence radiation carcinogenesis.

### Legal Rights of Pregnant Radiographers

Several court decisions have indicated that fetal protection policies restricting pregnant women from working in radiology departments are not valid. For example, a court case in Alabama disallowed a hospital's contention that termination of a technologist was appropriate and that a state of "nonpregnancy" was a bona fide qualification for employment.

The court's most important finding was that the pregnancy did not inhibit the technologist's ability to use x-rays. It was also found that two technologists had not been fired previously, even though they were pregnant. One was reassigned to the control desk. In this case, the first to test fetal pregnancy policies in radiology, the employee was awarded back wages as a settlement.

At the Supreme Court level, a decision made in 1991 has far-reaching implications, as it theoretically applies to all states. The Supreme Court found that a battery manufacturer, Johnson Controls, could not mandate that an employee be excluded from certain work areas as a means of fetal protection. Another implication of this case is that, so long as the employers warn the employee of risks involved, the employer has only a remote chance of being held liable. This is a decision of the mother, and attempts to mandate reassignment are seen as illegal sex discrimination. Reassignment would be appropriate only if it could be determined that pregnancy interferes with the ability of the individual to perform the job. Another court case, reported in 1990, indicated that a pregnant radiation worker could not be barred from overtime work simply because she was pregnant.

This means that students in radiography programs or employees in radiology departments cannot be forced to temporarily withdraw from the program, take sick leave, or be reassigned unless the pregnancy interferes with the ability of the employee to perform what is needed for that job or, in the case of a student, secure clinical competency. In the past, pregnant employees were sometimes asked to work in the film filing room at a lower wage until after the delivery. Students were sometimes asked to forgo certain rotations, such as fluoroscopy or portable radiography, and took longer to complete the program. Today, many departments have developed informal programs in which staff technologists switch assignments with nonpregnant staff.

Certainly, a program or department can offer advice when it is believed that the rotation will not be in the best interest of the unborn child. The employee or student can also be asked to sign waivers indicating an understanding and awareness of the potential effects of radiation to the fetus. Examples of such waivers are shown. Figure 10–11 is appropriate for new employees or students. Figure 10–12 would be used for pregnant employees or students.

---

Form 1
New Employee Waiver

This certifies that _____ , employed at New County Hospital
on _____ , has received:

1. A copy of the departmental pregnancy policy. This policy states that the employee must inform a
   department supervisor, should the employee become pregnant.

2. Documentation, including the article "Pregnancy in Diagnostic Radiology," that outlines potential
   risks to the fetus from radiation.

3. A session with a department supervisor to review understanding of the above.


_____              _____
Supervisor                         Employee


Date _____

---

**Figure 10–11** New employee waiver.


---

Form 2
Pregnant Employee Waiver

I, _____ , have received counseling from _____
regarding my legal rights and the potential risks to the fetus from ionizing radiation.

I realize that unless the pregnancy interferes with my ability to perform my assignments, that any
decision to be reassigned will be based on my own preferences. _____ has
discussed with me normal departmental procedure in securing potential reassignment.

I also certify that I have re-read the material initially provided to me regarding radiation work and
pregnancy upon employment.


_____              _____
Supervisor                         Employee


Date _____

---

**Figure 10–12** Pregnant employee waiver.

## CASE STUDIES FOR DISCUSSION: THE PREGNANT EMPLOYEE

1. Kim Smith is a radiography student in her second (senior) year. She has just learned that she is pregnant. Kim's options, according to her program's published policies, are to quit the program, or continue if she can secure a doctor's permission. She will have to make up her fluoro rotation at the end of the program, graduating after the other students.
   a. What would you do if you were Kim?
   b. Can the program require a doctor's permission or make her miss her fluoro rotation?
2. Hazel White is a radiology nurse who has just learned she is pregnant. If you were the RSO, what information would you have to collect in order to advise her on what she should do during her pregnancy? That is, what do you have to know about her job to give her the information she needs?
3. Jean Sheldrick is a nurse in the ER, working nights. Traditionally, when patients are judged unable to hold positions in radiology, the ER nurse comes and holds while the radiographer takes the radiographs. However, she is now telling her employer that she refuses to do so any longer until after she delivers. Is she within her rights?

## RADIATION PROTECTION DURING MOBILE RADIOGRAPHY

Mobile or portable radiography refers to bringing x-ray units to patients' rooms or areas such as the emergency department or surgery when the patient is unable to come to the department. Portable examinations are rarely able to provide the same kind of film quality that stationary units provide. Thus, portable radiography is not designed as an easy substitute for patients or health professionals. If the radiographer thinks that the patient is able to come to the depart-

ment, this individual should ask other health professionals, such as physicians, whether an examination in the department might not be more appropriate. Sometimes examinations are ordered at night for the next morning. At the time the examination is ordered, the patient is in a condition that definitely requires a portable examination. However, the condition of the patient may improve. In this case, it is in the patient's best interest to at least ask if the examination in the department might not be more appropriate. This is also part of the professional role of the radiographer.

The first rule of mobile radiography is the same as the first rule of regular radiography: establish communication with the patient. The mobile unit should be left in the hall, and the radiographer should assess the patient's condition and ability to cooperate, and should attempt to establish rapport. Before taking films, ask all nonessential individuals to leave the area. Individuals remaining, including the patient, should be shielded. Be certain to tell those individuals previously asked to leave when the procedure is complete.

Scatter from the patient is the main source of exposure to the operator and others present. This is normally very small. The intensity of radiation 1 meter from the patient in portable radiography is so small that a radiation worker standing at this distance in one study would have to have been exposed to 2000 films a month to reach the dosage allowed the general public. If the exposure for a portable chest x-ray is 40 mR, then scatter at 1 meter would equal 0.04 mR. At 2 meters, because of the inverse square law, exposure would be reduced to 0.01 mR. However, mobile radiography still constitutes a potential radiation hazard since, unlike the radiology department, patient rooms and surgical suites are not usually designed for radiation protection.

The percentage of scattered radiation at 1 m is greater for portable radiography than for undertable fluoroscopy because of the orientation of the tube. However, the amount of scatter produced is normally less for portable radiography (portable examinations, of course, use a much lower exposure than fluoroscopy). If a nurse were to ask about the amount of radiation received at 1 meter from a portable radiograph, a possible answer would be, "about the same as 1 hour of natural background radiation," although such comparisons always suffer a bit in the translation. As a general rule, encourage nurses and other health care personnel to stand 2 meters from patients receiving mobile examinations.

Distance is, as always, the most effective means of protection in mobile radiography for individuals other than the patient, especially when this is combined with appropriate methods of shielding. When performing mobile radiography, the radiographer is expected to stand 6 feet from the source, with the cord long enough to allow this distance. The NCRP regulations do not, as is sometimes assumed, specify that the cord length itself must be 6 feet. The use of cordless remote exposure systems has received mixed reviews. Such devices typically allow the radiographer to stand up to 36 feet from the the source (and will not expose if the device is less than 6 feet from the source). Possibly, as the "bugs" are worked out of the system, these devices will become more popular.

Radiographers sometimes try to stand behind the portable machine for protection. There is no guarantee that this constitutes sufficient protection from ionizing radiation, and in all such cases, a lead apron should be worn. If possible, it is best that the radiographer stand around a corner when making the exposure. Thus, any radiation that does reach the radiographer will have scattered at least twice—once from the patient and another time in a floor, ceiling, or wall. Generally, each scattering event reduces radiation exposure by a factor of 1000 (0.1%). Thus, if the dose at the patient is 100 mR, the two scattering events reduce exposure to 0.0001 mR, which is practically too small to be measured. However, there are, of course, operational issues associated with this (patient motion, getting the patient to hold his breath) that may preclude this safety measure.

## Personnel, Visitor, and Patient Protection

Radiographers and others who must remain in the room (such as patients who are not ambulatory or a respiratory therapist ventilating a patient) must be shielded with a lead apron, and, if necessary, lead gloves. Many state laws also require that either these individuals be provided with a dosimetric device of some type (e.g. a pocket dosimeter) or that the projections they hold for be recorded in a log. Health educators talk about "teachable moments"—situations in which individuals can be taught good health behavior. Use mobile examinations to show that a radiographer is a professional concerned with the radiologic health of the patient and others—family members, nurses, and physicians. When visitors ask to stay, for example, with an apron, explain to them the greater value of distance in radiation protection. Many people feel that lead aprons provide some sort of absolute protection against radiation, but, of course, they do not.

Physicians and nurses rarely want to stay. However, they may exhibit excessive anxiety. Experienced radiographers have probably heard the accusatory statement, "Don't take that film until I'm out of here!" more than once. The way the radiographer practices the teachable moment in this case is by reassuring these individuals that the radiographer will always exercise proper radiation protection practices.

In the July 13, 1992, issue of *RT Image,* Gregory Campbell makes the following comment about mobile radiography:

> Before you get on the rotor to make the exposure, double check for nearby staff members. Remember, most allied health professionals have little or no training in radiation safety. Other hospital employees don't really understand ionizing radiation and how to protect themselves, and they don't really believe technologists who say that six feet is a safe distance. There are too many movies and horror stories ingrained in their minds to be overcome by just a few words. You may consider them foolish because they run down to the main lobby while you make the exposure, but give them the choice.

This is an appropriate statement by an experienced technologist. Earlier in the article, Campbell notes that radiographers must realize that often the only contact a patient or family member has with the radiology department is through the technologist. The radiographer must seek to educate individuals who are apprehensive about radiation. Radiologic technologists are the group of individuals, along with radiologists and radiologic physicists, who are best able to educate the public about radiation safety practice.

## Holding Patients

The issue of radiographers and other workers holding patients is one that is always topical. Many states expressly forbid the holding of patients except in emergency situations, and some, such as California, expressly forbid students from holding. However, some radiographers have indicated that they have been threatened with losing their jobs if they do not hold patients.

This is a difficult issue and it will probably increase as the population ages and more frail elderly require medical imaging. It is important that radiographers present a unified professional front and hold only when absolutely necessary, and according to the laws of their jurisdiction.

## RADIATION PROTECTION DURING FLUOROSCOPY

Fluoroscopy is a dynamic imaging technique (see Chapter 2) that allows for the viewing of motion and location in real time. In addition to fluoroscopy in the radiology department, mobile fluoroscopy is often performed in the operating room for procedures such as nailing of long-bone fractures and fixation of hip fractures.

Fluoroscopic equipment is equipped with 5-minute reset timers to remind the operator that a certain recommended time limit has elapsed for beam-on time. This does not mean that it is illegal to exceed these 5 minutes. The timer is designed to serve as a reminder that this block of time has been exceeded. However, not setting the timer for each patient is poor radiation protection practice, as the physician will not know when 5 minutes has been reached on a patient. Also, a fluoroscopic foot switch, also known as a deadman switch, is designed to terminate the exposure once the foot is released from the switch.

The surface of the patient where the primary beam enters (the side *away* from the intensifier) should be considered a radiation source. The exposure at tabletop in fluoroscopy cannot exceed 10 R/min and should not exceed 5 R/min. The primary exposure to the technologist or radiologist will be from the scatter generated by the patient (Figure 10–13) when this primary beam passes through the patient. A drape or sliding panel (also called a *curtain*) of at least 0.25 mm of lead equivalent often hangs from the image intensifier to absorb scatter. When such a curtain cannot be used, such as when performing myelography, a retractable lead shield of at least 0.5 mm of lead equivalent should be used (Seeram, 1997). The majority of the dose from patient scatter to the technologist is at the level of the gonads.

Many U-arm and C-arm tubes (Figure 10–14) allow for both anteroposterior (AP) and posteroanterior (PA) fluoroscopy. AP fluoroscopy has the patient supine, the x-ray tube above the table, and the image intensifier below. The PA position has the x-ray tube below the table with the patient supine. AP imaging results in less magnification and less geometric unsharpness but increases the rate of scatter radiation to the neck, head, and upper extremities. This is similar to the operation of an undertable image intensifier (see Figure 10–13D), which also provides higher doses to the fluoroscopist—up to 10 times higher than conventional overtable intensification units.

A Bucky slot shielding device of at least 0.25 mm of lead equivalent is required to cover the Bucky slot opening with the Bucky tray positioned at the caudal end of the table. This provides additional protection at the level of the gonads from scatter.

A lead apron and lead gloves should be worn if the hands will be placed in the primary beam. Only those individuals required for the examination should be in the room, and they should be wearing lead aprons. Wearing lead aprons is important because about 80% of the active bone marrow in the body is covered with the normal lead apron. This reduces the possible oncogenic effect of radiation on bone marrow (the development of leukemia). Audible monitors are also available through Nuclear Associates of Carle Place, New York. They emit a chirping sound propor-

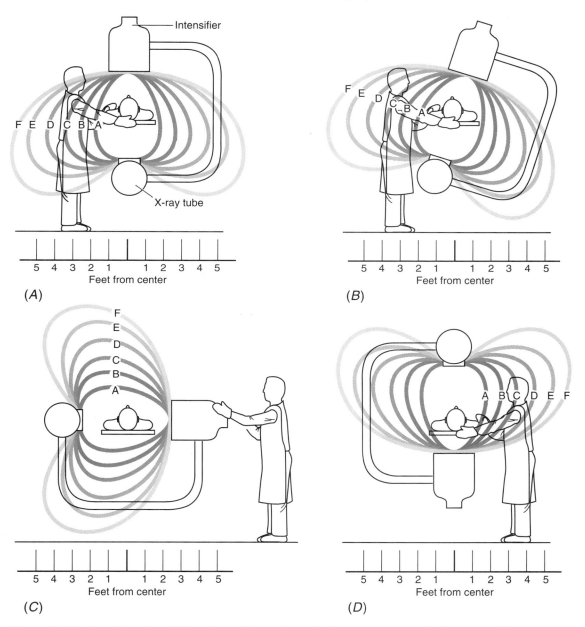

**Figure 10–13** The orientation of the tube and image intensifer has an impact on the dose rate of the person doing the fluoroscopy. Dose/rate line A is greater than 300 mR per hour, B is 100–300 mR per hour, C is 50–100 mR per hour, D is 25–50 mR per hour, E is 10–25 mR per hour, and F is less than 10 mR per hour. The fluoroscopy orientations shown in (A) and (D) are associated with both fixed and C-arm units, whereas orientations (B) and (C) are associated only with C-arm units. The normal fluoroscopy orientation is shown in (A). Note that the person operating the fluoroscopy does not receive a dose rate above 25 mR/hr to any unshielded area of the body in (A) or (B). In (C), the dose rate is at its lowest, but is useful only for lateral images. The orientation of (D) with the tube on top is not recommended because the dose rate can be as much as 10 times greater than the normal orientation.

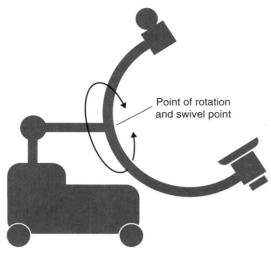

Point of rotation and swivel point

**Figure 10–14** C-arm image intensifier.

tional to the amount of scatter. These help the radiographer determine the ideal position during fluoroscopic procedures.

## Primary Means to Minimize Exposure

Distance is the best means of minimizing exposure to the operator in fluoroscopy. The second best means of minimizing exposure, which minimizes exposure to both operator and patient, is the use of higher kVp levels. As voltage increases, the penetration of the x-ray beam increases, and a greater fraction of the x-ray beam reaches the detector. The automatic brightness control (ABC) keeps the exposure at the image intensifier constant, and this decreases the entrance exposure with increasing kilovoltage.

Often, it is recommended that the technologist stand behind the radiologist during fluoroscopy to minimize exposure. The only problem with such a recommendation is that the movement of the radiologist cannot always be predicted. Certainly, it is one of the means by which exposure can be reduced; it should not be relied on excessively, however. Use distance as well.

Some fluoroscopic units are capable of both front and rear loading of spot film cassettes. It

## More Teachable Moments

Radiographers often work with other health professionals in a team—with speech–language pathologists for fluoroscopic studies of dysphasia (swallowing studies) and with cardiologists and nurses in the cardiac cath lab, for example. The advantage of a team approach is that each professional works for the best interest of all by bringing what he or she is best at to the team.

If a radiographer thinks that another health professional is not following proper radiation protection practices, he or she should not hesitate, in a professionally acceptable manner, to indicate that to other professionals. A speech–language pathologist who is leaving her hand in the useful beam too often while "feeding" the patient barium or who refuses to wear a thyroid shield, a nurse who "hangs her head" over the image intensifier during a cardiac cath, or an orthopedist who

leaves the beam of the C-arm in surgery on constantly instead of using intermittent pulses should all be appropriately educated about the consequences of their actions.

The issue of radiographers providing information to physicians should not be construed as "telling them what to do" or undermining their authority; if you think back to Chapter 1 and the ASRT Code of Ethics, you will recall that radiographers are ethically obligated to provide information to physicians that is in the best interests of patient care. You can try a brief reminder first: "Dr. Jones, we have now exceeded ten minutes of fluoro time." If that doesn't work, the chief or administrative technologist or head nurse for the OR might be a good resource. Remember, it is unethical to do anything that is not in the best interests of patient care. This includes just "letting it go."

is usually the radiographer's responsibility to load spot films. It is possible to operate the unit while the radiographer is loading films from the front or rear; however, there is rarely sufficient protection from radiation while rear-loading spot films. For this reason, the radiographer should indicate to the radiologist, with appropriate professional tact, that operating the unit while films are being rear-loaded is unacceptable practice.

## SUMMARY

Time and radiation exposure are directly proportional. The amount of time one is exposed to a source of radiation should be minimized. For the radiographer, this entails working with speed and efficiency in areas such as fluoroscopy and angiography.

Distance is the most effective means of reducing radiation exposure. For extended sources of radiation such as the patient, the intensity of radiation is reduced to 0.1% (one one-thousandth) of the original value at 1 meter. Point sources of radiation such as the primary beam (but not scatter sources) follow an inverse square relationship. Radiographers need to understand this relationship as well as to be able to solve formulas using the inverse square law for effective practice.

Shielding is the third method of reducing exposure. Shielding consists of fixed barriers (walls), as well as lead aprons, lead gloves, and mobile shields.

Radiographers have legal rights when pregnant; they may be asked to sign waivers and advised on radiation protection practice. In terms of rotation changes for the pregnant radiographer, the final decision rests with the radiographer. Radiographers cannot have their employment terminated because of pregnancy. The risk of carcinogenesis from radiation is much lower than other risks associated with pregnancy; however, this would not excuse unsafe operating practice.

The first rule of mobile radiography is the same as the first rule of regular radiography: establish communication with the patient. Radiographers should also realize that they are a professional role model and educator to individuals who are often apprehensive about radiation. For the radiographer and other health care workers, achieving a maximum distance is also the best means of protection, along with the above factors.

Doses to operators and patients can be reduced during fluoroscopy by using proper distance, positioning, and shielding. Also, because time is directly related to radiation dose, speed and efficiency are imperative in fluoroscopic studies.

## Questions

1. A lead apron covers about what percentage of the active bone marrow in the body?

   a. 25%               b. 50%
   c. 80%               d. 100%

2. When lead curtains cannot be used during fluoroscopy:

   a. the patient should be given a lead apron.
   b. the doses should be recorded.
   c. a retractable lead shield should be used.
   d. All of the above

3. The best means of minimizing exposure during fluoroscopy are:

   I. increased kVp.
   II. increased distance.
   III. standing behind the operator (radiologist).

   a. I and II only          b. I and III only
   c. II and III only        d. I, II, and III

4. Each scattering event reduces radiation intensity by what factor?

   a. 100               b. the inverse
                             square
   c. 1000              d. 1,000,000

5. If distance is doubled, intensity will be:

   a. reduced by half.       b. reduced by
                                four.
   c. increased by two.      d. increased by
                                four.

6. The second highest intensity to the fluoroscopist is at the level of the:

   a. gonads.           b. thyroid.
   c. skull.            d. clavicles.

7. Lead has a lessened ability to absorb radiation at which of the following energies?

    I. 40 keV
    II. 60 keV
    III. 80 keV

    a. I and II only
    b. I and III only
    c. II and III only
    d. I, II, and III

8. The most effective means of reducing exposure is:

    a. time.
    b. shielding.
    c. distance.
    d. wearing a film badge.

9. The minimum amount of lead equivalent required in an apron is:

    a. 0.25 mm.
    b. 0.5 mm.
    c. 0.75 mm.
    d. 1 mm.

10. In the case of a pregnant radiographer, it is best to:

    a. reassign the employee to the file room.
    b. rotate the employee voluntarily out of fluoroscopy and mobile radiography.
    c. terminate the employee.
    d. assign final decisions to the radiation safety officer.

11. In mobile radiography, the radiographer should:

    I. stand at least 6 feet from the source.
    II. stand behind a corner, if possible.
    III. use low-kVp techniques.

    a. I and II only
    b. I and III only
    c. II and III only
    d. I, II, and III

12. Exposure rate at tabletop in fluoroscopy cannot exceed:

    a. 1 R/min.
    b. 5 R/min.
    c. 10 R/min.
    d. 50 R/min.

13. If distance from the source is increased from 1.5 to 2 ft and the original exposure was 5 mrem/min, the new exposure will be:

    a. 3 mrem/min.
    b. 1.8 mrem/min.
    c. 8 mrem/min.
    d. 14 mrem/min.

14. To reduce intensity from 100 to 50 mrem, with an original distance of 1 foot, distance should change to:

    a. 4 feet.
    b. 2 feet.
    c. 1.41 feet.
    d. 0.41 feet

15. A thyroid shield will reduce dose by a factor of up to:

    a. two.
    b. five.
    c. seven.
    d. ten.

## Exercises

1. What are means of radiographer protection during mobile radiography?

2. What are the risks of exposure to a pregnant radiographer to the fetus?

3. What are the trade-offs in using an apron with a greater equivalency of lead?

4. What is the value to clinical practice of understanding and being able to presolve inverse square law problems?

5. Describe the use of increased kVp to minimize patient dose in fluoroscopy.

6. How should the working habits of pregnant radiographers be regulated?

7. What is the potential value of wearing leaded glasses or other types of protective face and eyewear?

8. What is the value of the "teachable moment" in mobile radiography? How might this be applied to other settings?

## Answers

Questions

| | |
|---|---|
| 1. c | 9. a |
| 2. c | 10. b |
| 3. d | 11. a |
| 4. c | 12. c |
| 5. b | 13. a |
| 6. b | 14. c |
| 7. c | 15. d |
| 8. c | |

Exercises

1. Distance and shielding are the most effective methods of radiographer protection during mobile radiography. The radiographer should stand at least 6 feet from the source (the patient), wear a lead apron, and stand behind a wall if possible.

2. The possibility of malformation of the fetus in one study was shown to increase from the normal level of 4 in 100 cases to 4.02 in 100 cases with an exposure of 1 rem. That same study estimated the probability of cancer would increase from the normal incidence of 4.07 per 100 cases to 4.17 per 100. Even at 5 rad, there appears to be little risk of congenital anomalies and malformations. The risk of carcinogenesis from radiation is much lower than other risks associated with pregnancy. However, as discussed in Chapter 1, we must be careful to not compound risk.

3. The main trade-offs in using an apron with a greater equivalency of lead are back strain and speed of motion due to the heavy lead. Some aprons weigh as much as 20 lb; the need to attenuate greater amounts of radiation must be balanced with these concerns.

4. Students with an understanding of the inverse square law will be able to presolve problems. This is valuable in clinical practice, where intuition is used more often than calculation.

5. The use of higher kVp levels is the second-best means of minimizing exposure and minimizes exposure to both operator and patient. As voltage increases, the penetration of the x-ray beam increases, and a greater fraction of the x-ray beam reaches the detector. The automatic brightness control (ABC) keeps the exposure at the image intensifier constant, and this decreases the entrance exposure with increasing kilovoltage.

6. The pregnant radiographer is the final decision maker in cases of pregnancy. Although this individual is often reassigned out of areas that have a high exposure potential such as angiography and fluoroscopy, she cannot be treated differently than other workers. She may be asked to read certain reference materials and sign a waiver indicating she intends to stay assigned to a certain area.

7. Protective face and eyewear may protect the radiographer or other operators from cataracts. The need for these items is not proved; each individual must decide if he or she wishes to wear them.

8. The "teachable moment" is a point when individuals are receptive to learning. In mobile radiography, there is often an opportunity to teach individuals such as patients, their families, physicians, and nurses about safe radiation protection practices. Radiographers should realize that each patient presents the opportunity to teach through example of safe radiation protection practices and the role of the radiographer as the professional primarily responsible for radiation protection.

## CHAPTER 11

# Protecting the Patient in Radiography

Steven B. Dowd   •   Elwin R. Tilson

## Chapter Outline

## Chapter Objectives

At the end of this chapter, the student should be able to:

1. Describe how technique selection can be used in radiation protection.

2. Describe the effect of filtration on the beam and patient dose.

3. Name one use of a compensating filter.

4. Describe the effect a grid has on radiation dose.

5. List examinations in which opposite projections (e.g., posteroanterior versus anteroposterior) can be used to minimize patient dose.

6. Describe the effect of film/screen combination on patient dose.

7. List means of collimation and their effect on patient dose.

8. Describe the appropriate use of gonadal shielding and types of shields.

9. Describe the value of immobilization and patient instructions in minimizing patient dose.

10. Develop personal means to communicate with the patient.

11. State how minimizing repeats decreases patient dose.

12. List recommendations from NCRP Report No. 102.

13. State the need for certification and education in reducing patient dose.

14. Develop well-constructed responses to patient inquiries regarding radiation dosage.

15. Evaluate means for protecting the pregnant or potentially pregnant patient.

## Important Terms

added filtration
compensating filter
fetal dose
film critique
fixed kVp
flat shield
geometric properties
gonadal shielding
image receptor
immobilization
inherent filtration
milliampere seconds (mAs)
optimum kVp
quality assurance
repeat rate
spectral matching
shadow shield
shaped shield
total filtration
variable kVp

## INTRODUCTION

The foundations of the profession of radiography are production of a diagnostic image and radiation protection of the patient. A variety of basic principles, many of which are under the control of the radiographer, can be used to minimize patient exposure while retaining a diagnostic image.

This chapter will use the term *exposure* as well as *dose*. It should be remembered, however, that the term *dose* is often confusing, as there are many different forms of dose—skin dose, integral dose, depth dose, organ dose, gonadal dose, and so on. After the description of the principles, their effects on exposure will be summarized. In most cases, when a factor is changed that influences patient exposure, it will have an effect on image quality as well. Often these changes work in opposition; that is, what improves image quality also provides additional exposure to the patient. However, in some cases, changes can be made that both improve the quality of the image and minimize patient exposure.

## TECHNIQUE SELECTION

Tube current (milliamperage; mA), time (seconds), and kVp (kilovoltage peak) should be selected in unison to produce an image that is diagnostically acceptable to the physician while maintaining good radiation protection practices. A high kVp is often preferred, but it should not be so high as to degrade image quality through excessively long-scale contrast from an increased amount of scatter reaching the film. Burns (1993) notes that, in general, images with a long scale of contrast produce less patient exposure than an equivalent image with a short scale of contrast. Remember that an increase in kVp does not increase scatter; it increases the amount reaching the film. Most examinations have an optimum kVp setting beyond which the contrast scale is degraded. Do not assume high kVp is always and in all cases good; learn the optimum kVp levels for various parts, part thicknesses, and examinations. In general, kVp changes are not recommended for controlling density, especially when using rare-earth screens.

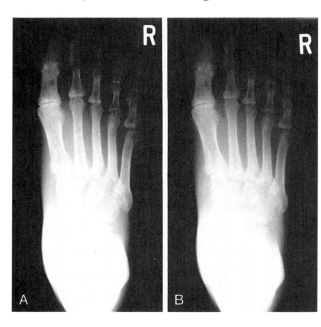

**Figure 11–1** Two films of equivalent density. (*A*) A variable-kVp technique was used. (*B*) A fixed-kVp technique was used.

An example of an incorrect use of high kVp would be using a 90-kVp technique on an intravenous pyelogram. Although this would lower patient exposure, a 90-kVp energy would not be consistent with the attenuation characteristics of iodinated contrast agents. Limiting the diagnostic efficacy while limiting dose is not in accordance with a wise use of risk versus benefit.

Fixed-kVp techniques, as opposed to variable-kVp-technique systems, allow a lower average mAs because kVp values are generally high. For example, equivalent density would be achieved using a fixed-kVp technique of 20 mAs and 80 kVp, whereas a variable-technique chart might require 40 mAs and 68 kVp. Using the fixed-kVp technique would reduce patient dose by about 56 mR. Figure 11–1 shows two radiographs, one using a fixed-kVp technique, the second using a variable-kVp technique. These exhibit equivalent density, with the fixed-kVp technique showing a reduction in patient exposure. Fixed kVp charts are also superior when using rare-earth screens.

Miller (1976) found that the use of 36 mAs and 90 kVp, instead of 75 mAs and 76 kVp, decreased male gonadal dose by 32% and female gonadal dose by 26%. These techniques are approximately equal in terms of overall density.

The relationship between mAs and density and intensity is direct: as mAs is doubled, density and intensity also double. This is due to the fact that doubling the amount of electrons in the tube doubles the amount of electrons that are converted into x-ray at the target. This is stated in a formula as follows:

$$\frac{mAs_1}{mAs_2} = \frac{I_1}{I_2}$$

where:

$mAs_1$ = the first mAs
$mAs_2$ = the second mAs
$I_1$ = the first intensity
$I_2$ = the second intensity

The relationship between kVp and intensity is more complex:

$$\left(\frac{kVp_1}{kVp_2}\right)^2 = \frac{I_1}{I_2}$$

where:

$kVp_1$ = the first kVp
$kVp_2$ = the second kVp
$I_1$ = the first intensity
$I_2$ = the second intensity

This formula states that intensity will increase or decrease as a result of the difference in the square of the kVp change.

If the variable technique of 40 mAs and 68 kVp provides an intensity of 180 mR, the intensity of the second technique can be calculated as follows:

Step 1: The mAs is being halved; therefore, the intensity due to mAs will decrease to half the original value.

$$\frac{mAs_1}{mAs_2} = \frac{I_1}{I_2}$$

$$\frac{40}{20} = \frac{180}{x}$$

$$x = 90 \text{ mR}$$

Step 2: kVp is being increased. Thus, intensity will now increase as follows:

$$\left(\frac{kVp_1}{kVp_2}\right)^2 = \left(\frac{68}{80}\right)^2 = \frac{90}{x}$$

$$x = 124.5 \text{ mR, a total decrease of about 56 mR.}$$

Students wishing further clarification of this topic should refer to Appendix A, which contains some examples of how to work these and other radiation protection problems. Note that this method and other methods presented here are estimates only of exposure calculation.

When manually selecting techniques, the time of exposure should be minimized to keep the degrading effects of motion as low as possible. Tube current (mA) can be increased to compensate in direct proportion. A technique of 200 mA and 0.1 seconds (20 mAs) is equivalent to 400 mA and 0.05 seconds (20 mAs). They provide equivalent density because of the reciprocity law. The reciprocity law basically states that "mAs is mAs"; that is, so long as the products of mA and time are equal, as in the above example, radiographic density also is equal.

When using automatic exposure control devices (AECs), it is important to use a balance between mA and the backup time that will not potentially overexpose the patient. For example, it is unwise to choose 400 mA and 1.0 second backup time for an abdomen. If a malfunction occurs, the patient would receive the full 400 mAs. Assuming that about 40 mAs is necessary, it would be wiser to select 400 mA and 0.5 second to minimize the possibility of grossly overexposing the patient. Some authorities recommend using only 1.5 times the expected mAs.

Another potential disadvantage of AECs is that they are not always as precisely reproducible as manual timing. If positioning is not duplicated exactly for the repeat exposure and the technical setting has been changed (e.g., density setting changed to 1¼), the film may be unacceptable because the amount of tissue over the detector has changed (Figure 11–2).

Some authorities recommend immediately switching to manual techniques when problems arise with AECs. In some European countries, the problem of incorrect positioning with AECs is solved by having the position of the detector show up on the radiograph. This solution, of course, leads to the negative outcome of having an artifact appear on the film.

See Table 11–1 for a summary of the effects of technique selection.

## FILTRATION

### Total Filtration

A filter is a device placed at the x-ray port to absorb low-energy radiation (Figure 11–3) that would not contribute to the diagnostic value of the image since this radiation would be

CORRECT

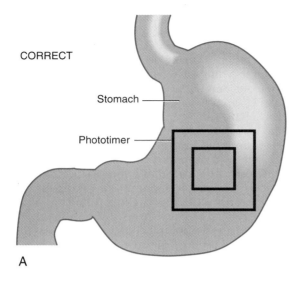

Stomach

Phototimer

A

INCORRECT

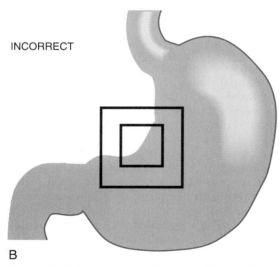

B

**Figure 11–2** Correct (*A*) and incorrect (*B*) use of a phototimer.

glass envelope and the cooling oil surrounding the tube.

Equipment operating at from 50 to 70 kVp must have 1.5 mm of aluminum equivalent total filtration. Equipment operating above 70 kVp must have 2.5 mm of aluminum equivalent total filtration. That amount of filtration will absorb all the photons of 10 keV or less, but only about 20% of those of 50 keV. For general radiography, filtration in excess of 3 mm of aluminum equivalent can be counterproductive, requiring additional exposure to produce a given density. Aluminum is a preferred absorber for filtration in general radiography because of its low atomic number of 13. It will absorb low-energy photons but not high-energy photons.

A study by Trout and colleagues found that, with an 18-cm pelvis, using 85 kVp, entrance skin exposure was 1225 mR without filtration. Intensity was reduced by 77% to 287 mR with the addition of 3 mm of aluminum equivalent filtration. To maintain film density, exposure would have to be increased by only 34%.

Mammography equipment often uses filters of holmium and gadolinium. These filters improve penetration and reduce the mean glandular dose in the dense breast. They remove photons of the lowest *and* highest levels in order to improve image contrast as well. Also, a glass window is not used in mammographic tubes because this would severely diminish contrast. Beryllium, which allows the relatively soft characteristic radiation generated by mammographic tubes to pass through and enhance subject contrast, is used instead. The atomic number of beryllium is 4.

If increases in filtration of the beam are compensated for by an increase in mAs, patient exposure increases if the increase in filtration is 1 mm of aluminum equivalent or less. Instead, the kVp should be increased to maintain image density, which will lower patient exposure. One effective means of reducing exposure to the pediatric patient is adding a copper filter of 0.2 mm and adjusting the kVp.

Increased uses of added filtration are primarily a result of the use of higher speed rare earth screens. Their acceptance in radiology departments has led to a variety of new means of patient protection.

absorbed within the patient. Removing these low-energy photons decreases overall patient skin dose (see below). As filtration is added to a tube, patient dose decreases, given equivalent techniques. Total filtration is a sum of that added to the tube (placed at the x-ray port) and inherent filtration of the tube itself. The components of inherent filtration include the

Table 11–1  Summary of Effects of Technique Selection

| Factor | Effect on Radiation Exposure | Effect on Image Quality |
|---|---|---|
| Increase mAs | → Increase in direct proportion | → Increased density (proportional) |
| Decrease mAs | → Decrease in direct proportion | → Decreased density (proportional) |
| Increase kVp | → Increase not in direct proportion | → Increased density; longer scale proportion of contrast |
| Decrease kVp | → Decrease not in direct proportion | → Decreased density; shorter scale of contrast |
| Increase kVp, decrease mAs using formula | → Decrease | → Density same; longer scale of contrast |

## Compensating Filtration

Compensating filters are used to compensate for variations in patient density. For example, wedge filters (Figure 11–4) are used in foot radiography, with the thick portion of the wedge over the toes and the thin portion toward the heel to provide for even density on the film. Trough filters are often used to even out density differences between the mediastinum and lungs in chest radiography. Figure 11–5 shows a variety of uses of compensating filters for spine radiography.

Correct use of compensating filters can cut the patient's exposure by half by reducing the need for two films. The largest disadvantage of compensating filters is that they cast an artifact onto the film.

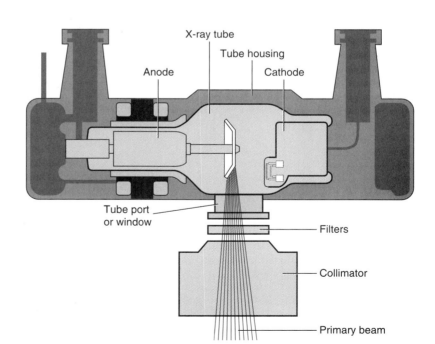

**Figure 11–3** Filtration in the x-ray tube.

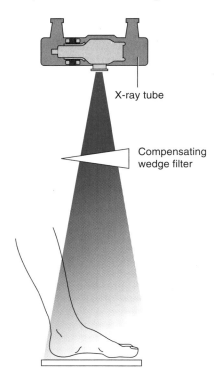

X-ray tube

Compensating
wedge filter

**Figure 11–4** Compensating (wedge) filter.

## More about Filters

Another type of filter is the compound, or K-edge, filter, which places materials of varying atomic numbers from greatest to least atomic number in a row to achieve maximum absorption of low-energy photons. One of these uses rare earth materials to achieve an energy (kVp) that is best suited for iodinated contrast studies.

Because of their absorption characteristics, these types of filters reduce both low- and high-energy photons. This reduces patient contrast and patient skin exposure, a rare combination.

Recently the role of compensating filters in reducing radiation exposure has been explored. Katsuda et al. (1996) compared radiation exposure levels with and without filters in a number of examinations, measuring the actual depth dose at 5 cm. They found that filters reduced exposure by 29% in skull radiography, by 47% in hepatic angiography, and by 80% in lower extremity radiography. This is an interesting line of research that should prove productive to the profession in the future.

**Figure 11–5** *(opposite)* Use of compensating filters for spine radiography. (Used with permission from Nuclear Associates, 100 Voice Road, Carle Place, NY 11514.)

# TYPICAL CLEAR-Pb FILTER POSITIONS

## AP Full-Spine (small to average patient)

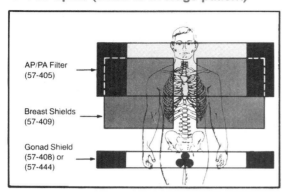

AP/PA Filter
(57-405)

Breast Shields
(57-409)

Gonad Shield
(57-408) or
(57-444)

## AP Full-Spine (large patient)

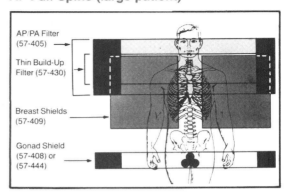

AP/PA Filter
(57-405)

Thin Build-Up
Filter (57-430)

Breast Shields
(57-409)

Gonad Shield
(57-408) or
(57-444)

## Lateral Full-Spine (single exposure)

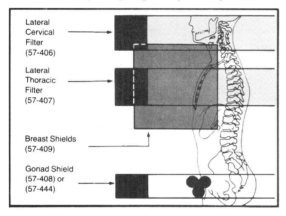

Lateral
Cervical
Filter
(57-406)

Lateral
Thoracic
Filter
(57-407)

Breast Shields
(57-409)

Gonad Shield
(57-408) or
(57-444)

## Lateral Thoracic Spine (sectional view)

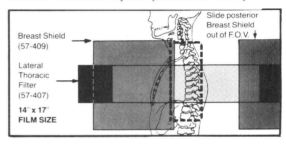

Slide posterior
Breast Shield
out of F.O.V.

Breast Shield
(57-409)

Lateral
Thoracic
Filter
(57-407)

**14" x 17"
FILM SIZE**

## Lateral Cervical Spine (sectional view)

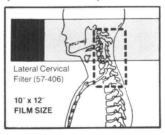

Lateral Cervical
Filter (57-406)

**10" x 12"
FILM SIZE**

## AP Cervical/Thoracic (sectional view)

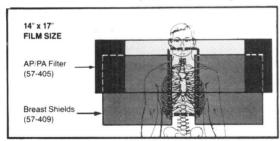

**14" x 17"
FILM SIZE**

AP/PA Filter
(57-405)

Breast Shields
(57-409)

## Lateral Lumbar Spine Including (L5-S1) Interspace (sectional view)

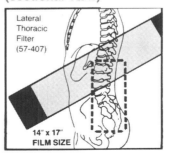

Lateral
Thoracic
Filter
(57-407)

**14" x 17"
FILM SIZE**

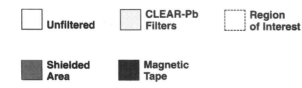

| | Unfiltered | | CLEAR-Pb Filters | | Region of Interest |

Shielded Area

Magnetic Tape

**Table 11–2** Summary of Effects of Filtration

| Factor | | Effect on Radiation Exposure | | Effect on Image Quality |
|---|---|---|---|---|
| Increased total filtration | → | Decreased entrance skin exposure (kVp should be increased to compensate) | → | Maintained* |
| Compensating filters | → | Decreases chances of repeats† | → | Artifact; may give a longer scale of contrast in thicker area of filter |

*It is theoretically possible that filtration can lengthen the scale of contrast.

†Fewer repeats will decrease overall patient exposure.

See Table 11–2 for a summary of the effects of filtration.

## GRIDS

Grids are placed between the patient and image receptor to absorb secondary scatter radiation (Figure 11–6). They are usually used when the thickness of a part exceeds 10 to 13 cm (depending on the preferences of the radiologist). Using a grid requires an increase in technique factors and thus dose; it is not a device to minimize radiation exposure. The factors that cause this increase in dose are summarized in the textbox. Grids do improve image quality by removing unwanted scatter secondary radiation.

If various grid ratios are available, it is the responsibility of the radiographer to choose

**Table 11–3** Average Percentage of Scatter Removed by Various Grid Ratios*

| Grid Ratio | Amount of Scatter Removed |
|---|---|
| 5:1 | 82% |
| 8:1 | 90% |
| 12:1; 16:1 | 96% |

*Varies based on technical and patient factors.

Data from Characteristics and Applications of X-Ray Grids. Cincinnati, Liebel-Flarsheim, 1983.

the lowest possible grid ratio that will reduce scatter yet not require overly high technical factors. Table 11–3 shows the amount of scatter removed by grids of different ratios. One example of how grid choice could lead to radiation protection of the patient would be using an 8:1 grid instead of a 12:1 grid on a child. Because of size, a child might not need as high a grid ratio. In the above change, mAs could be reduced by 20%, with an equivalent density and a 20% reduction in radiation exposure.

The use of an air-gap technique instead of a grid also provides for slightly lower patient dose than a grid technique. The air-gap technique uses an increased object-to-film (object-to-image receptor; OID) distance to remove scatter (Figure 11–7). Often, the SID (source-to-image receptor distance) is increased to overcome magnification. Increasing SID decreases patient exposure. A combination of doubling the SID and using a 6-inch air gap can decrease patient exposure by 70%.

See Table 11–4 for a summary of the effects of grids and air gap.

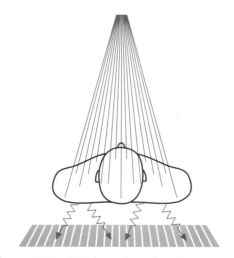

**Figure 11–6** Grid absorption of scatter.

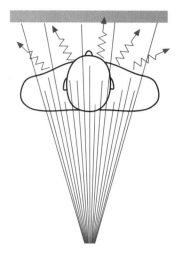

**Figure 11–7** Air-gap technique. Scatter is eliminated from the film through the use of greater object-to-image receptor distance (OID).

**Table 11–4** Summary of Effects of Grids and Air Gap

| Factor | | Effect on Radiation Exposure | | Effect on Image Quality |
|---|---|---|---|---|
| Adding a grid | → | Increased (with increased technique to compensate) | → | Shorter scale of contrast |
| Increasing grid | → | Increased (with increased technique to compensate) | → | Shorter scale of contrast |
| Using air gap | → | Decreased | → | Maintained* |

*Means that the quality of the image should not change.

## More Information:
## Grids' Influence on Exposure

There are many reasons why grids increase exposure, not simply due to the lead. Grids are actually fairly complex in their operation. In the delicate relationship between image quality and patient exposure, the following are important:

1. Grid ratio—as grid ratio increases, patient exposure increases.
2. Bucky (moving) grids absorb about 10% to 15% more radiation than the equivalent stationary grid, and thus require greater exposure.
3. Grid frequency—the density of lead strips. As this increases, relative exposure increases as well.
4. Interspace material—if aluminum is used rather than plastic, about a 20% increase in exposure will be needed. The encasing material for the strips also affects patient exposure; carbon fiber will reduce exposure by about 20%.
5. Selectivity of the grid, based on the grid ratio as well as the amount of lead used. Higher selectivity results, in general, in higher exposures.

## Grids' Influence on Exposure *(Continued)*

The ratio of remnant (image-forming) radiation exiting the patient to that exiting on the film side of the grid is called the Bucky or grid factor, and is often found in physics-based imaging texts. In general, as grid ratio increases the Bucky factor increases, as primary radiation should pass through and scatter radiation is increasingly absorbed with increasing grid ratios. Also, increasing kVp increases the Bucky factor as well. The excess scatter that exits the patient at higher kVp levels should be absorbed by the Bucky.

In addition to the Bucky factor's utility in determining how much additional radiation is required, it can also determine increases in patient exposure. Thus, increasing the Bucky factor increases the technical factors required to produce adequate density as well as patient exposure (Bushong, 1997). However, the concept of Bucky factor has little practical implication in regard to kVp since there are few or no examinations in which we use high-kVp and nongrid techniques. For example, in chest radiography, high-kVp techniques require a grid (standard departmental PA and lateral), whereas portable chest radiography uses low-kVp, nongrid techniques.

## POSITION AND PROJECTION

Certain projections are superior in terms of radiation protection. A 95% reduction in radiation exposure to the lens of the eye (important for preventing potential cataracts) is possible by using the posteroanterior (PA) projection of the cranium over the anteroposterior (AP). In a female patient undergoing an intravenous pyelogram (IVP) or a cystogram, the contrast-filled bladder will serve as a gonadal shield in the AP projection, whereas it will not in the PA projection. Using the PA rather than the AP projection for juvenile scoliosis examinations will reduce exposure to the breasts to 1% of the original value.

Figure 11–8 shows how proper use of collimation and positioning of the patient will reduce gonadal exposure on an upper extremity, an examination that is not typically associated with gonadal exposure, although it certainly can be if done incorrectly. The reduction in gonadal exposure has been cited as anywhere from 50 to 300 times by making such a change.

It has been stated that, because of the position of the AEC in relation to the anatomic parts, centering at T-6 rather than T-4 on a PA chest radiograph exposed with an automatic exposure control will provide a radiograph with a longer scale of contrast, less patient dose, and better visualization of cardiac outlines and fluid levels. This would make an interesting experiment for an energized lab—are the differences noticeable?

If the positions and projections used in the institution employing the radiographer do not make good use of radiation protection practices, it is the responsibility of that individual to *gently lobby* for their use. The term gently lobby means that the radiographer presents to responsible individuals (radiologist, chief technologist, and so forth) the reasons for changing protocol in a manner that shows that the patient is the primary concern. In many cases, this will involve a continued familiarity with the professional literature through continued education and self-directed learning.

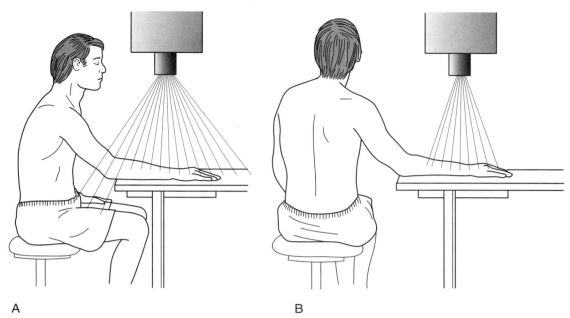

A                                                         B

**Figure 11–8** Effects of body positioning and collimation on gonadal dose. Gonadal dose of *A* is 50 times higher than that for *B*.

## Other Uses of Positions and Projections

Posteroanterior radiography of the chest and sternum is preferred to decrease the exposure to the sternum.

Scapulae are rotated out of view on a PA chest radiograph not only to improve image quality but also to decrease patient dose.

PA projections of the skull and facial bones are preferred to reduce the dose to the lens of the eye. However, image quality must be balanced with radiation protection. A projection such as the PA tangen-tial for the mastoids (Stenvers), which places the part of interest closest to the film, is preferred over the anteroposte-rior tangential (Arcelin) because it is superior from a radiation protection and image quality standpoint.

When working with nonradiologist physi-cians (e.g. on the night shift in the emer-gency department), the radiographer's knowledge of alternate projections can be especially valuable.

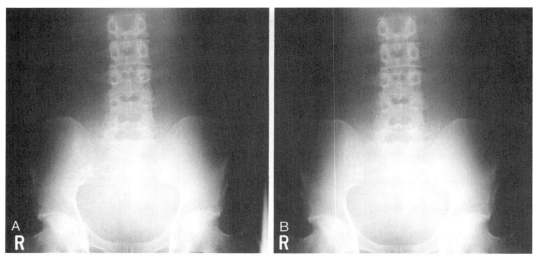

**Figure 11–9** Two anteroposterior radiographs on a phantom, equivalent density. Film *A* used a 100-speed film/screen; film *B* a 400-speed system. The exposure of *B* is 1/4 that of *A*.

## IMAGE RECEPTORS

As the speed of an image receptor increases, the amount of radiation needed to expose the film decreases. In x-ray images, intensifying screens are used to expose film with light and x-ray rather than just x-ray. About 95% of the density on a film is from the light generated by intensifying screens.

On a negative note, as the speed of the film/screen system increases, diagnostic quality decreases. The size of the crystals, the thickness of the layer, and the crystal concentration all influence both the speed and resolution of a screen. The highest possible film/screen combination still able to achieve the needed diagnostic quality should be selected in balance to minimize risk (radiation exposure) and maximize benefit (the quality of the examination).

As an example, changing from a 200-speed to a 400-speed system can decrease radiation exposure in terms of entrance skin exposures by 50%. On an AP abdomen, for example, entrance skin exposure can be reduced by 50%. After selection of peak voltage, the most effective technique for reducing patient dose is the use of faster film/screen combinations that will still allow the radiographer to obtain the desired image quality (Figure 11–9).

A factor also important in radiation protection of the patient, but not often under the control of the radiographer, is the spectral matching of screens and films. That is, if the screens have been designed to emit a certain wavelength of light, the film should be sensitive to that same wavelength. Many departments only have one type of screen speed, which also limits the radiographer's ability to use different film/screen combinations.

Recently, carbon fiber has been increasingly used as a front material for screens. These screens absorb about half as much radiation as conventional fronts, lowering patient dose. This material has also been used successfully in fluoroscopic and CT tabletops, as well as in grid interspace material. Plaut (1993) believes that these materials are of greatest use when used with lower kVp settings (85 and below).

Another relatively new innovation is the use of asymmetric intensifying screens, with slow screens on the front or tube side of a cassette

**Table 11–5** Summary of Effects of Image Receptors

| Factor | | Effect on Radiation Exposure | | Effect on Image Quality |
|---|---|---|---|---|
| Increased speed | → | Decreased (if mAs is decreased to compensate) | → | Decreased detail |
| Decreased speed | → | Increased (if mAs is increased to compensate) | → | Increased detail |
| Improper spectral matching | → | Increased (if mAs is increased to compensate) | → | Decreased |
| Carbon fiber front material | → | Decreased | → | Maintained |
| Asymmetric screens | → | Decreased | → | Increased* |

*An ideal but obviously rare result—less patient exposure and increased image quality.

and fast on the back. These screens have increased resolution as a result of the slow screen, and the fast screen increases the relative speed of the combination. Patient exposure is also reduced.

See Table 11–5 for a summary of the effects of image receptors.

## BEAM LIMITATION (COLLIMATION)

Most modern equipment is fitted with positive beam limitation (PBL), which automatically collimates or limits the beam to the size of the film when using the Bucky grid. However, in 1993 the FDA eliminated the PBL requirement, noting that "PBL is not a substitute for well-trained and supervised operators." Most such equipment allows the radiographer to further minimize the beam size. Proper collimation reduces patient exposure and improves image quality. See Figure 11–10 for an illustration of the differences in scatter due to beam size. Other means of collimation include cones and cylinders (Figure 11–11), which are attached to the tube housing to further limit beam size; aperture diaphragms, which are used for machines that lack collimators (found only on older equipment); and lead blockers and masks, which are placed in the beam to absorb primary and scatter radiation.

Lead blockers are sheets of lead-impregnated rubber. Commonly used with larger patients, they can be placed on the table during an examination of the lateral lumbar spine to absorb scatter produced in the patient's soft tissue. Lead masks (diaphragms), commonly used in cerebral angiography, are often cut to the desired

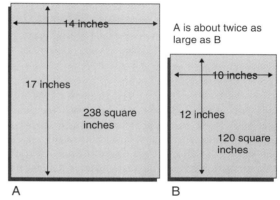

**Figure 11–10** Illustration of differences in scatter due to varying beam sizes. A is 14" × 17" field size (238 square inches), and B is 10" × 12" field size (120 square inches). A is about twice as large as B and will produce about 25% more scatter.

field size and secured to the collimator. These devices do not minimize patient dose directly; they improve the quality of the image, which may decrease the need for repeat exposures.

The area exposed in the body is actually larger than the collimated area shown in the light field. The radiographer must always limit the beam size to just the area of clinical interest. Collimating an exposure of the lumbosacral junction from an 8 × 10-inch field to a 6 × 6-inch field reduces exposure by more than 50%. Only a 2 × 2-inch field is needed for the open-mouth odontoid projection of the cervical spine. If the field is collimated to this size, the grid can be eliminated, decreas-

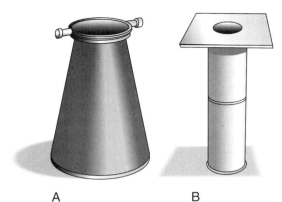

A        B

**Figure 11–11** Cones (*A*) and cylinders (*B*). A cone is preferred when exposing an entire film, since it more closely matches cassette size, limiting patient dose. A cylinder is best used to limit exposure to small, specific areas (e.g., the gallbladder).

ing patient exposure. The radiographer is often the sole individual responsible for correct collimation. This is especially acute when not using the Bucky grid (e.g., mobile radiography), or when using equipment not fitted with PBL. Collimation must be accurate by law to within 2% of the SID. Because proper collimation contributes to both image quality and radiation protection of patient and operator, the beam should always be collimated. In general, as field size increases, density increases and the scale of contrast lengthens.

See Table 11–6 for a summary of the effects of beam limitation.

## SHIELDING

One of the most important means of minimizing the potential effects of radiation exposure on future generations is shielding of the ovaries and testes (gonads). This is important for all individuals of reproductive age and younger. Some facilities recommend that all males, regardless of age, and all females younger than age 65 be shielded. A variety of examinations are associated with high gonadal doses, including barium enema, urography, and examination of the hip, femur, lumbar spine, sacrum, or coccyx. These examinations are also often associated with high bone marrow doses as well, making radiation protection a particular concern.

To minimize patient anxiety associated with radiation exposure, some facilities routinely use gonadal shielding unless it will interfere with the diagnostic quality of the beam. Often, gonadal shielding is an excellent public relations tool even when exposure to the gonads is minimal or nonexistent.

According to FDA recommendations, gonadal shielding should be used when the gonads are within 5 cm (2 inches) of the primary beam unless this would compromise diagnostic quality. It should be noted that improperly (or "sloppily") placed gonadal shielding is of no benefit, and may actually increase radiation exposure by necessitating repeats. According to Seeram (1997), the symphysis pubis is the best landmark to use when placing a gonadal shield on males; for females, the external landmark 2.5 cm medial to the anterior superior iliac spines (ASIS) will provide accurate shield placement for protection of the ovaries.

According to Statkiewicz-Sherer (1993), the correct use of gonadal shielding can result in a decrease of about 50% of the gonadal dose for females, and 90–95% for males. (See Figure 11–12.) Figure 11–13 shows the relationship between gonadal shielding and the dose to male gonads. There are three basic types of gonadal shields. Flat contact shields are usually made of lead-impregnated vinyl and are placed directly over the patient's gonads. They would

**Table 11–6** Summary of Effects of Beam Limitation

| Factor | | Effect on Radiation Exposure | | Effect on Image Quality |
|---|---|---|---|---|
| Collimation and other forms of beam limitation | → | Decreased | → | Increased |

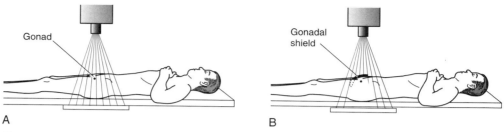

**Figure 11–12** Gonadal shields may be used to absorb up to 99% of the primary beam.

be placed under the patient during fluoroscopic examinations and over the patient for radiographic examinations.

Shaped contact shields are used for male gonadal shielding (Figure 11–14). They are cup-shaped to provide for maximum protection in a variety of settings, although they cannot be used to shield in PA projections.

Shadow shields cast a "shadow" in the beam and are mounted on the tube (Figure 11–15). Shadow shields have some definite advantages over other types. They are relatively easy to use, even when the patient is uncooperative. Also, they do not require the radiographer to touch a patient on or near a "private" area, preserving patient modesty. Finally, they are ideal for use during sterile procedures because the radiographer does not have to insert the shield inside a sterile field. Their main disadvantage is that they cannot be used during fluoroscopy.

Mobile shields, as described for personnel protection in the previous chapter, can also be used in some cases for patient protection. One example is the use of mobile pelvic shields for chest radiography. Although some authorities state that such shields are unnecessary (only about 1 mrad of gonadal dose is received during chest radiography, most of that from internal scatter), shielding as a public relations tool should not be underestimated (see "Tales from the Listservs: Gonadal Protection for PA Chest Radiography?" for a more in-depth discussion on this).

Unless it will interfere with the examination, male gonadal shielding should be used in examinations of pelvis, hip (except obliques),

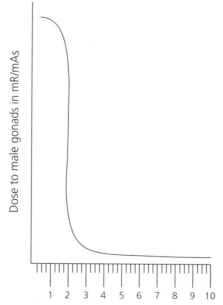

**Figure 11–13** A representation of exposure to male gonads related to the distance between the gonad and the primary beam.

and upper femur. Male gonadal shielding is not usually used on retrograde urethrograms, voiding cystourethrograms, and visualization of the rectum. It is more difficult to provide gonadal shielding to female patients because of the internal nature of the female gonads. One solution is the figleaf shield (Figure 11–16).

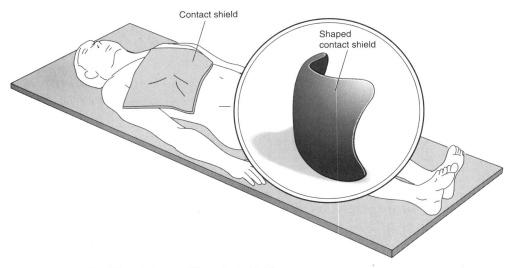

**Figure 11–14** Flat (A) and shaped (B) contact shields.

**Figure 11–15** Shadow shield. (Reprinted with permission from Buyer's Guide, vol 4. Mayfield Village, OH, Picker International, Inc.)

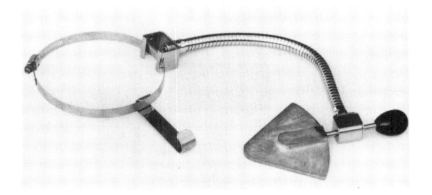

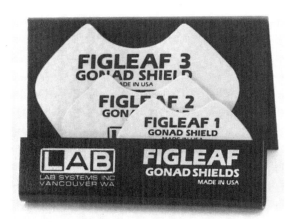

**Figure 11–16** Female figleaf shield. (Reprinted with permission from Buyer's Guide, vol 4. Mayfield Village, OH, Picker International, Inc.)

We have talked extensively about the different types of gonadal shielding and how they are used. Shielding is not the only way to protect gonads. Appropriate collimation of the beam is also a useful and often overlooked way to protect the gonads (refer to Figure 11–8). In the examples below (Figure 11–17), the impact of collimation can clearly be seen. When comparing Figures 11–17A to 11–17B, we see that collimation of the beam used for an abdominal series to exclude the gonads reduces the exposure by 250 times. Comparing Figures 11–17C to 11–17D, we see that proper collimation for a lateral knee reduces gonadal dose by a factor of 30. As can be seen in Figure 11–17E, lack of proper collimation for a chest examination can lead to a 25 times increase in gonadal dose.

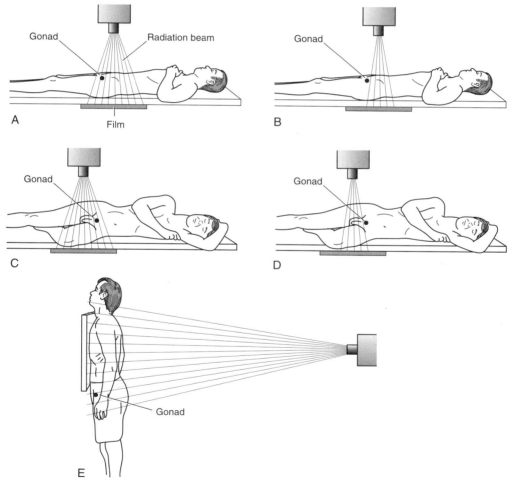

**Figure 11–17** The impact of collimation on gonadal dose. (*A* and *B*) Poor and good collimation for abdomen. (*C* and *D*) Poor and good collimation of extremity. (*E*) Impact of improper collimation for chest radiograph.

Other types of shielding include contact lens shields for the lens of the eye (Figure 11–18) and breast shields for juvenile scoliosis examinations. It has also been suggested that breast shields be used during other examinations (Plaut, 1993) such as examinations of the humerus and shoulder girdle. This might be a particularly acute issue with young females because, as we saw in the radiobiology chapters, the developing and young female breast is the most sensitive to ionizing radiation. Shielding can be used in conjunction with other methods to further minimize exposure; for example, a combination of fast rare earth screens, compensating filters, patient positioning, and breast shields will lower patient dose during juvenile scoliosis radiography. Remember that a shield is effective in protecting the patient only from the primary beam; it does not provide protection from internally generated scatter radiation.

See Table 11–7 for a summary of the effects of shielding.

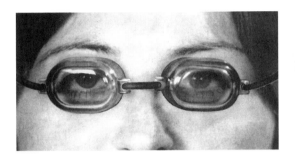

**Figure 11–18** Lens shielding for eyes. (Courtesy of Nuclear Associates, 100 Voice Road, Carle Place, NY 11514.)

**Table 11–7** Summary of Effects of Shielding

| Factor | | Effect on Radiation Exposure | | Effect on Image Quality |
|---|---|---|---|---|
| Shielding | → | Decreased; may also increase patient confidence in the radiographer | → | None if properly used |

## Tales from the Listservs: Gonadal Protection for PA Chest Radiography?

One of the issues that arose in the summer of 1997 on the RadSci Internet listserv was whether gonadal shielding is necessary for PA chest radiography, and if it is, where should it be placed? As can be seen in Table 11–8, chest radiography generates very little gonadal exposure: about a millirad for the male and about half that for a female patient. What are the relevant issues here? Most of the gonadal exposure from a PA chest x-ray, of course, is from internally generated scatter, not the primary beam.

However, it was noted on the listserv that the upright chest unit (Bucky, etc.) provides a certain amount of backscatter that can result in gonadal exposure—thus the question, "Should the gonadal shield be placed in front of the patient then? Or in back?" Of course, x-rays of chests that are taken at 120 kVp should generate less backscatter. Is it more of an issue for males than females, due to the external nature of the former's gonads and thus their increased vulnerability to backscatter? A number of individuals indicated that

## Tales from the Listservs: Gonadal Protection for PA Chest Radiography? (Continued)

they had taken multiple measurements in their facilities or energized labs, and found negligible readings all around. This led some to conclude that no type of shielding at all was necessary. The discussion then fragmented off into whether there were *ever* any circumstances in which one should not shield the patient—including trauma cases.

Although it seems that this discussion came to no conclusion, it educated all on the list and made them think more about shielding—if you are not going to shield, you need to have a good rationale why, and if you are, you need to do so in the way that best benefits the patient. "Sloppy" or improperly applied shielding can be worse than no shielding at all.

**Table 11–8** Representative Exposures for Radiologic Examinations

| Examination | Skin Dose | Gonadal Dose | |
|---|---|---|---|
| | | Male | Female |
| Posteroanterior chest | 10–20 mrad | 1 mrad | <0.5 mrad |
| | 0.1–0.2 mGy | 0.01 mGy | <0.005 mrad |
| Anteroposterior abdomen | 250–400 mrad | 100 mrad | 225 mrad |
| | 2.4–4 mGy | 1 mGy | 2.25 mGy |
| Lateral skull | 100–200 mrad | <0.5 mrad | <0.5 mrad |
| | 1–2 mGy | <0.005 mGy | <0.005 mGy |
| Extremity | 10–200 mrad | | |
| | 0.2–2 mGy | | |
| Lower extremity | | 15 mrad | <0.5 mrad |
| | | 0.15 mGy | <0.005 mGy |
| Upper extremity | | <0.5 mrad | <0.5 mrad |
| | | <0.005 mGy | <0.005 mGy |

## CASE STUDY

Sally Jones, the radiographer in a busy orthopedic office, is responsible for everything regarding radiography there. She is debating with one of the orthopedists about the best way to radiograph a patient for scoliosis—that is, will AP erect or PA erect provide a diagnostic radiograph while keeping the patient's dose low?

The doctor contends that doing the film in the PA erect position will reduce the dose to the breast, especially important in adolescent girls. Sally did it this way for several years, but after acquiring breast shielding, reversed her position and that of the patient.

The AP projection offers the ability to better shield the patient as well as providing less deformity and enlargement of the vertebrae due to dorsal kyphosis, and thus a better image. Although the PA projection might provide a superior protection to the breasts (without shielding), the issue is whether the bone marrow or the breasts are more radiosensitive, and some authorities feel that the bone marrow is more sensitive. The spine in both projections is unshielded, but making the spine the exit point rather than the entrance point for the beam reduces the exposure to the spine from the primary beam.

The issue of scatter is also there; in Sally's estimation, using the AP projection exposes the breasts to more of the forward-directed primary beam and reduces their scatter exposure. Of course, her choice also increases the scatter exposure to the spine, but this may be counterbalanced by making the spine the exit, rather than the entry point, for the primary beam.

Like most clinical practice issues, there is no one right answer here. Given the evidence presented here, which method would you lobby for? Is there additional evidence that needs to be considered?

## CASE STUDIES: "BUT IT WORKS!"

Are there technologists who "can't be bothered" with radiation protection? Certainly, although fortunately they are few in number. We have noted, though, in recent years, with the trend to more automated equipment, that there are technologists who never learned or who have forgotten some of the radiation protection implications of the actions they perform. Let's look at a very bad day in the life of Wanda Jones, a radiography student on clinicals at Heaven Help Me Hospital.

### Case 1

Having recently learned about kVp and mAs, and their effect on image density and exposure, Wanda asks a portable technologist about the mAs that should be used on a computed radiography (CR) system using photostimulable phosphor plates (PSPs). "It doesn't matter!," he brags. "You can use one thousand mAs if you want," and promptly proceeds to do so. He then shows her how one can postprocess just about any image to get an acceptable film.

Of course, if this film would normally have required 100 mAs (a very large amount), using 1000 mAs would expose the patient to ten times the amount of radiation normally used, and although one certainly can postprocess these images to make them acceptable, as Burns (1993) notes, such systems are designed to handle changes of plus or minus 30%. Even though gross density can be altered, techniques 30% above the needed exposure will show excess scatter and thus long-scale contrast. Techniques more than 30% below the needed exposure will show excess quantum mottle.

Some technologists use this to justify overexposing images—after all, most radiologists will accept a radiograph that has slightly longer scale contrast more readily than a mottled radiograph—but technologists should still know manual techniques for such images to provide proper radiation protection and optimal image quality.

### Case 2

Late, Wanda proceeds to "swap out" the grid normally found in the upright Bucky (which is focused for 48″ to 72″) for one focused for 36″ to 40″ for an upright abdomen. "We don't have time for that," the technologist exclaims, "we'll just use that grid!" As Wanda then says, "Well, won't we get grid . . . ," asking about cutoff, the technologist anticipates her question, and states, "The phototimer will take care of that! Didn't your instructors teach you anything about phototimers?" Warner's (1998) research clearly showed that even phototimed exposures will show losses in optical density when the wrong grid is used (improperly focused); he also found that such images could show both losses in optical density and increases in patient exposure. Thus, one could get a "bad film" and overexpose the patient, and probably have to expose the patient again, probably using even higher density settings.

## Case 3

Wanda is trying to collimate to the best of her ability on a PA chest radiograph. "Get back here," the technologist yells, "I want to get to my break!" When Wanda gets back to the control panel, the technologist (mercifully enough, in a low voice this time so the patient can't hear) says, "What the heck were you doing?" Wanda tries to explain that since this was a large patient, she was having some trouble collimating properly, and her teacher had told her last week that proper collimation was the best way to get a good film and provide a low dose. "When a patient is that fat," the technologist says, "there is no way you will get an optimal film, and her size is the main factor that will increase her dose!"

Later, on another large patient, the same technologist gets a light radiograph. She keeps increasing the density settings—first to 1¼, then to 1½, and so on. Eventually, it dawns on her to try manual techniques. "Where is that chart?" she says with an exasperated tone, "I know we have one here somewhere!" Unable to find it, she writes, "machine malfunctioned repeatedly" on the requisition and sends the patient to another room.

In reality, the research of Chu, Parry, and Eaton (1998) showed that patient exposure only weakly correlated with size, and that, as they state, "the effective dose and therefore the radiation risk can be reduced by limiting the radiographic field size." Thus, it is not a foregone conclusion that a large patient must have a poor film and an increased dose.

Also, automated exposure systems still require occasional manual techniques, and every technologist should know those techniques and know the locale of the technique charts when an automated exposure fails. It is the policy of some departments that, when an automated technique fails, the technologist must take all repeats using manual techniques—a good practice since it is often difficult to isolate the problem (e.g., has the phototimer "drifted" in this case?—there are many possibilities), and since many automated exposure problems must be fixed by a service engineer.

## Case 4

Even later that same bad day, Wanda is working with another technologist who is getting ready to do an abdominal x-ray on a very obese patient. The technologist grouses that all abdomen film on this patient were going to be "just awful. I don't even know why they bother to order these examinations" continues the technologist, "the images are so gray that you can't see anything! Not only that, but the radiologists almost always make me repeat the film two or three times."

Wanda notices that the technologist has overridden the recommended abdominal kVp setting of 80 for large patients and raised it to 105 kVp. When asked why, the technologist informed Wanda that higher kVp was necessary to "get through" such a large patient, it reduced the chance of motion because the automatic timer would shut off quicker, and besides, it lowered the patient's dose.

The technologist was correct in stating that increasing the kVp reduces the chance of motion and tends to lower the patient's dose. However, in this case, it has the exact opposite effect because of the need for repeat exposures. When a large body part or large patient is exposed, more scatter and secondary radiation is produced than with a thinner body part or patient. This can significantly reduce the contrast and, consequently, the visibility of the radiograph's information because of fog formation. It is rarely necessary to increase the kVp above the recommended "optimum" levels in order to penetrate. Doing so increases the likelihood of needing a repeat exposure because the first image was not diagnostic.

Although Wanda's stories are of course far beyond the norm, and we hopefully have no hospital like Heaven Help Me Hospital, these examples show how technologists who don't stop to think can consistently overexpose patients.

## IMMOBILIZATION

Immobilization is sometimes needed to prevent the image-degrading effects of voluntary motion. Another type of motion, involuntary (physiologic) motion of organs, is best handled by shortening the time of exposure. For example, cardiac motion of the heart is best handled on chest radiographs by using a short time of exposure in conjunction with a high mA setting.

Far superior to immobilization is the use of effective communication (described in the next section) and positioning aids such as sandbags, angle sponges, foam pads, and the radiographer's standby, tape. Caution must be taken to not exercise more restraint than an adult patient is willing to allow. Some patients are allergic to tape, so it is best to use hypoallergenic tape with the sticky side twisted so that it is not in contact with the skin. On pediatric patients, sheets, towels, compression bands, and tape all also make excellent immobilizers.

However, patients unable to cooperate must be immobilized. The patient's ability to cooperate must be ascertained by the radiographer, who will then decide on appropriate means of immobilization. An adult may be unable to hold the forearm still and may need sandbags applied to each end of the arm to prevent image-degrading motion. Obviously, a 6-month-old infant will be unable to cooperate and may need immobilization in the form of a Hugger (Figure 11–19) for examinations.

The radiographer should ascertain the patient's ability to cooperate by evaluating the following factors:

* Patient's ability to hold still for the exposure
* Patient's ability to follow instructions

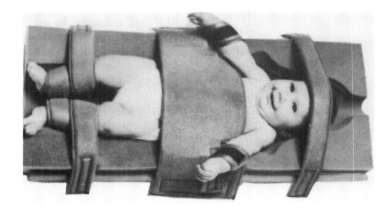

**Figure 11–19** Hugger immobilizer. (Reprinted with permission from Buyer's Guide, vol 4. Mayfield Village, OH, Picker International, Inc., p 212.)

Table 11–9  Summary of Effects of Immobilization

| Factor | | Effect on Radiation Exposure | | Effect on Image Quality |
|---|---|---|---|---|
| General immobilization | → | Decreases chances for repeat exposures | → | Increased |
| Compression band | → | Decreased | → | Increased |

- Type of examination (e.g., it is more difficult to hold still for a lateral decubitus abdomen than for an AP supine position)

Since assistance often is needed for patients who may need immobilization, it is best to determine these factors in consultation with another radiographer if possible. This helps to ensure that all options are considered.

Human immobilizers are the last resort. Radiographers are the last choice for holding patients, and no one should be responsible for routinely holding patients. Relatives, especially males, are the first choice for holding patients. Males are the first choice because they cannot be pregnant. After that, nonradiology hospital personnel, such as patient transporters, are the next choice over other radiology personnel.

Human immobilizers must be provided with shielding, minimally lead aprons and gloves. They should wear a monitoring device. The ICRP also recommends that the individual holding be older than the normal reproductive age. The ideal device for "guests" would be a pocket dosimeter. If this is not available, the procedure and the specific exposures should be documented. Also, take the time to explain some of the basic principles of personnel protection to the individual assisting in immobilization. This display of professional concern will be appreciated and will be helpful if problems arise in the future.

One positive aspect of immobilization is the use of compression bands in abdominal radiography. This results in less tissue density and less scatter radiation, which minimizes patient dose and gives a more appropriate scale of contrast. A few words of caution are appropriate here, however. There are definite possible legal ramifications to using a restraint device such as a compression band. Patient consent should be secured before restraining the patient. Also, the

patient should not be left alone or in the erect position because of problems that may result, such as patient falls. A compression band, when used for restraint, should never be the sole restraining device.

See Table 11–9 for a summary of the effects of immobilization.

## PATIENT INSTRUCTIONS

It is extremely important that the patient who is able to cooperate be allowed to do so. Experienced radiographers know the value of securing patient cooperation and the extent to which this minimizes the need for repeat examinations. Taking a few extra seconds to secure patient cooperation and consent and to instill a sense of trust in the radiographer can easily save the radiographer 15 minutes on repeat films. In fact, securing cooperation and communicating with the patient should be the first rule of radiography.

Radiographers need to adopt a professional approach to patient instruction giving, which involves a combination of visible technical competence, a caring, patient-oriented attitude, and effective communication skills. The following activities will establish a communication process that will facilitate patient cooperation:

- *Listen effectively.* Always listen first. Moving through an examination without listening can cause patient resentment and a loss of cooperation.
- *Use appropriate vocabulary.* Some patients may not understand more complicated terms. On the other hand, talking down to patients will minimize cooperation. For example, individuals with a college education would resent being told that they are here for a "picture of their tummy."
- *Organize your thoughts.* The radiographer

Table 11–10  Summary of Effects of Patient Instructions

| Factor | Effect on Radiation Exposure | Effect on Image Quality |
|---|---|---|
| Proper patient instructions $\rightarrow$ | Increases patient cooperation $\rightarrow$ | Possible decrease in repeats |

should have a preplanned routine that can be altered as needed. Never ramble or appear to be unprepared for the patient. On the other hand, it is easy to allow rehearsed explanations to sound too impersonal.

• *Use appropriate voice tone and volume.* Experienced radiographers know that some elderly patients become uncooperative when spoken to in a loud voice because they resent the assumption that they are deaf. Other patients may resent a health care worker they find acts too familiar or "chipper," and thus, by assumption, unprofessional.

Patients have the right to refuse examinations (with certain exceptions such as minors and individuals who have had their civil rights removed), but the radiographer cannot advocate refusal to the patient. Advocating refusal may be seen as diagnosis by indicating that the patient does not need the examination, which is not within the scope of practice of a radiographer (see Chapter 1). On the other hand, the radiographer must support patient decisions to not have an examination. This is a delicate balance.

The radiographer may, first of all, question the validity of the request for the examination with the appropriate personnel involved in the care of the patient. In many cases, this is in the patient's best interest. For example, the patient may have pain in the right wrist but a left wrist radiograph was ordered. In this case, the referring physician, the radiologist, or the nurse assigned to the patient may be questioned as to the validity of the request. Other examples include radiographs ordered for malpractice or "placebo" purposes, or when a series of radiographs are ordered—for example, a hand, wrist, and forearm when there is evidence only of wrist pain.

This obligation also extends into additional views. Radiographers often know of additional views, based on their training, that would better visualize certain anatomic structures. A radiographer cannot simply perform these views but may indicate to the patient's personal physician or the radiologist that such a view may be of value. Since this involves exposing the patient to more films, with the resultant increase in exposure, this responsibility should never be taken lightly.

Second, the radiographer may provide the patient with information that indicates that the benefits of diagnostic examinations tend to outweigh the risks (e.g., the information relative to patient doses given in this chapter and earlier ones). Don't overdo it, however; just provide information relevant and understandable to the patient. Probably the most important piece of information to the patient is the radiographer's credibility as a certified, competent professional who understands both the needs of the patient and the proper use of equipment to produce a diagnostic film. This is discussed in more detail in Chapter 14.

See Table 11–10 for a summary of the effects of patient instructions.

## REPEAT EXPOSURES

An "average" repeat rate for radiographs ranges from about 4% to 15%, although authorities give a variety of rates. Many factors influence repeat rate, including the experience level of the radiographer and the radiologist's view of image quality. The purpose of a departmental quality assurance program is to reduce repeats and to improve image quality. Abdominal and thoracic or lumbar spine radiographs are usually cited as the source of the most repeats, although some authorities cite chest radiography. This again depends on the experience level of the radiographer.

An analysis of 49 studies by Adler, Carlton, and Wold (1992) found that the mean repeat rate was 8%. Exposure errors accounted for about half of all repeats, with positioning errors accounting for just under 30%. Motion was an infrequent cause of repeat films, although it is often thought to be a major cause of repeats.

It is particularly important to analyze repeats by type of examination. For example, abdominal examinations are a common area for repeats. They also are examinations that tend to provide higher bone marrow and gonadal doses, as mentioned earlier. Thus, they should form as few repeats as possible; any departmental repeat analysis and follow-up (continuous quality improvement) program should seek to determine the causes for such repeats and how they can be minimized.

A very low repeat rate can indicate a highly competent staff; however, it also might indicate that poor-quality films are being passed. For example, some departments have radiographers with long job tenures of 10 years or more; such a department might have a repeat rate of 3%. However, in some departments, overexposed and underexposed films are kept, even if repeated, because some radiologists believe that these films still contain some diagnostic information. In that case, the reported repeat rate will be artificially low. Repeat rates in specialized areas such as mammography are much lower than those in general radiography (2–5%).

Repeat exposures due to improper film processing, poor positioning, improper exposure factors, and poor patient instruction are under the control of the radiographer. In line with risk-versus-benefit analysis, radiographs should be repeated only when the quality of the film is unacceptable. For example, although not marking or improperly marking films is contrary to professional practice, it is not grounds for exposing a patient for another film.

Film critique is a method to determine the acceptability of a film. Ultimately, proper use of film critique reduces patient dose. Although the radiographer never attempts to diagnose, to produce the best possible image for the radiologist, the radiographer must understand the needs of the radiologist in terms of a diagnostic image. The basic signs used by the radiologist to determine pathology on a radiograph are:

- Alterations in size of organ
- Alterations in number
- Changes in density
- Changes in shape from normal
- Changes in position from normal
- Changes in internal and external environment
- Alterations in organ functioning
- Changes with respect to time (sequential radiographs)
- Changes due to treatment

Film critique for the radiographer involves the use of critical thinking skills and technical knowledge. Together, these constitute creative thinking on the part of the radiographer—the use of logic and technical knowledge to solve a patient problem.

A technologist performing radiography must be attuned to a variety of image factors. For example, are changes seen in the regular 6 A.M. portable chest x-ray on a patient in the intensive care unit due to pathology, patient improvement, or improper technique? In trauma radiography, Drafke (1990) has applied educational principles of critical thinking and problem solving to film evaluation:

- *Define the problem.* What are the constraints or limitations? Why did the usual solution (method) not work?
- *List alternatives.* List all the possibilities without judging them. List the opposite for each: many problems that cannot be solved in one way can be solved by turning the image 180 degrees.
- *Evaluate each.* Look for things that would make a solution work or would prevent a solution from working.
- *Select the best solution and try it.*
- *Critique the results.* If it worked, make a note of it. If it did not work, find out why, reevaluate the method for the remaining alternatives, and try again.

The above can work well for all types of radiography. In terms of potential problems, there are four basic signals to which the radiographer must be attuned when critiquing the image:

- Photographic properties such as density and contrast and factors that affect these

Table 11–11 Summary of Effects of Repeat Exposures

| Factor | Effect on Radiation Exposure | Effect on Image Quality |
|---|---|---|
| Fewer repeats → | Fewer repeats will decrease overall patient exposures → | Fewer repeats will improve film quality |

properties such as selection of mA, time, kVp, SID, grids, and beam restrictors.

- Geometric properties are well represented through the appropriate use of factors such as SID, object-to-film distance, focal spot size, and alignment of part, film, and beam.
- Positioning demonstrates the anatomy required; projections meet standard evaluation criteria; markers and collimation are evident.
- Equipment malfunction. The radiographer should be able to suspect possible equipment malfunctions (as opposed to, for example, improper technique selection) to report to the appropriate individual.

Combining the above gives a film critique process that, in a step-by-step manner, would go as follows:

1. The radiographer always evaluates the entire image.
2. The image is evaluated in terms of photographic and geometric properties, positioning, and possible equipment problems.
3. The image is accepted, or causes for the substandard image are theorized.
4. This theory is tested.
5. From these tests of theory, the most plausible causes are accepted.
6. The image is repeated with appropriate corrective factors.

Proper use of film critique is one important means by which the radiographer can ensure diagnostic quality and patient radiation safety. The radiographer with an understanding of why films need to be repeated and with the knowledge to correct the factors that lead to substandard films will provide the best possible films at the lowest possible patient dose.

See Table 11–11 for a summary of the effects of repeat exposures.

## EQUIPMENT

The radiographer should report all equipment problems as soon as possible. The radiographer may also be involved in quality assurance checks of equipment. For some procedures, a medical radiation physicist assesses the radiation safety characteristics of the machine. One study found that in a 1-year period the output of about one third of the fluoroscopic machines studied varied by as much as 100%. This is, it is hoped, no longer true with mandatory state inspections of radiology equipment.

Many states have a variety of equipment regulations and recommendations for safe practice. For example, the Illinois Department of Nuclear Safety recommends that all operators of equipment be aware of the following operational controls and emergency procedures:

- Emergency off switch/electrical power switch
- Source-to-image distance indicator and beam-limitation devices
- Proper operation of the beam-on indicator
- The recommended manufacturer's operating procedures

At the national level, the Safe Medical Devices Act of 1990 requires radiographers to report any accidents caused by the malfunctioning of equipment. Radiographers may also report the "potential danger" of apparently defective equipment anonymously to the Food and Drug Administration. Since civil penalties can be as high as $15,000 for each violation, radiographers who report apparently defective equipment to their supervisor and see no response may wish to consider this route.

Processor maintenance and proper darkroom procedure, including the proper balance of time, temperature, and replenishment, help to keep patient doses low, although it is not usually possible to increase these factors to minimize patient dose. A study by Burns and Turner (1983) indicated that decreased processor activity could increase patient exposure by three times as much as it would be under normal conditions. Also, the darkroom must be kept light-tight, and safelight illumination must be enough for viewing but not enough to fog the film. These types of quality control are often seen only as affecting image quality; they also affect exposure to the patient.

Some authorities claim that using three-phase equipment, because it allows for production of a higher average kVp, will result in radiation protection of the patient. That is, higher average kVp techniques result in lower patient dose. Others (e.g., Carlton and Adler) claim that, once techniques are adjusted for, there is no appreciable difference in the exposure dose. This issue was also discussed in Chapter 2.

Equipment and some other recommendations are listed in Table 11–12, which reviews some of the material presented in Chapter 9 as

| Table 11–12  Summarized Recommendations from NCRP Report No. 102 | |
|---|---|
| Thickness of fluoroscopic curtain | 0.15 mm Pb equivalent |
| Maximum tabletop thickness over Bucky tray | 1 mm Al equivalent |
| Maximum fluoroscopic tabletop exposure rate | 10 R/min |
| Minimum thickness of fluoroscopic aprons | 0.5 mm Pb equivalent |
| Minimum thickness of gloves | 0.25 mm Pb equivalent |
| Minimum source-to-skin distance for mobile equipment | 30 cm (12 inches) |
| Posting of a warning sign | 5 mR/hr |
| Maximum leakage radiographic tube housing | 100 mR/hr at 1 m |

well. See Table 11–13 for a summary of the effects of equipment.

### Table 11–13  Summary of Effects of Equipment

| Factor | | Effect on Radiation Exposure | | Effect on Image Quality |
|---|---|---|---|---|
| Improperly calibrated equipment | → | Increase either directly or through additional repeats | → | Decreased |
| Improper use of processing | → | Increase | → | Decreased or maintained |

### More Information:
### The Pursuit of Quality and Protecting the Patient

Quality management (QM) refers to all efforts to bring about quality in an institution. The term *quality assurance (QA)* is rarely used anymore, as it is difficult to assure quality; more commonly the term *continuous quality improvement (CQI)* is used. CQI programs in hospitals typically are geared toward the pursuit of customer satisfaction. The maintenance of technical quality in the radiology department is called *quality control (QC)*. CQI and QC are not wholly separate; they are interrelated and together compose a comprehensive program of quality management.

The primary goal of a radiology QC program is to enhance accurate diagnosis (Seeram, 1997). However, an associated goal is to reduce radiation dose. The primary

## More Information:
## The Pursuit of Quality and Protecting the Patient (Continued)

means by which QC programs reduce patient dose is through the elimination of unnecessary repeats; however, QC also optimizes the operation of equipment. The dose reduction of a comprehensive QC program was estimated by Cohen (1985) as reducing the mean whole-body dose equivalent by half.

There are a number of guidelines for QC in radiology. The most authoritative in the US is NCRP Report No. 99, *Quality Assurance for Diagnostic Imaging Equipment*. The guidelines are summarized below.

| Section | Area | Limits |
|---------|------|--------|
| 7.1.1 | HVL | minimum of 2.3 mm Al at 80 kVp |
| 7.1.2 | Light/beam congruency | ±2% of SID |
| | CR alignment | ±2% of SID |
| | PBL/cassette congruency | <3% of SID |
| | Beam area indicator on collimator | ±2% of SID |
| 7.1.3 | SID indicators | ±2 % of SID |
| 7.2.2 | kVp | ±3 kVp accuracy for cassette measurement |
| | | ±2 kVp accuracy for electronic measurement |
| | | ±0.5 kVp reproducibility for electronic measurement |
| 7.2.3 | Timers | ±5% accuracy electronic measurement |
| | | ±1 dot accuracy for manual measurement above 1/20 sec |
| | | ±0 dots accuracy for manual measurement 1/20 sec and down |
| 7.2.6 | mA linearity | ±10% between adjacent stations and ±50% overall |
| 7.2.7 | mA reproducibility | ±5% |
| 7.3.1 | Grid uniformity | ±10% variation in density anode to cathode |
| 7.3.2 | Grid alignment | Highest density on exposure centered to midline |

## PATIENT DOSES

The radiographer should be familiar with estimated doses of representative examinations. Since the radiographer is able to control factors that lead to this dosage and patients may be interested in their exposure, this information is valuable to the professional.

Patients vary greatly in the amount of infor-

mation they want to know about their examination. Often, the trigger to wanting more information is a recent television program or magazine article on the hazards of radiation. Sometimes college students have recently covered the topic of radiation exposure in a course and want to know more out of curiosity, not resistance to an examination. Never confuse curiosity with refusal of an examination.

The radiographer's not knowing the information or appearing incompetent may make the patient have second thoughts about the examination, however.

A variety of means exist to inform patients about the doses they receive. In some departments, this information is released only by the radiologist or physicist. In any case, the radiographer should know what type of information is to be provided to patients about dose and who provides it to the patient, as well as representative dose values for professional use. Some of these values are listed in Table 11–8. Table 11–14 lists some ranges of expected patient entrance exposures based on data collected in Washington state (Warner, 1993).

Some advocate informing patients of their dose in a variety of equivalencies. For example, a chest x-ray can be compared to a certain number of hours in the sun. The value of doing this is not fully clear—it can cause as much misunderstanding as clarification. Patients may not want to know the specific information; in some cases they may just want to be sure that the individual performing their examination knows the amount of radiation produced by a certain examination. These issues are discussed in greater detail in Chapter 14.

There is a growing trend to measure and record patient doses as part of dose reduction programs. All institutions accredited by the Joint Commission on Accreditation of Healthcare Organizations (JCAHO) must monitor doses from diagnostic radiology procedures. Many states also have requirements on acceptable ranges of exposures, typically for representative examinations such as chest, abdomen, and so on. Finally, the Center for Devices and Radiological Health (CDRH) recommends that diagnostic radiology facilities be aware of the amount of radiation received by a patient. If these exposures do not fall into acceptable levels, appropriate action must be undertaken.

The entrance skin exposure (ESE) for radiographic projections is a common method of calculating patient dose and can be estimated by using a digital dosimeter (ionization chamber). The dosimeter is exposed using the technique required for a certain project. The following formula will calculate an estimated ESE dose:

**Table 11–14  Ranges of Expected Patient Entrance Exposures***

**AP supine abdomen**

| | |
|---|---|
| Upper quartile | 4 mGy (400 mrad) |
| Median | 3 mGy (300 mrad) |
| Lower quartile | 2.5 mGy (250 mrad) |

**PA upright chest @ 115 kVp and grid**

| | |
|---|---|
| Upper quartile | 0.20 mGy (20 mrad) |
| Median | 0.16 mGy (16 mrad) |
| Lower quartile | 0.12 mGy (12 mrad) |

**PA upright chest @ 80 kVp, nongrid**

| | |
|---|---|
| Upper quartile | 0.12 mGy (12 mrad) |
| Median | 0.08 mGy (8 mrad) |
| Lower quartile | 0.05 mGy (5 mrad) |

**AP supine lumbar spine**

| | |
|---|---|
| Upper quartile | 4.5 mGy (450 mrad) |
| Median | 3.5 mGy (350 mrad) |
| Lower quartile | 2.7 mGy (270 mrad) |

**AP cervical spine**

| | |
|---|---|
| Upper quartile | 1.1 mGy (110 mrad) |
| Median | 0.8 mGy (80 mrad) |
| Lower quartile | 0.5 mGy (50 mrad) |

**PA and lateral knees, with 8:1 grid**

| | |
|---|---|
| Upper quartile | 0.30 mGy (30 mrad) |
| Median | 0.20 mGy (20 mrad) |
| Lower quartile | 0.10 mGy (10 mrad) |

**AP and lateral forearm, with 100-speed detail screens**

| | |
|---|---|
| Upper quartile | 0.25 mGy (25 mrad) |
| Median | 0.18 mGy (18 mrad) |
| Lower quartile | 0.10 mGy (10 mrad) |

*Based on data collected in Washington state.

From Warner R: Using Technique Factors to Predict Patient ESE. Radiol Technol 65(1):25, 1993. Used by permission.

$$\frac{\text{Dosimeter exposure (mR)}}{\text{ESE (mR)}} = \frac{\text{SSD}^2}{\text{SDD}^2}$$

where:

SSD = source-to-skin distance
SDD = source-to-detector distance

The SSD is calculated for Bucky techniques by subtracting the sum of the part thickness and the distance from part to film from the source-to-image distance (SID). For tabletop techniques, it is simply the SID minus the part thickness.

For Bucky techniques, the SDD is calculated by subtracting the sum of the detector thickness and the detector-to-film distance from the SID. For a tabletop technique, it is the SID minus the detector thickness.

From the ESE, tissue doses may be calculated with the computer program described in Chapter 4. Remember that these are estimates or approximations of dose. Another means of approximating patient dose is through the Du Pont Bit System of technical factor selection. For more information on the Bit System, contact E.I. Du Pont DeNemours at 1-800-527-2601. The excellent article by Warner (1998) also indicates how nomograms (a graph plotting the range of exposure rates [mR/mAs] as a function of beam filtration, kVp, and anode-to-skin distance) can be used to predict patient ESE. An example of a similar type of graph is also found in the section "Protecting Children." Knowing the mR/mAs of a machine is an extremely valuable tool for a radiographer—then when questions are asked about exposure, it is relatively simple to calculate the ESE. For example, if the mR/mAs at 70 kVp is 1.5, then a technique of 20 mAs and 70 kVp provides an ESE to the patient of 30 mR.

## CERTIFICATION AND EDUCATION

As professionals, radiographers should only engage in performing procedures for which they have received education, are certified, and in some cases have received specialized training. The ICRP (1982) has stated that the operation of radiologic equipment requires "technical competence," as well as "adequate knowledge of the physical properties and harmful effects of ionizing radiation." Such knowledge is achieved through formal training, not quick "OJT." Various reports have shown the value of training in radiation protection to the patient. For example, it has been found that radiographers who voluntarily engaged in continuing education were more likely to provide radiation protection to patients.

Another study found that limited radiography in small-practice settings as performed primarily by nurses led to a 55% rejection rate by radiologists. Although only 18% of these radiographs were completely undiagnostic, it stands to reason that patients should be provided only with films that are completely diagnostic. These rates are much higher than those seen even with novice radiographers.

Wochos and Cameron found that, except in the case of chest radiography, certified radiographers delivered significantly lower exposures to patients. The variance in chest radiography was due to the fact that radiographers used grids much more often than untrained operators (look back at Table 11–15 for a comparison of high-kVp, grid versus low-kVp, nongrid chest radiography). Additionally, radiographers practiced collimation better, further lowering patient dose.

The purpose of state licensing of radiographers and voluntary certification by the American Registry of Radiologic Technologists (ARRT) is to ensure that patients are provided with competent practitioners able to protect the patient from excess radiation. The overall effect is to increase the health of the population.

Student radiographers engaged in a program accredited by the Joint Review Committee on Education in Radiologic Technology (JRCERT) are taking advantage of a system of education that does not stop at training them in proper methods of positioning and exposure for good diagnostic films. They also learn the why of their practice through courses in radiologic physics, radiobiology, and pathology (to name but a few); the ethical value of providing radiation protection to the patient; and the long-term value of continuing to learn imaging and patient care throughout their career.

It only stands to reason that the best mammographers, for example, are those who undertake additional training and experience in this area and who attempt to become certified as advanced practitioners in this field through the ARRT examination in mammography. Recently the ARRT also began offering other examinations, including one in quality management (QM) that stresses the role of the technologist in providing quality imaging. In the long run, it is the patient who benefits the most from this process.

**Table 11–15** Summary of Effects of Certification and Education

| Factor | | Effect on Radiation Exposure | | Effect on Image Quality |
|---|---|---|---|---|
| Radiographer certified by ARRT | → | Decreased | → | Increased* |
| Radiographer engaged in continued education specific to radiography | → | Decreased | → | Increased* |

*Two additional rare examples of decreased patient exposure with increased image quality. No amount of physical resources can, at this time, replace a radiographer skilled in radiation protection. It is still the person operating the equipment, not the equipment, that is of greatest importance.

See Table 11–15 for a summary of the effects of certification and education.

## THE PREGNANT OR POTENTIALLY PREGNANT PATIENT

As noted earlier, at low doses (below 1 rad [0.01 Gy]), the risk to the fetus is considered minimal to nonexistent. For patients, who may receive upward of 1 rad (1 cGy), the risk is greater. Still, NCRP Report No. 54, *Medical Radiation Exposure of Pregnant and Potentially Pregnant Women* considered the risk of 5 rad to be negligible when compared with other risks of pregnancy, with the risk of malformation increasingly significant above 15 rad (cGy). This report concluded that radiation exposure is rarely cause for terminating a pregnancy. These cases require a variety of considerations. The most vulnerable time for the fetus is from the 10th day to the 10th week after conception. Some women might consider abortion with a fetal exposure of 25 rad (0.25 Gy) 4 weeks after conception. Others would never consider such an option. Certainly, a dose of 5 rad (0.05 Gy) in the 20th week would rarely suggest termination of a pregnancy. Baker and Dalrymple believe that three pieces of information must be gathered before a decision to terminate a pregnancy can be made:

1. The exact gestational time of radiation exposure must be known.
2. A reasonably accurate estimate of fetal dose is needed.
3. A variety of patient factors such as the age and general health of the patient and attitude toward pregnancy and abortion must be gathered.

The 10-day rule seeks to eliminate potential radiation exposure to the embryo by postponing elective abdominal x-rays of fertile women until the 10-day period following the onset of menstruation. This rule has not found much favor recently. Instead, the potential pregnancy status of female patients is determined, with steps taken to minimize fetal and embryonic exposure (see Chapter 9 for additional material on radiation exposure and pregnancy). Often, a radiation physicist will calculate the potential fetal dose when procedures are deemed absolutely necessary.

The radiographer is often responsible for ascertaining that a pregnancy test has been performed on female patients and questioning patients relative to their pregnancy status. This is the most effective means of avoiding fetal exposure. Other means include patient consent forms and wall posters. Combinations of these methods are also used in departments.

Pregnant and potentially pregnant patients must be handled professionally and must be reassured that appropriate safety measures are always taken, regardless of pregnancy status. The radiographer should be extremely cautious, and patients wanting specific information should be referred to the institution's radiation safety officer.

Following the Chernobyl accident, a large number of women in Denmark underwent therapeutic abortions due to miscommunications over risk. That can happen in diagnostic radiology as well. Radiographers need to realize that what they tell one patient will probably be communicated to others as well.

## PROTECTING CHILDREN

In many ways, protecting children is one of the most difficult aspects of radiation protection.

However, it is also one of the most important. Children can be extremely uncooperative, but because of their greater radiosensitivity, a high repeat rate is unacceptable. The radiosensitivity of children to leukemia, for example, has been estimated to be as high as twice that of adults.

Immobilization, securing patient cooperation, and shielding have been discussed in previous sections of this chapter. These are extremely important in pediatric radiography.

Pediatric radiography is another example of the art of radiography. Each department of radiology must commit to limiting doses to as low as reasonably achievable. Specific solutions will come from a combination of this commitment and the artistic application of scientific principles by the practitioner. Using a lower-ratio grid and some other factors were mentioned earlier. Other means of limiting dose include:

- *Use of faster speed screens.* This must be balanced with image quality.
- Some individuals, especially younger students and practitioners, have difficulty working with babies. Children sense the apprehension level of adults well. To improve their ability to work with younger patients, a course or inservice program on child psychology combined with working with a practitioner experienced in working with younger patients is invaluable.
- *Limiting comparison views.* Some departments still require routine comparison views on orthopedic examinations of children. The rationale is that it is difficult to determine pathology on unformed bones. Ideally, comparison views should be obtained only when necessary—that is, after the radiologist has reviewed the first set of films.
- *Optimum use of kVp.* It is too easy to assume that a high kVp level is always good. Because of the size of a child, too high a kVp level will overpenetrate the part and degrade the quality of the image. In fluoroscopy of children, the kVp level used should be about 20% to 25% less than that of the equivalent adult technique. This varies somewhat with the age and body habitus of the child. Also, always note all technical factors used on a child; that child may return.

- During fluoroscopy of a baby (except barium enemas), place a piece of lead under the baby's pelvis.

One special case involves portable radiography of neonates (newborns) in the neonatal unit. The following recommendations will help to protect neonates from excessive radiation:

1. Align the patient, tube, and film such that the long axis of the patient is perpendicular to the x-ray anode-cathode direction. This can reduce dose by 10%.
2. For babies undergoing radiography in an incubator, the best method of shielding must be determined by the institution. This issue is discussed in the textbox "Neonatal Radiation Protection."
3. The congruence of the x-ray field and light field (variance of 2% of SID maximum) must be checked regularly.
4. Each unit should have a calibration curve determined by a radiologic physicist that plots voltage versus exposure in mR/mAs (Figure 11–20). This allows the radiographer to determine skin exposure based on technical factor changes.
5. Thermoluminescent dosimeter monitoring will allow regular follow-up of neonatal exposures.

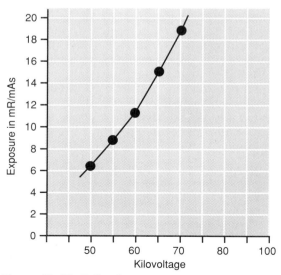

**Figure 11–20** Calibration curve.

## Neonatal Radiation Protection

One issue in the profession has been whether shadow shielding or contact shielding is the best method of protecting babies radiographed in the neonatal unit. The doses are of course small and, some might argue, not perceptibly larger than background radiation—and thus, not an issue. However, if one accepts potential cumulative damage (due to multiple radiographs while in the unit; some also argue that neonates tend to have more radiographs throughout their lives), the fact that neonates are twice as radiosensitive as an adult, and the difficulties involved in exactly collimating to "the chest" on neonates, who have a body habitus quite unlike an adult, there may be reason to be concerned about radiation exposure of the neonate. Thus, whereas on an adult, gonadal exposure is minimal and easy to keep low, the "rounded" nature of neonates plus their inability to "assume the position" may cause gonadal exposure on examinations that should have none, such as portable chests x-rays.

An additional issue in contact shielding is the potential for cross-contamination. That is, if multiple infants are radiographed and the same piece of lead rubber is used, then there is a potential to cross-infect other infants. The shadow shield of course avoids this problem, but there are also other solutions: having a dedicated piece of lead for each isolette that is sterilized after each patient, for example.

The study by Yoshizumi et al. in 1987 found that shadow shielding was the best method; a more recent study by Barcham et al. (1997) using more up-to-date dosimetry methods found that the contact method was the best. However, the issue is not solved there.

Probably the best solution is to determine the best method for each hospital or facility. The Barcham et al. article gives a method for determining exposure using containers of water that mimic the size and shape of a neonate. Armed with the dosimetry data for their own facility, a radiographers can work with other members of the health care team, particularly neonatal nurses, in determining the best method, contact shielding or shadow shielding, based on dosimetry, cross-contamination threats, and the availability of materials such as sterilized lead. The method that appears to be operationally sound and best for the patient should prevail.

## FLUOROSCOPY

Means of reducing patient dose in fluoroscopy include:

1. Exposure rate at tabletop cannot exceed 10 R/min and should not exceed 5 R/min.
2. Perform fluoroscopy intermittently rather than continuously to minimize dose. The use of pulsed fluoroscopy with videodisc memory provides reductions in dose of up to 80%.
3. Use a minimum focal distance of at least 30 cm for mobile units and 38 cm for fixed units.
4. Collimate the beam to expose only the clinical area of interest.
5. Optimize technical factors, using appropriate mA and kVp.
6. Provide sufficient beam filtration to meet regulatory requirements. Because fluoroscopy units are operated at 90 kVp or higher, 3 mm of aluminum equivalent or more is considered optimal.

Distance is the best means of minimizing exposure to the operator in fluoroscopy. The second-best means of minimizing exposure, which minimizes exposure to both operator and patient, is the use of a higher kVp level. As kilovoltage increases, the penetration of the x-ray beam increases, and a greater fraction of the x-ray beam reaches the detector. The

Increase or decrease in dose is approximately equal to ratio of area of input phosphor used.

Area at 6 inches = 36 inches
Area at 9 inches = 81 inches
36 ÷ 81 = 0.44

44% of exposure at 9 inches compared with 6 inches. Exposure has been reduced by 56%.

9-inch mode

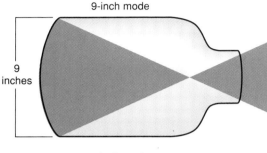

9 inches

6-inch mode

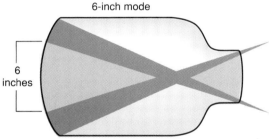

6 inches

**Figure 11–21** Illustration of the inverse square effect in reducing exposure through the image intensifier mode.

automatic brightness control (ABC) keeps the exposure at the image intensifier constant, and this decreases the entrance exposure with increasing kilovoltage.

Spot film cassettes require approximately three times the dosage 70- or 105-mm spot films do. This also depends on other factors, such as filming methods of the fluoroscopist.

Another means by which patient entrance exposure can be reduced in fluoroscopy is through the use of the image intensifier mode. As the image area changes from a large field of view to a small field of view, object magnification increases (Figure 11–21). When a small field size is used, the same amount of radiation is necessary to form the image as when a large field size is used and must be compensated for

by an increase in exposure rate. With a small field size, the radiation is concentrated into less tissue, causing more damage. Because the area of a fluoroscopy field is based on the square of the diameter, the increase in exposure rate is theoretically proportional to the decrease in area, an inverse square law type of relationship. Larger fields of view should be used whenever possible to minimize patient exposure.

Some authors (e.g., Gray and Swee, 1982; Rudin and Bednarek, 1991) have recommended not using a grid during some fluoroscopic procedures. Grids are used to remove scatter and improve contrast. Grids increase patient dose by a factor of anywhere from two to ten, depending on the grid ratio. Higher ratio grids, as discussed earlier, because they remove more scatter and primary radiation, require an increased technique and thus a higher dose to the patient.

Gray and Swee found that fluoroscopic exposure was reduced by 35% and spot image exposure was reduced by 48% by not using a grid. Rudin and Bednarek found that dose could be reduced by a factor of ten during fluoroscopic nasoenteral tube insertions. Some authors claim that this procedure is best limited to children (Drury and Robinson). A variety of factors must be considered; for example, if a high kVp without a grid is used, many generators may not provide an adequate time of exposure.

### Appropriate Uses of Fluoroscopy

Many states have restrictions on the use of fluoroscopy. The state of California allows radiographers to become certified in the limited use of fluoroscopy. Illinois law does not allow for anyone not licensed to practice medicine to operate fluoroscopic equipment, except for static functions (spot filming) under the direct supervision of a radiologist who is physically present. Because fluoroscopy is a dynamic technique that often involves diagnosis, radiographers are not usually considered qualified to perform fluoroscopy. This would violate the radiologic technology Code of Ethics. However, some states are experimenting with advanced practice licenses to allow some specially trained radiographers to perform fluoroscopy. This is a move supported by the ASRT.

Another action that would definitely violate the Code of Ethics is the use of fluoroscopy as a localization device by radiographers to determine the centering point for overhead films. Because the dose to the patient would exceed that of a normal repeat rate for films, this violates the principle that patient dose should be kept as low as possible, as well as the fact that the radiographer is unnecessarily exposed to radiation.

### Angiography

Angiographic studies are modified fluoroscopic studies. Catheters are placed in the patient and monitored under fluoroscopic control. Patient doses tend to be high because of the long fluoroscopic times required for catheter insertion and the many images needed to record anatomic structures.

Cardiac cineangiography is one example of a high-dose study. Typically, 13 minutes of fluoroscopy and 110 seconds of cinefluorography are used. The entrance skin dose for cinefluorography is about 2 mR per frame. If 60 frames are used per second, this translates into about 7.2 R/min or about 13.2 R total, assuming 110 seconds of cinefluorography. Because the tabletop dose is about 1 to 3 R/min for most fluoroscopic equipment (with a maximum of 10 R/min), patient dose could easily range from 26 to 52 R. For this reason, speed and efficiency are imperative in cardiac cinefluorography.

---

## More Information:
## Fluoroscopy and Radiation Injuries

Because of improvements in radiation protection methods, reports of radiation-induced erythemas and other skin damage from diagnostic radiology had become very rare, with almost no cases from the 1930s through the 1980s. Unfortunately, since the late 1980s, there has been a dramatic increase in the number of these reports. This has been in part because of the development of procedures that require very high levels of fluoroscopy time such as percutaneous transluminal angioplasty, radiofrequency cardiac catheter ablation, vascular embolization, stent and filter placement, thrombolytic and fibrinolytic procedures, percutaneous transhepatic cholangiography, endoscopic retrograde cholangiopancreatography, transjugular intrahepatic portosystemic shunt, percutaneous nephrostomy, biliary drainage, and urinary/biliary stone removal. Another aspect of this unfortunate situation is the growth of imaging suites (particularly in the cardiac area) that are not staffed by anyone with a through understanding of radiation

protection. Often, these suites are managed by a cardiologist and normally no RTs, radiologists, or physicists are there to assure good radiation protection. Because fluoroscopy is often seen as "safe" by many nonradiology professionals, very long fluoroscopy times are used for some procedures. See the FDA advisory titled "Avoidance of Serious X-Ray-Induced Skin Injuries to Patients During Fluoroscopically-Guided Procedures" in Appendix B for specific information of dose levels associated with these skin injuries.

So many of these cases have appeared in the last decade that the U.S. Food and Drug Administration had issued warning about this problem and has presented research finding at meetings. Below is an excerpt from one warning.

September 30, 1994
To:   Healthcare Administrators
      Risk Managers
      Radiology Department Directors
      Cardiology Department Directors

## Fluoroscopy and Radiation Injuries *(Continued)*

The Food and Drug Administration (FDA) Center for Devices and Radiological Health (CDRH) has received reports of occasional, but at times severe, radiation-induced skin injuries to patients resulting from prolonged, fluoroscopically-guided, invasive procedures. Physicians performing [high-dose flurosocopy] procedures should be aware of the potential for serious, radiation-induced skin injury caused by long periods of fluoroscopy during these procedures. It is important to note that the onset of these injuries is usually delayed, so that the physician cannot discern the damage by observing the patient immediately after the treatment.

The absorbed dose in the skin required to cause skin injury depends on a number of factors, but typical threshold doses for various effects are about 3 Gy (300 rad) for temporary epilation, about 6 Gy (600 rad) for main erythema, and 15 to 20 Gy (1,500 to 2,000 rad) for moist desquamation, dermal necrosis and secondary ulceration.

The absorbed dose rate in the skin from the direct beam of a fluoroscopic x-ray system is typically between 0.02 Gy/min and 0.05 Gy/min (2 to 5 rad/min), but may be higher, depending on the mode in which the equipment is operated and the size of the patient. Even typical dose rates can result in skin injury after less than one hour of fluoroscopy.

FDA suggests that facilities performing fluoroscopically-guided procedures observe the following principles:

Establish standard operating procedures and clinical protocols for each specific type of procedure performed. The protocols should address all aspects of the procedure, such as patient selection, normal conduct of the procedure, actions in response to complica-

tions, and consideration of limits on fluoroscopy exposure time.

Know the radiation dose rates for the specific fluoroscopic system and for each mode of operation used during the clinical protocol. These dose rates should be derived from measurements performed at the facility.

Assess the impact of each procedure's protocol on the potential for radiation injury to the patient.

Modify the protocol, as appropriate, to limit the cumulative absorbed dose to any irradiated area of the skin to the minimum necessary for the clinical tasks, and particularly to avoid approaching cumulative doses that would induce unacceptable adverse effects. Use equipment which aids in minimizing absorbed dose.

Enlist a qualified medical physicist to assist in implementing these principles in such a manner as not to adversely affect the clinical objectives of the procedure.

Physicians should know that radiation-induced injuries from fluoroscopy are not immediately apparent. Other than the mildest symptoms, such as transient erythema, the effects of the radiation may not appear until weeks following the exposure. Physicians performing these procedures may not be in direct contact with the patients following the procedure and may not observe the symptoms when they occur. Missing the milder symptoms in some patients can lead to surprise at the magnitude of the absorbed doses delivered to the skin of other patients when more serious symptoms appear. For this reason, we recommend that information be recorded in the patient's record which permits estimation of the absorbed dose to the skin. Patients should also be advised to report signs and/or symptoms

---

## Fluoroscopy and Radiation Injuries *(Continued)*

of radiation-induced injury to their attending physician.

The Safe Medical Devices Act of 1990 (SMDA) requires hospitals and other user facilities to report deaths, serious illnesses and injuries associated with the use of medical devices. Follow the procedures established by your facility for such mandatory reporting. Practitioners who become aware of any medical device related adverse event or product problem/malfunction should report to their Medical Device User Facility Reporting person. If it is not reportable under the SMDA, it may be reported directly to MedWatch, the FDA's voluntary reporting program. Submit these reports to MedWatch, Medical Product Reporting Program, by phone at 1–800-FDA-1088 (also call for MedWatch information); by FAX at 1–800-FDA-0178; by modem at 1–800-FDA-7737; or by mail to MedWatch, HF-2, Food and Drug Administration, 5600 Fishers Lane, Rockville, MD 20857.

If you have questions concerning radiation injuries from fluoroscopy appropriate for the FDA, or for a copy of a more detailed communication from the FDA on this topic, contact Paula Simenauer, Division of Device User Programs and Systems Analysis, CDRH, HFZ-230, FDA, 1350 Piccard Drive, Rockville, Maryland 20850 or FAX 301-594-0067.

Sincerely yours,

D. Bruce Burlington
Director Center for Devices and Radiological Health

### REFERENCE

1. Wagner LK, Eifel PJ, and Geise RA. Potential Biological Effects Following High X-ray Dose Interventional Procedures, Journal of Vascular and Interventional Radiology 1994; 5:71–84.

---

## MOBILE RADIOGRAPHY

The first rule of mobile radiography is the same as the first rule of regular radiography: establish communication with the patient. The mobile unit should be left in the hall, and the radiographer should assess the patient's condition and ability to cooperate, and should attempt to establish rapport. Before taking films, ask all nonessential individuals to leave the area. Individuals remaining, including the patient, should be shielded. Be certain to tell those individuals previously asked to leave when the procedure is complete.

Drafke also notes that the patient can be protected during mobile radiography by reducing repeat exposures, shielding, collimating, and selecting the proper grid, screen, and technical factors. He cites the following three factors as leading to the reduction of repeats in mobile radiography:

1. Checking positioning.
2. Checking previous radiographs or records to determine the technical factors that should be used. Portable techniques should be recorded so that sequential films can be repeated in the same manner as the original film. mAs, kVp, SID, screen speed, and grid ratio (if used) should all be recorded, as well as any description of nonroutine positions.
3. Using relatively high-kVp techniques, which have a wider margin for exposure error.

Shielding certainly should not be neglected

during mobile radiography. All patients should be shielded, if possible. Collimation should not be ignored in mobile radiography simply because it is more difficult to provide exact collimation. Also, a source-to-skin distance of at least 12 inches (30 cm) must be used. A short source-to-skin distance increases entrance dose, which is of course not desirable.

The primary difficulty in using a grid during mobile radiography is that although larger parts (except chests) and higher kVp settings require a higher ratio grid, increasing grid ratio gives less margin for error in positioning.

Intensifying screen selection is dependent on the size of the part: larger parts, in general, require faster screens. Faster screens require less mAs, which allow for a shorter exposure time, reducing the possibility of motion. For chest radiography of very obese or muscular patients, it is sometimes necessary to return to slower speed screens as the patient already exhibits a naturally long-scale contrast through body habitus. This, of course, requires an increase in technical factors, which increases patient dose. Thus, the decision to use slower speed screens must be carefully thought out, which is not usually possible—for example, when doing a set of 20 portable chest radiographs in the hectic morning hours. Martin recommends that if the "average" technique is 4 mAs and 85 kVp, then any patient that would require a technique of greater than 6 mAs and 95 kVp should be radiographed using slower speed screens. This may not be appropriate for all departments, but certainly some standardization of technique is appropriate whether one is using different speeds of screens or not.

Technical factors can be adjusted to reduce patient dose. Don't forget that reducing patient dose can have the effect of reducing the dose of the radiographer as well.

## SUMMARY

Various factors were described in this chapter that the radiographer can use to limit patient dose. The application of these scientific principles is part of the professional practice of the radiographer.

Technique selection is the primary means by which the radiographer can minimize patient dose. Both mAs and kVp must be selected in unison to produce an acceptable image while protecting the patient. Phototiming must be selected with care because of the possibility of grossly overexposing the patient with excess mAs and the lack of precisely reproducible exposures.

Filtration absorbs low-energy (low-kV) radiation that would not contribute to the image. When filtration is increased, kVp should be increased to maintain density. Compensating filters are used to adjust for variations in patient density.

Grids absorb scatter and require an increase in technical factors. The radiographer must choose the grid that will not require overly high technical factors and provide the desired scale of contrast.

Flexibility in the use of alternative positions and projections can decrease exposure to sensitive organs such as gonads, eyes, and the juvenile breasts to less than 1% of original value. Using a higher speed film/screen system can reduce patient exposure. The loss in image quality with faster speeds must be balanced with the decrease in patient dose in accordance with risk-versus-benefit analysis.

The radiographer must seek to secure patient cooperation by exhibiting professional competence, a caring, patient-oriented attitude, and effective communication skills. The first rule of radiography should be to establish communication with the patient. If this does not produce the desired result, immobilization may be necessary as a last resort. Immobilization devices should always be used before the use of personnel to hold patients.

The radiographer must strive for a repeat rate in accordance with department and professional standards. The radiographer is a professional who uses scientific knowledge of image factors with critical thinking skills (film critique) to produce a diagnostic image that provides the least exposure to the patient. Equipment problems must be reported to appropriate personnel as soon as possible.

Familiarity with estimated doses of examinations further establishes the radiographer as a knowledgeable professional. This professional should also engage only in examinations for which he or she is educated, licensed, and competent as determined by outside authorities.

The most vulnerable time for the fetus is from the 10th day to the 10th week after conception. Above 15 rad (15 mGy) the risk of potential malformations increases significantly. The radiographer does not advocate specific actions for the patient but reassures the patient and refers her to the radiation safety officer if she wishes additional information.

Protecting children is one of the most difficult yet important aspects of radiation protection. Each department and each practitioner must develop individualized methods of reducing pediatric dose.

## Advanced Information: Radiation Protection in Computed Tomography

Radiographers performing CT rarely receive any significant exposure because they are rarely in the room when the exposure is being made. If this does occur (remember, technologists should be the last to hold, with male relatives preferred, then female relatives, then nonradiology personnel), a lead apron and other protective equipment should be worn. However, exposures are still low. Scatter at 1 meter from the patient is usually less than 5 mrad (0.05 mGy).

Dose to the patient in CT is difficult to compare to the comparable radiographic examination of that area. Due to the way in which CT images are produced, the estimation of dose is much more difficult than in conventional radiography. However, in general, CT exposures to the patient are higher than radiographic examinations of the same area.

According to Seeram (1997), CT dose is dependent on the following:

1. *Slice thickness.* This is an inverse proportion; halving the slice thickness requires an doubling of dose to maintain contrast resolution.

2. *Contrast resolution.* This is a direct proportion to the square of the contrast resolution; thus, to double contrast resolution requires a 4× increase in dose.

3. *Spatial resolution.* This is an inverse proportion to the square of the cube; thus, to double spatial resolution requires an 8× increase in dose.

## Advanced Information: Radiation Protection in Mammography

Patient dose can be minimized in mammography by observing the following:

1. *High tube output.* A single-phase-voltage unit with a high-frequency generator should be used.
2. *Grids.* Exposure is about doubled with a grid. Fatty breasts require less radiation and no grid.
3. *Screen/film combinations and developer time*

*and temperature.* Judicious use of screen/film combinations and extended developer time can reduce patient exposure by up to 40%. Old cassettes should be compared with new cassettes to ensure that they are providing equivalent density.
4. *Compression.* This can reduce dose, on average, by about 20%.
5. *Mobile units.* Processing should be available

## Radiation Protection in Mammography *(Continued)*

(same day at latest) to reduce the possibility of latent image fading, which can reduce image quality.

6. *Using large cassettes on large-breasted women can reduce the need for two exposures.* Mammography also allows for an expanded role of the radiographer in patient care and radiation protection. Kimme-Smith and colleagues make the following observation in the June 1992 issue of *Administrative Radiology:*

A patient who objects to additional views may consent to them when she is shown her initial mammograms. This should not increase anxiety if the technologist uses an easily understood phrase like, "This area is not spread out enough, so we are going to change your position to see the area more clearly." By making the patient a partner in the examination, rather than an object, the technologist may gain more cooperation and achieve a better diagnostic study.

## *Advanced Information:*
## Research Papers

Maybe you just were curious about one of the assertions made in this chapter, or just performed one of the experiments listed in the back. Your results may have confirmed what was said, or you may have had a different result.

Is the best thing to do to just put it in a notebook and forget about it? No! One thing radiologic science needs is more people engaged in and especially reporting on research, including students. Your view might be that your study certainly is no cure for the common cold or AIDS. However, what this profession really needs is focused studies that solve clinical problems for staff technologists. Sometimes the simplest problems are the hardest to solve.

You might be surprised to know that the Barcham et al. article on neonatal gonadal shielding discussed earlier started as a student project. The professional journal *Radiologic Technology* also publishes a column titled "Student Scope" in which student papers are published. You wouldn't be doing this just for the profession, you would also be doing it for yourself as well, to get your "name in

lights" and possibly win a cash prize of $1000, awarded to the best paper each year.

So now you ask, how do I write my results up? A summary follows:

1. *Title and abstract.* These appear first, but are best written last. The title should simply and concisely describe your project, for example: "A Comparison of AP versus PA Gonadal Shielding for PA Chest Radiography." The abstract should be a summary of the project, ideally written in four sentences, one that summarizes the introduction, one for the methods/materials, one for results, and another for conclusions. For example: "This study investigates the use of AP versus PA gonadal shielding for PA chest radiography. Using MDH dosimeters and an upright torso phantom, measurements were taken at the level of the gonads using AP and PA shielding. Readings were negligible at both sites, but PA shielding provided the best protection overall."

2. *Introduction.* Here you state the research problem. Typically you begin with a para-

## Research Papers *(Continued)*

graph or two that discusses the issues surrounding the research problem, then you state the problem directly. After that, a few paragraphs are devoted to a brief review of the relevant literature surrounding the issue. Don't just cite anything and everything, and don't ramble about. Keep it focused to the research problem. In some cases, this can be broad (for example, you might want to talk about dose–response curves in a protection article to show exactly *why* it is important to shield), but it is usually best to think and write this section in a focused manner.

3. *Methods/materials.* Here you describe what you did. The general rule for writing this section is to write it in such a way that another individual in your profession would be able to replicate it. This is often called the Materials and Methods section, since you will often spend some time discussing the materials you used—in a radiation protection study, for example, you will spend some time discussing the equipment you used and the type of dosimeter. Remember how earlier chapters discussed the difference between single-phase and three-phase equipment, the differences in waveforms, and so on?

All this is important to the reader of your study, who may choose to disagree with it based on a methodologic issue or may wish to try the study as well.

4. *Results.* If you are familiar with the old television show "Dragnet," you will remember Joe Friday, who always intoned, "Just the facts, ma'am." The Results section is similar. There should be no hint of bias or preference in this section. As we tell students, "Although your paper may be interesting, there should be nothing interesting about your results." Just state facts, and don't use phrases like, "Interestingly, it was found that. . . ." This section provides mostly data.

5. *Conclusions.* In this section you are allowed a bit more latitude. However, the conclusions must also be based on the facts you have presented—you cannot now pursue some interesting sideline. You need to discuss your conclusions in reference to previous studies and assertions, and your expectations for the study. Whereas the Results section provided data, here you provide information by placing the data in its relevant context.

Good luck! We hope to be seeing *your* name in print soon.

## Questions

1. In general, patient dose may be reduced (while maintaining density) through the use of _____ techniques.

   a. high-kVp, low-mAs
   b. high-kVp, high-mAs
   c. low-kVp, low-mAs
   d. low-kVp, high-mAs

2. The greatest radiation exposure, given otherwise identical technical factors, would result from which of the following primary beam sizes?

   a. 5 × 5 inches     b. 6 × 6 inches
   c. 8 × 10 inches     d. 10 × 12 inches

3. Which of the following structures would receive the least exposure from an AP abdomen?

   a. stomach     b. small bowel
   c. liver     d. kidney

4. The basic types of gonadal shields are:

   I. flat contact.
   II. shaped contact.
   III. shadow.

   a. I and II only     b. I and III only
   c. II and III only     d. I, II, and III

5. Total filtration is the sum of _____ filtration.

   a. inherent plus innate
   b. inherent plus added
   c. innate plus added
   d. wedge plus compensated

6. Most of the density on the image results from:

   a. x-ray.
   b. gamma rays.
   c. light from the screen.
   d. patient thickness.

7. How is voluntary motion best controlled?

   I. limiting exposure time
   II. immobilization
   III. patient cooperation

   a. I only
   b. II and III only
   c. I and II only
   d. I, II, and III

8. Which of the following is not a radiation protection measure?

   a. high-speed screens
   b. shielding
   c. grids
   d. high-kVp techniques

9. An expected patient dose for a PA chest might be:

   a. 10 mrad.
   b. 100 mrad.
   c. 1000 mrad.
   d. 10 rad.

10. By law, collimation must be accurate to within:

   a. 2% of the SID.
   b. 5% of the SID.
   c. 2% of the beam size.
   d. 5% of the beam size.

## Exercises

1. Calculate the reduction in exposure from switching from a technique of 20 mAs and 70 kVp to 10 mAs and 80 kVp. The original exposure was 100 mR.

2. What are the two most effective factors for reducing patient dose? List examples of how these could be used in actual clinical practice.

3. What is the ultimate goal of state licensing and voluntary certification?

4. Why is establishing communication important in radiation protection?

5. What factors influence repeat rate?

6. Who can refuse a radiograph? How can the radiographer best indicate to the patient the need for an examination?

7. What are the dangers of a radiographer's advocating refusal of an examination to a patient?

8. How can the potential disadvantages of using AECs (in relation to radiation exposure) be minimized?

9. What is the public relations value of a lead apron?

10. What is the role of the radiographer with a pregnant patient?

## Activities

The laboratory activities listed here are described in greater detail in the instructor's manual for this course. Your instructor will be able to provide more specific details when these labs are assigned.

1. Choose a technique that will provide a minimal exposure (e.g., 10 mR on a 100-mR dosimeter) on a dosimeter. Experiment first with providing mAs values that will conform to the reciprocity law (give the same mAs). Then experiment with doubling the mAs. What are the recorded results to exposure?

2. Using a phantom, expose one abdominal film using the normal technique with a dosimeter attached to the top of the abdomen. If a manual technique is used, double the mAs and reduce kVp by 15%. If an automatic exposure control (phototimer) is used, drop the kVp setting by 10. Shoot a second film at this setting. Record the observed results to the image and to exposure.

3. Using a penetrometer and a dosimeter, record the effect on films and on dosage by

shooting five films, beginning with 0 mm of aluminum equivalent filtration and adding 1 mm of filtration up to 4 mm. Record the results to the image and to exposure.

4. Experiment with a phantom part such as a foot by using paper as a compensating filter. Experiment with different colors of paper. Does any one work better than the others?

5. Secure an 8:1 and a 12:1 (or any other two) stationary grid. Using a phantom part and a dosimeter, shoot a diagnostic film of the same part using both grids and equivalent density. Vary the mAs to compensate. What is the resultant change in exposure?

6. Using a phantom part, shoot a pelvis with and without (male) gonadal shielding, with the dosimeter at the level of the gonads. Record the resultant change in exposure.

7. Observe graduate radiographers while in clinical. Pay special attention to their patient instruction. Write a short paper (keep it confidential; this is not an exercise designed to criticize staff) on how you believe these radiographers have secured patient cooperation and could improve their ability to do so.

## Answers

### Questions

| | |
|---|---|
| 1. a | 6. c |
| 2. d | 7. b |
| 3. d | 8. c |
| 4. d | 9. a |
| 5. b | 10. a |

### Exercises

1. Step 1: mAs is being halved; therefore, the intensity due to mAs will decrease to half the original value.

$$\frac{mAs_1}{mAs_2} = \frac{I_1}{I_2}$$

$$\frac{2}{1} = \frac{100}{x}$$

$$x = 50 \text{ mR}$$

Step 2: kVp is being increased. Thus, intensity will increase as follows:

$$\left(\frac{kVp_1}{kVp_2}\right)^2 = \frac{I_1}{I_2} = \left(\frac{70}{80}\right)^2 = \frac{50}{x}$$

$$x = 65.3 \text{ mR, a total decrease of}$$
$$34.7 \text{ mR.}$$

2. Selection of kVp level is the most effective method of limiting patient dose of those items easily selectable by the radiographer. This is illustrated in exercise 1. The second most effective technique for reducing patient dose is the use of faster film/screen combinations. Doubling screen speed will effectively limit patient dose (cut it in half), but this technique is not as often under the control of the radiographer.

3. The ultimate goal of state licensing and voluntary certification is protection of the patient. By providing patients with competent practitioners who understand and are able to practice safe radiation protection, the health of the population is protected. Students who have entered accredited programs recognize the need for education that results in sound radiation protection practice.

4. By establishing communication, it is easier to secure patient consent. If patients understand the reason behind procedures and are included in the examination, they will cooperate. Another aspect of communication is the provision of information to the patient. Some patients want very specific information about their examination; others may only want reassurance that the individual performing their examination is a competent professional. Although radiographers must have certain standard information prepared, they must also be sure that they can adapt to the individual needs of the patient to secure cooperation for maximum radiation protection.

5. The factors that will influence repeat rate include the experience level of the radiographer and the radiologist's view of image quality. Also, a departmental quality assurance program is designed to minimize repeats, which results in higher image quality and patient protection.

6. Adults (unless they have had their civil rights removed) can refuse an examination. The radiographer should never advocate refusal to a patient but should instead gently try to emphasize the concept of safe radiation protection and risk being counterbalanced by the benefit of radiography.

7. The radiographer cannot advocate refusal to the patient. Advocating refusal may be seen as diagnosis by indicating that the patient does not need the examination, which is not within the scope of practice of a radiographer. The radiographer is also a patient advocate, however, which means that the radiographer must support patient decisions to not have an examination. This is a delicate balance. The radiographer may question the validity of the request for the examination with the appropriate personnel involved in the care of the patient. Radiographers also often know of additional views, based on their training, that would better visualize certain anatomic structures. Since this involves exposing the patient to another film, with the resultant increase in exposure, this responsibility should never be taken lightly.

8. The balance between mA and backup time is extremely important using automatic exposure controls. To minimize the possibility of grossly overexposing the patient, some authorities recommend using only 1.5 times the expected mAs. Also, phototiming is not always as precisely reproducible as manual timing. Positioning must be duplicated exactly for the repeat exposure.

9. Providing a lead apron establishes the radiographer as a professional by showing concern for the well-being of the patient. This apron may not always be needed, but how people feel about their health care experience is often more important than the actual technical care received.

10. The radiographer is often responsible for making sure that a pregnancy test has been performed on female patients. The radiographer also often questions the patient about her pregnancy status. This is the most effective means of avoiding fetal exposure. The radiographer must be sure to maintain professional decorum, since this is often a sensitive issue. The patient must be reassured that appropriate safety measures are taken. Patients wanting specific information should be referred to the institution's radiation safety officer.

## CHAPTER 12

# Radiation Protection in Nuclear Medicine

**Ann M. Steves**

## Chapter Outline

## Chapter Objectives

At the end of this chapter, the student should be able to:

1. Give specific examples of how a technologist's radiation exposure can be minimized through the use of time, distance, and shielding.

2. State the guidelines for avoiding internal radiation contamination.

3. Describe the precautions for working with radioiodine solutions.

4. State the limit set by the Nuclear Regulatory Commission for radiation exposure to the fetus of an occupationally exposed worker.

5. Describe how the radiation dose to a fetus is monitored and enumerate steps a worker could take to minimize this exposure.

6. Describe the ways in which a nuclear medicine technologist protects other personnel from radiation exposure or contamination.

7. Describe the steps in handling a major and a minor radioactive spill.

8. Identify the methods of radioactive waste disposal.

9. Describe the safe handling of radioactive gases and aerosols.

10. Identify the information to be given to hospital personnel who come in contact with patients who have received diagnostic amounts of radioactivity.

11. Identify the instructions to be given to housekeeping and maintenance staff who access restricted areas.

12. Identify the information in the patient medical record that should be reviewed prior to administration of a radiopharmaceutical to a patient.

13. Describe the technologist's responsibilities in preparing and administering a patient dose.

14. Describe the value of instrumentation quality control, immobilization, and patient instruction in minimizing patient radiation dose.

15. Suggest some questions that could be asked to elicit information about the pregnancy status of a female patient.

16. List the radiation safety precautions to be followed by the patient after radioiodine therapy.

17. Describe the preparation of the patient, the isolation room, and nursing personnel prior to the initiation of radioiodine therapy.

18. Describe the radiation safety precautions to be followed for P-32, Sr-89, and Sm-153 therapy.

19. State the Nuclear Regulatory Commission regulations regarding:

    a. shielding of vials and syringes containing radiopharmaceuticals

    b. the definition of restricted and unrestricted areas

    c. posting of restricted areas

    d. area surveys

    e. required quality control tests and their frequency for a dose calibrator

    f. assay of patient doses

    g. limits for release from isolation of a patient receiving radioiodine therapy

## Important Terms

aerosol
ALARA
becquerel (Bq)
bioassay
biohazardous
bremsstrahlung radiation
critical organ
decontamination
Department of Transportation
dose-equivalent
Geiger-Mueller (GM) meter
gigabecquerel (GBq)
gray (Gy)
health physicist
ionization chamber
L-block shield
megabecquerel (MBq)
microcurie (μCi)
millicurie (mCi)
millirem (mrem)
millisievert (mSv)
negative pressure
nonoccupationally exposed individual
Nuclear Regulatory Commission (NRC)
occupationally exposed worker
paracentesis
quality management program
rad
restricted area

| | |
|---|---|
| Standard Precautions | unrestricted area |
| thermoluminescent dosimeter (TLD) | volatile |
| thoracentesis | wipe test |

## INTRODUCTION

Nuclear medicine technologists are responsible for keeping their own radiation exposure as low as reasonably achievable, the ALARA concept, as well as that of patients, visitors, and other hospital personnel. Radiation safety practices are incorporated into almost every task performed by the technologist to minimize radiation exposure to self and to others. This chapter reviews the principles of radiation protection and the implementation of those principles into clinical nuclear medicine practice.

## PROTECTING THE NUCLEAR MEDICINE TECHNOLOGIST

Although the Nuclear Regulatory Commission (NRC) has set limits of radiation exposure for radiation workers, the ALARA concept requires that nuclear medicine technologists use any reasonable means to lower their exposure. Monitoring personnel radiation exposure is one way to assess that radiation safety practices and the ALARA concept are being observed. Therefore, it is important that personnel monitors be used consistently and handled properly to ensure that the readings are an accurate reflection of a technologist's radiation exposure. The body badge, which records exposure to the whole body, should be worn between the shoulder and the waist in the area most likely to receive the greatest radiation exposure. Radiation exposure to the hands is best assessed with a thermoluminescent dosimeter designed to be worn as a ring. The ring should be worn on the dominant hand with the thermoluminescent crystal facing the palm, since the palm will be receiving the greatest radiation exposure when manipulating radioactive materials or positioning patients. When not in use, the ring and body badges

should be stored in an area away from radiation sources. Abnormally high readings, even those within NRC limits, recorded on either the body or ring badge should be investigated to ensure that radiation safety practices are being used to the fullest extent possible to minimize personnel radiation exposure. Consistent with ALARA, reasonable and cost-effective means of decreasing radiation exposure and protecting the technologist include the use of time, distance, and shielding.

### Shielding

One of the most effective means of decreasing radiation exposure is to absorb most of the radiation through the use of shielding around the radioactive source. The NRC requires that syringes be shielded during radiopharmaceutical kit preparation and administration to the patient, unless the use of the shield is contraindicated for a particular patient. It is estimated that the dose equivalent to the index finger tip from an unshielded syringe containing 20 mCi (740 MBq) of technetium-99m (Tc-99m) is about 22 rem/hr (220 mSv/hr). This results in significant radiation exposure to the technologist's hands that may exceed occupational limits, depending on the number of radiopharmaceutical administrations performed and the length of time the technologist holds the syringe. Likewise, according to the NRC, all vials containing radiopharmaceuticals must be shielded.

Specially designed lead shields that fit around radionuclide generators are necessary because a generator's internal shielding is intended only to meet Department of Transportation regulations for shipment of radioactive materials. Additional shielding is required once the generator is set up for operation in the nuclear medicine department. Lead bricks

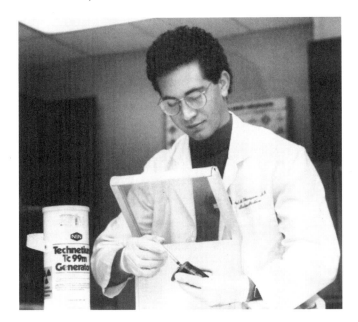

**Figure 12–1** A nuclear medicine technologist using L-block shielding during dose preparation.

can also be used to provide extra shielding around generators and other areas where radioactive materials are stored. An L-block shield should be used during the preparation of radiopharmaceutical kits and unit doses (Figure 12–1). The leaded glass window permits the technologist to see the manipulation of the equipment while affording some protection to the eyes and torso.

Although lead provides appropriate shielding for most of the gamma-emitting radionuclides used in nuclear medicine, it should not be used for beta-emitting radionuclides such as phosphorus-32 (P-32). Placing a beta source in a lead shield causes the production of bremsstrahlung radiation, which results from the deceleration of beta particles as they approach the nuclei of the lead atoms in the shielding. As the beta particles slow down, they lose energy that is emitted in the form of x-radiation. Therefore, placing a beta-emitting source in a lead shield can actually increase the amount of radiation emitted. Low-density materials such as plastic or Lucite are recommended to absorb beta radiation and to prevent the production of bremsstrahlung radiation.

**Time and Distance**

In some instances, the use of shielding is not practical. Minimizing the time spent working with the radiation source and maximizing the distance from the radiation source are other practical methods of reducing radiation exposure. These methods are particularly useful when working with patients who have been administered radiopharmaceuticals. Table 12–1 shows some average whole-body radiation exposures to technologists when performing selected imaging procedures. The reported exposures do not include exposure from the preparation or administration of radiopharmaceuticals, but only the exposure received while escorting the patient back and forth from the waiting area and during the imaging itself. The greatest radiation exposures were obtained during daily flood phantom imaging and during gated cardiac studies. Other procedures yielded exposures four to six times less than these two procedures. Not surprisingly, the investigators found that difficult patients could as much as double the radi-

Table 12–1  Technologist Radiation Exposures from Selected Imaging Procedures

| Procedure | Radiopharmaceutical | Administered Activity (mCi) | Mean Time (minutes) | Mean Exposure (mR) |
|---|---|---|---|---|
| Bone (whole-body imaging) | Tc-99m medronate | 20 | 51 | 0.15 |
| Gated heart (rest only) | Tc-99m pertechnetate | 20 | 43 | 0.45 |
| Flood phantom quality control | Tc-99m pertechnetate | 5–8 | 26 | 0.58 |
| Gallium imaging | Ga-67 citrate | 4 | 61 | 0.06 |
| Liver tomography | Tc-99m sulfur colloid | 5 | 32 | 0.09 |
| Lung perfusion | Tc-99m MAA | 3 | 13 | 0.11 |
| Lung ventilation | Xe-133 gas | 10–20 | 16 | 0.13 |
| Myocardial perfusion | T1-201 thallous chloride | 2.2 | 32 | 0.04 |
| Thyroid imaging | I-131 sodium iodide liquid | 0.05 | 13 | 0.01* |
| Thyroid uptake | I-131 sodium iodide liquid | 0.05 | 6 | 0.01* |

*Values consistent with zero.

Reprinted with permission from Sloboda RS, Schmid MG, Wills CP: Technologist radiation exposures from nuclear medicine imaging procedures. J Nucl Med Technol 15:16–24, 1987.

ation exposure to the technologist for a given imaging procedure.

Obviously, the condition of the patient will dictate the proximity of the technologist and the amount of time it will take to complete an imaging study. However, technologists need to keep in mind that even a short distance can significantly reduce radiation exposure from the patient, without conveying a fearful or uncaring attitude on the part of the technologist. Small imaging rooms filled with ancillary equipment, such as cardiac monitors or exercise equipment, can make keeping a distance from patients more difficult. The size of imaging rooms, from a radiation safety point of view, should be taken into consideration when planning a nuclear medicine department.

Technologists also should become adept in using appropriate restraint devices to hold patients in the correct position for imaging, rather than holding or having other personnel hold patients in position. Such devices are also more effective in maintaining a given position than holding the patient and can decrease the number of repeat acquisitions due to patient motion. This action will be less likely to be per-

ceived as punitive or uncaring if the technologist explains the reasons for restraining the patient.

Using long-handled tongs to move unshielded radioactive material is another way to use distance for radiation protection. Likewise, working efficiently with radioactive materials, practicing new procedures with non-radioactive materials, and remaining in the "hot lab" only for the time necessary all decrease radiation exposure by minimizing the time the technologist is exposed to radiation.

### Internal Exposure

Technologists can receive internal radiation exposure by inhaling or ingesting radioactivity or by absorbing it through the skin or wounds. Since internal exposure is not detected by a personal radiation monitor or routinely monitored through bioassay, it is controlled primarily by eliminating potential causes of internal contamination. This type of contamination may be avoided by abstaining from eating, drinking, smoking, or applying cosmetics in areas where radioactive materials are used. Food should not be kept in the same refrigerators where radioactive materials are stored. Also, pipetting of radioactive solutions by mouth must be strictly prohibited. Protective clothing, especially gloves, can minimize absorption through the skin and simplify decontamination if spills occur.

Radioiodine solutions require special handling because of the ease with which the iodide ion is oxidized to iodine. Since iodine is not very soluble in water, it comes out of solution, forming an iodine vapor that can be inhaled. Exposure to air or the use of diluents containing oxidants, such as tap water that contains chlorine, causes iodine to volatilize. Once iodine is airborne, it is readily inhaled and eventually localizes in the thyroid. Given that 1 µCi (37 kBq) of iodine-131 ($^{131}$I) delivers a radiation dose of 1.3 rad (0.013 Gy) to the thyroid, based on a 25% thyroid uptake, stringent precautions should be taken to avoid this type of contamination.

It had been thought that radioiodine capsules lessen the potential for iodine vaporization, thereby decreasing the radiation hazard associated with radioiodine solutions. However, Hackett and associates (1995) found significant radioiodine contamination on the absorbent packets of activated charcoal packaged with $^{131}$I capsules. Based on the results of their study, they recommend that radioiodine capsules be vented in a fume hood before the capsules are assayed. This will remove any volatile $^{131}$I not trapped by the absorbent as well as any Xe-131m gas produced by $^{131}$I decay. The charcoal packets should not be assayed with the capsules and should be disposed of as radioactive waste.

Opening all packages and vials containing iodine solutions and capsules in a fume hood, wearing gloves and ensuring that the skin of the lower forearms is covered, and using only distilled water to dilute radioiodine solutions will help minimize internal contamination from airborne iodine. Also, wipe testing the outside of shipping containers and lead shields will indicate where contamination is present and will help ascertain the extent of iodine volatility. Finally, to ensure that the precautions have been successful in preventing internal contamination, the thyroid gland of any person handling radioiodine solutions should be assayed the day after handling the radioiodine

to estimate the amount of radioiodine uptake. Using an uptake probe, external counts of the thyroid are obtained. The formula for calculating the amount of I-131 in the thyroid is:

$$\text{activity in thyroid } (\mu Ci)$$
$$= \text{activity of known } ^{131}\text{I standard } (\mu Ci)$$
$$\times \frac{cpm_{neck} - cpm_{thigh}}{cpm_{std} - cpm_{bkg}}$$

Ventilation studies performed with xenon-133 (Xe-133) are another potential source of internal radiation exposure through inhalation. Properly functioning exhaust and gas-trapping systems can minimize technologist exposure should a release of Xe-133 occur. Familiarizing the patient with the equipment and the breathing technique required to complete the study may increase patient cooperation and thereby decrease the likelihood of accidental xenon release during the study.

### The Pregnant Technologist

Since nuclear medicine technologists are routinely exposed to radiation during the performance of their work responsibilities, they are considered to be occupationally exposed workers, according to the NRC. However, a fetus is limited to receiving not more than 500 mrem (5 mSv) during the gestation period. Consequently, determining and limiting radiation dose to the fetus become important considerations for the pregnant and potentially pregnant technologist.

Technologists who are considering pregnancy or who are of childbearing age may wish to review their monthly radiation exposure records. Individuals who receive more than 100 mrem (1 mSv) to the whole body per month should monitor their gonadal radiation exposure and use all appropriate precautions to minimize this exposure. In this way, exposures that may exceed the 500 mrem (5 mSv) limit can be reduced before pregnancy occurs. Also, by surveying the workplace, sources of radiation that may contribute to radiation exposure more significantly than other sources can be identified. For example, hot lab duties such as eluting the radionuclide generator and assisting in the administration of radioiodine therapy may produce more radiation exposure than routine imaging procedures. Also, more stringent precautions against the inhalation, ingestion, or absorption of radioactivity should be implemented to prevent possible incorporation of radioactive material into a developing fetus.

An employee should notify her supervisor as soon as she suspects that she may be pregnant or has confirmed that she is pregnant so that radiation exposure to the fetus can be monitored. It is important to remember that it is the radiation exposure to the fetus, not the mother, that must remain below 500 mrem (5 mSv). Thermoluminescent badges rather than film badges are recommended for monitoring radiation exposure, as TLDs provide a more accurate reading. Changing badges more frequently than once a month is not recommended since the badges do not give reliable readings below radiation exposures of 50 mrem (0.5 mSv). Double badging—placing one TLD at the waist, underneath the lead apron if the technologist wears one, and the other at the collar on the outside of the apron—is one way to record the dose to the fetus. In determining the radiation dose to the fetus, however, the effects of wearing a lead apron and attenuation of the overlying maternal tissue and amniotic fluid should be taken into account. Therefore, the exposure to the surface of the mother's abdomen overestimates the true radiation exposure to the fetus.

The pregnant employee should also be counseled by an appropriate individual (e.g., the nuclear medicine supervisor, radiation safety officer, nuclear medicine physician). The counseling session should be documented and include a review of the employee's previous radiation exposure record and methods for decreasing future radiation exposure. Also, the employee should be aware that up to 3% of all births involve serious defects and that the adverse effects of radiation exposure at low dose levels, such as those experienced by a nuclear medicine technologist, are extremely small in comparison with the normal risks of pregnancy. If there is a possibility that the fetus will receive more than 500 mrem (5 mSv), the employee's options should be addressed.

## PROTECTING OTHER PERSONNEL IN THE WORK ENVIRONMENT

Nuclear medicine technologists employ certain radiation safety practices to protect other personnel who may or may not be classified as occupationally exposed workers. The intent of such practices is to limit radiation exposure to others and to confine radioactivity to designated restricted areas and prevent its spread to other areas.

### Area Posting

Areas are classified as unrestricted or restricted. Unrestricted areas are accessed by the general public, so anyone who occupies such an area must receive not more than 2 mrem (0.02 mSv) in any single hour, not more than 100 mrem (1 mSv) in 7 consecutive days, and not more than 500 mrem (5 mSv) in a year. If these radiation limits are exceeded, access to the area must be controlled and the area is considered to be restricted. According to the NRC, restricted areas must be identified with one of the following signs.

*Caution: Radioactive Materials.* This phrase identifies any area in which radioactive materials are used or stored in amounts exceeding exempt quantities. A sign of this type is most often seen on nuclear medicine imaging rooms and storage areas.

*Caution: Radiation Area.* These words indicate an area in which a major part of the body could receive greater than 5 mrem (0.05 mSv) in any 1 hour or more than 100 mrem (1 mSv) in 5 consecutive days. Isolation rooms used for radioiodine therapy and radiopharmacy hot labs are areas that often require this sign.

*Caution: High Radiation Area.* This phrase indicates an area in which a major part of the body could receive more than 100 mrem (1 mSv) in any 1 hour. This sign has few nuclear medicine applications.

*Grave Danger: Very High Radiation Area.* These words indicate an area in which an individual could receive an absorbed dose of more than 500 rads (5 Gy) in 1 hour. This sign has few nuclear medicine applications.

## Area Surveys

Surveys of areas in which radioactivity is used or stored are required by the NRC to monitor external radiation exposure levels as well as removable surface contamination. Daily monitoring with a Geiger-Mueller (GM) counter or ionization chamber is required in areas where radiopharmaceuticals are prepared and administered. Weekly monitoring is required in areas where radioactive materials are stored. Places where higher than background levels of radiation are detected should be wipe tested to determine whether the contamination can be removed. Decontamination of sites should be carried out if the wipe tests indicate that the radioactivity is removable and should be continued until the background radiation level is reached or until no more contamination can be removed. If all contamination cannot be removed, taping a sheet of paper over the area will remind others in the area about the contamination and discourage them from walking or working in the area. NRC regulations require that records of area surveys and wipe tests be maintained for 3 years.

## Radioactive Spills

Spills of radioactive materials should be cleaned up promptly and thoroughly to prevent the spread of contamination to other areas or to personnel. Minor spills, involving only a small area or low level of radioactivity, can be handled as outlined here:

1. Inform other people working in the area that a spill has occurred and clear that area.
2. Put on protective clothing, such as gloves and shoe covers, before attempting to clean the spill.
3. Confine the spill to as small an area as possible. Placing absorbent paper over a liquid spill will soak up the spill as well as contain it in the absorbent material.
4. If personnel are contaminated, they should be decontaminated as soon as possible to prevent absorption or inhalation of the radioactivity. Decontamination may involve simply the removal of contaminated clothing or washing affected areas of the skin with mild soap and warm water. Harsh or abrasive cleaners and brushes should not be used because they may cause breaks in the skin, promoting internal absorption of the radioactive material or infection. Serious injuries should be treated before decontamination begins.
5. Place all materials used to clean up the spill in plastic bags for monitoring and disposal.
6. Monitor the area of the spill with a GM meter and start decontamination if necessary.
7. When decontamination is finished, remove all protective wear and discard with other contaminated materials. Monitor personal clothing, remove any that is contaminated, and place it in storage until the contamination has decayed to background levels.
8. Label all discarded materials as radioactive, and dispose of them properly or place in decay storage.
9. Notify the radiation safety officer about the spill.

Major radioactive spills involving high levels of radiation exposure or widespread contamination require special handling. Guidelines for dealing with major spills include the following:

1. Shut off ventilation, air conditioning and heating systems, and fume hoods to contain the spread of airborne contamination.
2. Remove contaminated clothing before leaving the area of the spill.
3. Evacuate personnel from the affected area and close and lock all doors to the area.
4. Post warning signs to inform others of the contamination.
5. Begin personnel decontamination. Again, medical treatment takes precedence over decontamination activities.
6. Notify the radiation safety officer immediately. Do not attempt to clean up or decontaminate major spills without direction from radiation safety personnel.

## Radioactive Waste Disposal

Decay in storage is an inexpensive method of disposal for short-lived, low-level radioactive waste, such as that generated in a nuclear medicine department. The waste is separated according to half-life and allowed to decay to background levels. Following decay, the waste is monitored and all radiation symbols are removed or defaced. The waste is then discarded along with other nonradioactive trash. Radioactive waste that contains potentially biohazardous materials, such as used needles and syringes, is incinerated after it has decayed to background radiation levels. The NRC requires that records of waste disposal by decay in storage be kept for 3 years.

Disposal of certain soluble materials through the sewer system is allowed, providing the amounts do not exceed calculated limits. The allowable limits vary for each institution since they are based on the rate of waste-water discharge from that facility. No limit is placed on patient excreta; therefore, all such material can be discarded through the sewer system. Limited quantities of radioactive gases may be discharged into the atmosphere. NRC regulations indicate the maximum permitted airborne concentrations. Typically, a health physicist calculates the limits of gas release into the atmosphere or soluble material release into the sewer for a facility.

Long-lived (half-life greater than 65 days) radioactive waste is disposed of by transfer to licensed commercial waste handlers. Such companies are authorized by the NRC to bury radioactive waste at an approved site or to incinerate it. All materials transferred for disposal must be labeled and packaged according to Department of Transportation requirements.

Care should be taken to keep radioactive and biohazardous waste separate from ordinary trash. Radioactive waste disposal records must be maintained, regardless of the method of disposal, to verify compliance with regulations.

### Handling Radioactive Gases and Aerosols

Radioactive xenon gas and Tc-99m DTPA aerosol are both used for lung ventilation imaging. Both require special handling to prevent the spread of radioactive contamination. Radioxenon is administered to the patient from a closed system through a mouthpiece, making the patient a part of the system. For the system to remain closed, patient cooperation is essen-

tial. The patient must maintain a firm grip on the mouthpiece and wear a nose clamp to prevent the gas from leaking out through the nose or around the mouth. Certain patients may not be able to cooperate or may attempt to remove the mouthpiece during the procedure, releasing the radioactive gas into the imaging room. The technologist should assess the patient's ability or willingness to cooperate before the xenon is administered and should explain the reasons for the breathing apparatus. Also, leading the patient through a practice run will acquaint him or her with what is expected as well as the sensations experienced in breathing into a closed system. The patient should be reassured that adequate oxygen will be supplied to the system.

Imaging rooms in which xenon ventilation studies are performed should be equipped with a ventilation system that maintains negative pressure within the room. Should a leak occur, such a system will contain the xenon inside the room and vent it out into the atmosphere. The room's ventilation system should be activated whenever a xenon ventilation study is performed. Xenon leaks can occur from the administration apparatus itself, as well as from the patient. Therefore, the equipment should be routinely checked for leaks by collecting an air sample during a ventilation study. Any evacuated tube designed for the collection of blood samples can be used. During the imaging procedure, the stopper of the evacuated tube is pierced with a needle. The vacuum in the tube causes room air to be drawn through the needle and into the tube. Samples should be collected around the tubing of the gas administration apparatus or other areas where a leak may occur. Following the ventilation study, the technologist counts the tubes in a well counter to determine that there are no leaks in the closed system. Also, the charcoal filter contained in the apparatus to absorb exhaled xenon should be replaced periodically. It becomes saturated with xenon, which decreases its trapping effectiveness.

During the administration of Tc-99m DTPA aerosol, it is important that the nebulizer into which the radiopharmaceutical is introduced is shielded and kept sealed to prevent the release of aerosol particles into the air. There have been reports that significant contamination can occur during the performance of aerosol studies. McGraw and colleagues found that the primary source of contamination is the exhaust vent of the aerosol administration device. The filter in the device is not able to trap all the exhausted aerosol adequately enough to prevent airborne contamination. Crawford and associates found that patient cooperation affected the amount of contamination in the air and on the floor. However, a patient's ability to cooperate did not always correlate with the amount of contamination found. Instead, patient practice and coaching by the technologist during the aerosol administration most strongly correlated with lower levels of contamination.

### Instructions to Hospital Personnel

Hospital employees such as nurses, patient escort personnel, and housekeeping staff are not considered occupationally exposed workers but often enter restricted areas or care for patients who have been administered radiopharmaceuticals. Housekeeping and maintenance staff should be informed that certain areas they enter contain radiation and instructed about the meaning of signs posted in those areas. Housekeeping staff should be told that contents of containers marked with the radioactive symbol and the phrase *Radioactive Materials* must not be discarded with other ordinary trash. Also, these containers will be handled by the nuclear medicine staff and should not be removed by housekeeping. Nuclear medicine personnel should ensure that housekeeping and maintenance staff will not be exposed to radiation and should not expect these staff members to assess radiation hazards.

Escort personnel frequently transport patients from the nuclear medicine department to patient rooms. The exposure to the escort is minimal because of the relatively brief association with the patient. However, if an escort is assigned to the nuclear medicine department, it may be appropriate for the escort to wear a radiation dosimeter.

Nurses often are assigned to care for patients who have received diagnostic amounts of radioactivity. Several studies have measured radiation exposure to nurses from such patients. Burks and colleagues monitored radiation expo-

sure from ambulatory patients over one calendar quarter to a group of nurses. All of the nurses received exposures much lower than the maximum permissible dose for nonoccupationally exposed workers, that is, less than 100 mrem (1 mSv) in a year. The highest cumulative quarterly exposure was 32.5 mrem (0.32 mSv) for one individual; the average cumulative quarterly dose was 11.2 mrem (0.11 mSv). Jankowski studied radiation exposure to critical care nurses over a 3-year period from portable X-ray machines, fluoroscopic units, and patients injected with radiopharmaceuticals. She concluded that radiation is not a significant occupational hazard for critical care nurses, since no cumulative exposures measured over the period exceeded 80 mrem (0.8 mSv). Contamination with radioactive body fluids is eliminated if Standard Precautions, designed to protect hospital personnel from the biologic hazards of human excreta, are followed. Nurses should also be advised that radioactive excreta can be disposed of through the sewer system.

Additional, special precautions are needed for handling patients who have received therapeutic amounts of radioactivity. These precautions are addressed in the section titled Radionuclide Therapy.

## PROTECTING THE PATIENT

For purposes of radiation protection, the conservative assumption is that there is no "risk-free" level of radiation. However, the risk or probability that an individual will develop a radiation-induced effect as a result of low-level radiation exposure is very small. Nevertheless, radiation is not used for diagnostic or therapeutic purposes unless the patient receives some medical benefit from its application. Many of the activities of nuclear medicine technologists directly influence the outcome of a nuclear medicine procedure and determine whether a particular procedure supplies appropriate, valid information to the physician to direct patient management. These activities provide radiation protection for patients by ensuring that they receive the minimum amount of radioactivity necessary to complete a test and by deriving the maximum benefit from the small amount of radiation received.

Table 12–2  Dose Calibrator Quality Control Tests

| Quality Control Test | Frequency* | Action |
|---|---|---|
| Constancy | Daily | Repair or replace instrument if error exceeds 10% |
| Linearity | At installation and quarterly | Correct readings if error exceeds 10% |
| Accuracy | At installation and annually | Repair or replace instrument if error exceeds 10% |
| Geometry | At installation | Correct readings if error exceeds 10% |

*All tests should also be performed following adjustment or repair of the dose calibrator.

## Patient Records

The medical record of every patient for whom a nuclear medicine test is ordered should be reviewed before any part of the test begins. First, the physician's order for a particular test should be verified, followed by confirmation of the reason, the clinical indication, for the test. Technologists should not be reluctant to seek additional information if the clinical indication for the test is not clear. This may spare the patient from undergoing an unneeded procedure or may identify a more appropriate test for the patient's condition. Asking questions should not be interpreted as questioning a physician's judgment but rather as performing the best test in the interests of the patient. Also, it is unrealistic to expect referring physicians to know the technical details of all diagnostic tests that they order. Obviously, information gathering of this type must be carried out with tact. In some instances, enlisting the help of the nuclear medicine physician may be more prudent than contacting the referring physician directly.

Certain diagnostic tests, therapies, and medications may cause an alteration of the radiopharmaceutical distribution in the patient. Knowledge of any of these in advance of the nuclear medicine procedure may cause the study to be postponed, suggest that additional views be performed, or add relevant detail to the interpretation of the study's results.

## Patient Doses

It is the technologist's responsibility to ensure that the correct patient receives the prescribed

radiopharmaceutical in the prescribed dosage and by the appropriate route of administration. First, the technologist must verify the identity of the patient. Quality management programs advocate a system in which two individuals independently confirm the patient's identity before any drug is administered or procedure initiated. Next, in preparing the prescribed patient dose, the technologist must ensure that the correct radiopharmaceutical is furnished by carefully reading the label on the radiopharmaceutical vial or unit dose syringe. Many of the radiopharmaceuticals used in nuclear medicine are tagged with the same radionuclide, Tc-99m, so it is important to read the entire radiopharmaceutical name including the compound. Before administering the dose to the patient, the NRC requires that it be assayed in a dose calibrator to confirm that the prescribed amount of radioactivity is being administered. A record of these measurements must be retained for 3 years. To ensure that the dose calibrator reading is valid, dose calibrator quality control must be performed as outlined in the NRC regulations and the records must be maintained for 3 years. Table 12–2 summarizes the required dose calibrator quality control tests and their frequency.

It is important to remember that when radiopharmaceuticals are administered to a patient, many organs of the body are irradiated, not only the organ being imaged. In many instances, the critical organ, the organ receiving the greatest radiation exposure, is not the organ being imaged. However, the radiation dose to the critical organ strongly governs the recommended range of radioactivity to be administered for a

Table 12–3  Estimated Absorbed Radiation Doses to the Target Organ
for Selected Radiopharmaceuticals

| Radiopharmaceutical | Target Organ | Absorbed Radiation Dose to Target Organ (rad/mCi [mGy/MBq]) |
|---|---|---|
| Ga-67 gallium citrate* | GI tract | |
| | Stomach | 0.22 (0.059) |
| | Small intestine | 0.36 (0.097) |
| | Upper large intestine | 0.56 (0.151) |
| | Lower large intestine | 0.90 (0.243) |
| T1-201 thallous chloride† | Kidney | 1.2  (0.32) |

*MIRD Dose Estimate Report No. 2. J Nucl Med 14:755–756, 1973.

†Atkins HL, et al: Thallium-201 for medical use. Part 3. Human distribution and physical imaging properties. J Nucl Med 18:133–140, 1977.

particular agent. For this reason, it is important that only the prescribed amount of radioactivity be given to minimize the radiation dose to the critical organ as well as other target organs. Table 12–3 lists several radiopharmaceuticals, their target organs, and the absorbed radiation dose to the target organs to illustrate this point.

### Instructions to Patients

Appropriate instruction of the patient is another way in which the technologist applies the ALARA concept to minimize radiation exposure to the patient. Giving inadequate directions or failing to determine the patient's understanding of the directions may result in the study's having to be repeated, increasing the patient's radiation exposure. Failure to discontinue certain medications, to abstain from certain foods, or to return for delayed images are examples of not following instructions that affect the outcome of a test. Some instructions are designed to reduce exposure by hastening the transit of the radiopharmaceutical through the body. Encouraging patients to drink fluids following injection of a bone-imaging agent and prescribing laxatives or enemas after administration of Ga-67 gallium citrate remove excreted radiopharmaceutical from the body and decrease radiation exposure to the bladder wall and gastrointestinal tract wall, respectively.

In certain situations, the instructions should include precautions to reduce radiation expo-

sure to others the patient may come in contact with, such as members of the same household, particularly children. Such instructions are most important following radionuclide therapy and are discussed in that section of the chapter. However, when radiopharmaceuticals are administered to nursing mothers, their babies receive external gamma radiation as it is emitted from the mother and may ingest radioactivity contained in the breast milk. Since data are limited on the uptake and excretion of radiopharmaceuticals in infants, recommendations for discontinuing breastfeeding following radiopharmaceutical administration vary from one author to another. Some recommended times for selected radiopharmaceuticals are shown in Table 12–4.

### Equipment

As discussed in the section on patient doses, dose calibrators are used to verify the amount of radioactivity administered. Clearly, it is important that these instruments provide accurate readings. Too much administered radioactivity will increase the patient's radiation exposure beyond what is necessary to obtain a technically satisfactory study. Conversely, too little administered radioactivity can compromise the quality of images because of inadequate counting statistics or lengthy imaging times for which the patient may not be able to cooperate or during which the patient may move. Not only will the patient probably not

Table 12–4 Recommendations for Discontinuing Breast-Feeding Following Radiopharmaceutical Administration to Nursing Mothers

| Radiopharmaceutical | Administered Activity (mCi [MBq]) | Time Interval |
| --- | --- | --- |
| I-123 sodium iodide (without radiocontaminants)* | 0.3 (11) | 4 days# |
| I-123 sodium iodide (with I-124 or I-125)† | 0.3 (11) | Discontinue |
| I-131 sodium iodide* | 10 (370) | Discontinue |
| Tc-99m MAA* | 3 (111) | 12 hours# |
| Tc-99m medronate‡ | 11 (400) | 4 hours# |
| Tc-99m pertechnetate§ | 20 (740) | 24 hours# |
| Tc-99m labeled RBCs‡ | 15 (550) | 4 hours# |

*Wagner LK, Fabrikant JI, Fry RJM, et al: Radiation Bioeffects and Management Test and Syllabus. Reston, VA, American College of Radiology, 1991.

†Dydek GJ, Blue PW: Human breast milk excretion of iodine-131 following diagnostic and therapeutic administration to a lactating patient with Graves' disease. J Nucl Med 29:407–410, 1988.

‡Ahlgren L, Ivarsson S, Johansson L, et al: Excretion of radionuclides in human breast milk after the administration of radiopharmaceuticals. J Nucl Med 26:1085–1090, 1985.

§Romney BM, Nickoloff EL, Esser PD, et al: Radionuclide administration to nursing mothers. Radiology 160:549–554, 1986.

#During this interval, all milk should be expressed and discarded.

benefit from a suboptimal study, he or she also may be exposed to a second dose of radioactivity if the study must be repeated.

Likewise, proper scintillation camera performance is necessary to produce diagnostically accurate images. Scintillation camera systems must be assessed for uniformity, spatial resolution, and linearity on a routine basis. Tomographic cameras require additional quality control tests to assess their ability to perform as tomographic devices. Table 12–5 summarizes the recommended scintillation camera quality control tests and their frequencies. Improperly functioning imaging equipment can introduce artifacts into diagnostic images that may lead to misinterpretation of a study's results. This misinterpretation may adversely influence the patient by falsely suggesting that no treatment is necessary or by suggesting unnecessary treatment. And again, such a study may necessitate its repetition, exposing the patient to additional radiation. It is important for the technologist to remember that the physician is often far removed from the assessment of equipment function and the technical performance of a study. Therefore, the nuclear medicine technol-

Table 12–5 Scintillation Camera Quality Control Tests

| Quality Control Test | Frequency |
| --- | --- |
| Planar scintillation camera | |
| Field uniformity | Daily |
| Spatial resolution and linearity | Weekly |
| Sensitivity | Annually |
| Tomographic scintillation camera | |
| Center of rotation correction | Weekly |
| Uniformity correction | Weekly |

ogist is obligated to perform instrumentation quality control conscientiously, to obtain the necessary service for equipment when indicated, and to inform the physician about any conditions that could compromise the diagnostic accuracy of a procedure.

## Immobilization Techniques

Patient restraint devices have already been discussed as one method of using distance to reduce radiation exposure to the technologist from a radioactive patient. Immobilization devices and techniques also benefit the patient by preventing motion that could lengthen imaging time or compromise image quality. Immobilization has become increasingly important with the growth of tomographic imaging. Tomographic imaging times are lengthy and patients must maintain the same position for the entire imaging time. Certain patients may not be able to cooperate throughout a second acquisition, so acquiring data on the first try without movement is critical. Also, having to repeat lengthy acquisitions can seriously upset a department's imaging schedule. More importantly, the technologist should strive to obtain the best quality study to justify the patient's radiation exposure and to minimize the possibility of having to repeat the images with a second dose of radioactivity.

### The Pregnant or Potentially Pregnant Patient

At low radiation doses, below 1 rem (0.1 Sv), the risk to a fetus is thought to be minimal and outweighed by the medical benefit of the procedure to the mother. However, most nuclear medicine procedures exceed this radiation dose, so the pregnancy status of women of childbearing age is established before the administration of radionuclides.

Along with reviewing the medical record, the nuclear medicine technologist is often responsible for gathering additional medical information by interviewing the patient. In the case of female patients of childbearing age, it is always important to question the patient about whether she may be pregnant. This is a sensitive subject and may be better addressed toward the end of the interview after the technologist has established a rapport with the patient. The technologist should explain the necessity of obtaining this information. If 4 weeks or more have passed since the patient's last menstrual period, the nuclear medicine physician should be told, because this may indicate the need for a more extensive menstrual history and a pregnancy test.

Pregnancy is a contraindication to radioiodine therapy. Any female patient scheduled for radioiodine therapy should have a pregnancy test immediately before therapy.

## RADIONUCLIDE THERAPY

### Radioiodine Therapy

Iodine-131 sodium iodide is used to treat hyperthyroidism and thyroid cancer. The special handling and precautions required when working with radioiodine have been discussed earlier in this chapter. Administration of the radioiodine may take place in the nuclear medicine department away from imaging and waiting areas, or in a hospital isolation room, if the situation indicates. The patient should be asked to remove any dental appliances to which the radioiodine may adhere, such as removable bridges and dentures, thereby increasing radiation exposure to the oral cavity. The patient should be fasting to enhance absorption of the radioiodine from the stomach and to minimize the volume of vomitus should the patient develop nausea. An emesis basin should be at hand to minimize contamination of the area should vomiting occur. If a patient vomits, all personnel in the immediate area should be monitored for contamination. Anyone known to be contaminated should receive oral potassium iodide or another blocking agent immediately to prevent radioiodine uptake in the thyroid. Thyroid counting should be performed on the following day on all personnel in the area of contamination to determine any thyroid uptake of radioiodine.

Arrangements for radioiodine therapy requiring isolation of the patient include preparation of the isolation room, the patient, and selected nursing personnel. The isolation room should be a private room at the end of a hall or in some other area where traffic from other patients, visitors, and personnel is at a minimum. It should be prepared to minimize contamination and facilitate decontamination of the space after discharge of the patient. The floor and other flat surfaces such as countertops and dressers should be covered with plastic-backed absorbent paper. The mattress and chairs should also be covered with plastic. Door knobs, drawer knobs, television knobs, handles, and the telephone receiver should be covered with plastic wrap secured with tape or rubber bands. A container for dirty linen should be placed in the patient's room. All linen should be monitored for contamination before it is sent to the hospital laundry, as should the patient's disposable eating utensils and uneaten food before disposal.

Once the radioiodine has been administered to the patient, the isolation room must be posted with a sign reading "Caution: Patient Contains Radioactive Material." Following the patient's discharge, the room should be decontaminated and monitored by either nuclear medicine personnel or the radiation safety officer before the room is released for cleaning and assigned to another patient.

It is important that the patient be informed about what is expected during the isolation period. Patient cooperation is essential if radioactive contamination and external radiation exposure to staff and visitors are to be minimized. The patient should be briefed about the sources of contamination from radioiodine therapy. In addition to the radiation safety precautions noted earlier, the patient should be advised that routine nursing care will be kept to a minimum. Reassurance that any necessary medical or nursing care will be provided as necessary is appropriate to decrease any feelings of abandonment or rejection the patient may feel. Such feelings may be compounded since visitation by family members must also be restricted. Children and pregnant women should not be allowed to visit the patient. The length of visits and the distance to be maintained between visitors and patients should be thoroughly explained to both the patient and the visitors.

Many patients experience feelings of boredom and isolation while confined to one small area, even though they have verbal contact with others. Diversional activities may make the time spent in isolation feel shorter and perhaps more productive. Access to a television, radio, and telephone can decrease feelings of being cut off from the world. Patients should also be encouraged to bring their own materials to occupy their time. It must be stressed that at no time can the patient leave the isolation room since this may spread radioactivity into other areas of the hospital and expose others to radiation emitted from the patient. Because most radioiodine is excreted in the urine, the patient should be encouraged to drink fluids and instructed to flush the toilet several times after each use. The technologist should be extremely cautious in predicting when the patient will be released from isolation. However, the technologist should offer reassurance that the patient's radiation level will be monitored daily, so that the patient will be hospitalized for the shortest time necessary.

All nursing staff who will be caring for the patient must be issued either film or thermoluminescent dosimeters. They should be instructed how and when to wear them. No pregnant personnel should be assigned to care for the therapy patient. Nursing staff should be instructed to minimize the time spent in direct contact with the patient. However, it should be stressed that emergency care should be given immediately if needed. Nursing personnel should be instructed that following Standard Precautions will reduce the possibility of external contamination. Gloves should always be worn if contact with the patient, patient's body fluids, or other objects in the isolation room is a possibility. The only additional protective clothing necessary is shoe covers, which should be worn whenever a nurse enters the therapy patient's room and removed immediately outside the door.

The names and telephone numbers, both home and work, of the nuclear medicine physician, radiation safety officer, and nuclear medicine technologists should be posted along with other detailed instructions in the front of the patient's medical record. Nursing personnel should be encouraged to contact any of these individuals with their questions or if any unusual circumstance arises. Nuclear medicine personnel need to keep in mind that handling radioactivity is a daily routine for them but it is an unfamiliar, and perhaps apprehensive, experience for the personnel assigned to provide nursing care to the therapy patient. All questions should be answered in an informative, nonpatronizing way that respects the inquirer as a colleague.

The radioiodine dose should be transported to the isolation room in a shielded container for administration. Since the radionuclide will be transported through unrestricted areas, adequate shielding should be used so that individuals in these areas are not exposed to more than 2 mrem (0.02 mSv). The patient should be fasting before the radioiodine is administered.

After administration of the radioiodine, the

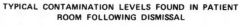

TYPICAL CONTAMINATION LEVELS FOUND IN PATIENT
ROOM FOLLOWING DISMISSAL

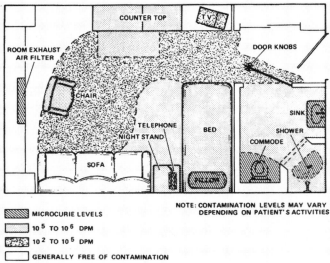

NOTE: CONTAMINATION LEVELS MAY VARY
DEPENDING ON PATIENT'S ACTIVITIES

MICROCURIE LEVELS
$10^5$ TO $10^6$ DPM
$10^2$ TO $10^5$ DPM
GENERALLY FREE OF CONTAMINATION

**Figure 12–2** Typical contamination levels found in the patient room following dismissal. (Reprinted with permission from Miller KT, Bott SM, Velkley DE, Cummingham DE: Review of contamination and exposure hazards associated with therapeutic uses of radioiodine. J Nucl Med Technol 7:163–166, 1979.)

patient is monitored with a portable ionization chamber at a distance of 3 meters to determine the initial dose rate. Daily measurements collected using the same counting geometry are compared to the initial dose rate and may be used to determine when the patient can be removed from isolation. The dose rate measurements are related to the amount of radioactivity retained by the patient:

$$\frac{\text{initial dose rate}}{\text{mCi administered}} = \frac{\text{subsequent dose rate}}{\text{mCi retained}}$$

For example, a patient receives 200 mCi (7.4 GBq) of $^{131}$I. Immediately following the administration, the dose rate at 3 meters measures 200 mrem/hr (2 mSv/hr). Forty-eight hours later, the dose rate at 3 meters measures 50 mrem/hr (0.5 mSv/hr). How many mCi (GBq) remain in the patient?

$$\frac{200 \text{ mrem/hr}}{200 \text{ mCi}} = \frac{50 \text{ mrem/hr}}{\text{x mCi}}$$

$$\text{x} = \frac{200 \text{ mCi (50 mrem/hr)}}{200 \text{ mrem/hr}}$$

$$\text{x} = 50 \text{ mCi (1.85 GBq)}$$

The measured dose rates are also used to determine exposure times for personnel, visitors, and patients in adjacent rooms. According to NRC regulations, the radiation exposure of nonoccupationally exposed individuals, which includes nurses, must be limited to 2 mrem (0.02 mSv) in any 1 hour, or 100 mrem (1 mSv) in 7 consecutive days. Since the measured exposure rates from therapy patients always exceed these limits, the length of time visitors and nursing personnel can remain in the room must be calculated.

Patients in rooms adjacent to the isolation room also should not exceed the radiation exposure limits stated above. Therefore, following administration of the radioiodine, the radiation dose rate to nearby patients should be measured and recorded.

Following discharge of the therapy patient, the isolation room must be decontaminated before it can be released for use by another patient. Figure 12–2 illustrates the level and location of radioiodine contamination in a typical therapy isolation room. Prior preparation of the room should make decontamination easier. Special attention should be given to the bathroom floor and fixtures, the telephone

**Table 12–6** Summary of NRC Regulations for Patients Receiving Therapeutic Doses of I-131

| Basis for Release | Criteria for Release | Instructions Needed? | Release Records Required? |
| --- | --- | --- | --- |
| Administered activity | Administered activity ≤33 mCi (1221 MBq) | Yes, if administered activity >7 mCi (259 MBq) | No |
| Retained activity | Retained activity ≤33 mCi (1221 MBq) | Yes, if retained activity >7 mCi (259 MBq) | Yes* |
| Measured dose rate | Measured dose rate from patient ≤7 mrem/hr (0.07 mSv/hr) | Yes, if measured dose rate from patient >2 mrem/hr (0.02 mSv/hr) | Yes* |
| Patient-specific calculations | Calculated dose to others ≤5 mSv (0.5) rem | Yes, if calculated dose to others >1 mSv (0.1 rem) | Yes* |

*These records must include a patient identifier that preserves the patient's confidentiality, the radioactive material administered, the administered activity, and the date of administration. Additional information specific to the basis for release is also required.

receiver, and the bed pillow. Air filters collect airborne $^{131}$I and should be monitored and replaced. The contaminated filters should be decayed in storage before reuse or disposal. If housekeeping staff are involved in the decontamination process, they should be supervised by the radiation safety officer. When decontamination is complete, all participants should be monitored. The patient's personal effects that were brought into the isolation room should also be monitored before they are released to the patient.

The NRC regulations regarding the release of $^{131}$I therapy patients from isolation have changed recently. The new regulations apply to any patient receiving therapeutic doses of $^{131}$I. The need for isolation or the release from isolation are both based on the potential radiation dose to individuals with whom the patient may come in contact. If the estimated radiation dose to any of these individuals will likely exceed 5 mSv (0.5 rem), then the patient must be isolated. The four criteria that may be used to determine whether a patient can be released from isolation are summarized in Table 12–6. All four criteria are based on members of the public receiving no more than 5 mSv (0.5 rem) from the patient.

Based on the new regulations, in most instances, instructions regarding radiation safety precautions must be given to $^{131}$I therapy patients. In practice, these instructions were typically given to therapy patients anyway, but now they are specifically required by the NRC regulations. It is best to review these instructions when $^{131}$I therapy is suggested, so that the patient will have a full understanding of the procedure and be able to make a more fully informed decision about the therapy. However, it is important to discuss them again following the therapy.

The technologist should inform the patient about the most likely routes of radioiodine transfer and should review the following guidelines:

1. Intimate personal contact should be avoided. Spouses should not occupy the same bed. Children, especially, should not be held or kissed.
2. Minimize time in public places such as grocery stores, theaters, sporting events, and restaurants.
3. The toilet should be double flushed after each use.
4. Thorough handwashing is essential.
5. Eating utensils, cups, and glasses should not be shared with the patient.
6. Breastfeeding should be discontinued.

The technologist should be reassuring and should seek to alleviate any anxiety or fear the patient may have regarding the safety of the family members.

Jacobson and associates monitored the family members of patients who received radioiodine therapy. His group recorded external radiation exposure to these relatives, as well as internal radiation exposure to their thyroids. His findings showed that transfer of radioiodine from patient to family members does occur and that adherence to certain guidelines did minimize external and internal radiation exposures to family members. For the first few days after treatment, iodine that is not bound to thyroid hormone is present in urine, saliva, perspiration, and the breath. Eventually, the unbound iodine is eliminated. During this interval of about 1 week, therapy patients should be instructed to adhere to the guidelines listed above.

### Phosphorus-32 Therapy

Phosphorus-32 (P-32) is used in several chemical forms for therapeutic purposes. Sodium phosphate P-32 is administered intravenously in amounts ranging from 4 to 15 mCi (148 to 555 MBq). Typically, this administration is performed on an outpatient basis in the nuclear medicine department. P-32 is a pure beta emitter and should be shielded accordingly. Beta particles cause the production of bremsstrahlung radiation when they interact with a high-density shielding material such as lead. Therefore, effective shielding includes the radiopharmaceutical vial itself or the syringe into which it is withdrawn. External and internal contamination should be avoided by the standard methods already discussed. This agent is taken up into the bone marrow almost completely within 2 days of administration. Patients should be informed about the potential for contamination from urine in the week following P-32 injection. They should be advised to flush the toilet twice after each use and to wash hands thoroughly after voiding.

Chromic phosphate P-32 is a colloidal suspension used for treating pleural or peritoneal effusions. Five to 20 mCi (185 to 740 MBq) of the radiopharmaceutical is introduced into the pleural or peritoneal space. Patients receiving this type of therapy are usually hospitalized because thoracentesis or paracentesis is necessary to inject the material into the body cavity. The radioactivity remains in the body space and leaves the body only through physical decay. All equipment used to administer the P-32 should

**Table 12–7** Physical Characteristics of Selected Radionuclides Used for Therapy

| Radionuclide | Half-Life (days) | $E_{max\ \beta-}$ (MeV) | $E_\gamma$ (keV) |
|---|---|---|---|
| Phosphorous-32 | 14.3 | 1.71 | None |
| Strontium-89 | 50.5 | 1.43 | 910 (<1%) |
| Samarium-153 | 1.9 | 0.81 | 103 (29%) |

be handled as radioactive waste. Since some of the fluid containing the radionuclide may leak from the body cavity, personnel responsible for changing bed linens or bandages covering the puncture site should be instructed to wear gloves and to keep potentially contaminated materials separate for monitoring and disposal by nuclear medicine personnel.

### Strontium-89 and Samarium-153 Therapy

Strontium-89 (Sr-89) chloride and samarium-153 (Sm-153) lexidronam are used to relieve the pain of bone metastases. They are administered intravenously and the excess radiopharmaceutical not taken up into the bone is excreted into the urine. Table 12–7 outlines the physical characteristics of these radionuclides along with P-32, which has also been used to treat bone pain. Note that Sr-89 is essentially a pure beta emitter; hence, the same shielding considerations should be observed as previously described for P-32. Samarium-153 emits, in addition to beta particles, a gamma photon with an abundance that requires lead shielding. A lining of low atomic number material such as plastic may be used between the Sm-153 container and the lead shield. The plastic lining will absorb the beta particles emitted by the Sm-153 and prevent their interaction with the lead shield, thereby minimizing the production of bremsstrahlung radiation.

The technologist should be aware of a few other important technical considerations. Since beta particles have short ranges in tissue, infiltration of these radiopharmaceuticals can cause localized radiation damage to the soft tissue. Therefore, it is recommended that a patent intravenous line be established through which the agent is administered. Urinary excretion of these agents is greatest for the first 24 hours following administration. Incontinent patients should be catheterized to prevent radioactive contamination of clothing, bed linens, and the surrounding environment. Finally, all materials contaminated with Sr-89 or Sm-153, such as those associated with their administration, should be handled as radioactive waste, typically by placing them in storage and allowing the radionuclides to decay to background levels.

## SUMMARY

This chapter addresses radiation protection techniques applicable to the practice of nuclear medicine. Nuclear medicine technologists are responsible for incorporating the ALARA philosophy into daily practice to minimize radiation exposure to themselves, their patients, members of the general public, and other personnel in the work environment.

Nuclear medicine technologists minimize their occupational radiation exposure by shielding radioactive sources whenever practical. Maximizing the distance from radioactive sources and reducing the length of time spent working with radioactivity are two other methods to decrease exposure. Guidelines to reduce the potential for internal contamination include methods to prevent the ingestion, inhalation, or absorption of radionuclides through the skin. The pregnant technologist should notify her supervisor as soon as she suspects or confirms the pregnancy so that radiation exposure to the fetus can be monitored and kept below the regulatory limit of 500 mrem during the gestation period.

Nuclear medicine technologists use many radiation safety practices to protect other hospital personnel as well as themselves. The intent of such practices is to limit external radiation exposure to others and to prevent radioactive contamination of restricted and unrestricted areas.

The goal of nuclear medicine technologists is to administer the minimum amount of radioactivity to achieve the maximum medical benefit for the patient. The accuracy of patient doses, proper instruction of patients, regular instrumentation quality control testing, and

attention to the technical detail of nuclear medicine procedures all contribute to this goal and minimize the radiation exposure to the patient. Technologists must make an effort to establish the pregnancy status of all female patients of childbearing age before a radiopharmaceutical is administered.

Radioiodine therapy involves higher amounts of radioactivity than is used for diagnostic examinations. The patient should be instructed in the special precautions to be followed to minimize radiation exposure or contamination of family members. If the patient must be placed in isolation, special preparation of the patient, the isolation room, and the nursing staff is necessary prior to administration of the therapy dose. Additional radiation safety precautions must be followed by visitors and hospital personnel while the patient is in isolation. Following discharge of the patient, the isolation room must be decontaminated. Phosphorus-32, Sr-89, and Sm-153 are also used therapeutically and require special handling because they are beta emitters.

## Questions

1.  All of the following activities will reduce radiation exposure *except:*

    a. wearing a ring thermoluminescent dosimeter on the dominant hand
    b. using syringe shields at all times
    c. occupying the hot lab only when preparing patient doses
    d. employing immobilization devices to hold patients in position

2.  Which of the following materials provides the best shielding for a beta-emitting radionuclide?

    a. lead syringe shield    b. plastic syringe
    c. glass vial             d. b or c

3.  Thyroid counting should be performed how long after workers have handled radioiodine solutions?

    a. immediately    b. 4 to 6 hours
    c. 24 hours       d. 1 week

4. Which of the following is the best method of immobilizing a patient?

   a. verbal encouragement
   b. restraint by another technologist
   c. taping the patient in position
   d. b or c

5. Which of the following signs should be posted in an area where radiation levels are less than 2 mrem/hr?

   a. Caution: Radioactive Materials
   b. Caution: Radiation Area
   c. Caution: High Radiation Area
   d. No sign is required

6. All of the following radionuclides can be decayed in storage *except:*

   a. Cs-137      b. Ga-67
   c. $^{131}$I      d. Tl-201

7. Patients who are having bone imaging performed are instructed to drink fluids and to void frequently to:

   a. increase bone uptake of the radiopharmaceutical
   b. prevent visualization of the kidneys on the bone image
   c. enhance clearance of the tracer from the body
   d. ensure proper biodistribution of the radiopharmaceutical

8. Radioiodine is excreted from the body in which of the following body fluids?

   a. urine
   b. saliva
   c. perspiration
   d. all of the above

9. Following radioiodine therapy, the greatest amount of contamination will most likely be found on the:

   a. table and dresser tops
   b. floor
   c. door knobs
   d. bathroom fixtures

10. Chromic phosphate P-32 is administered by what route?

   a. orally
   b. intraperitoneally
   c. intrathecally
   d. intravenously

## Exercises

1. Outline the key elements of an ALARA program associated with hot lab duties (generator elution, radiopharmaceutical kit and unit dose preparation).

2. Identify steps to minimize the spread of radioactive contamination when performing lung ventilation studies with radioxenon or radioaerosol.

3. What instructions should be given to nursing personnel who routinely care for patients who have received diagnostic doses of radioactivity?

4. As part of a quality improvement program, identify items to be placed on a checklist designed to assist technologists in gathering the appropriate information from the patient and the medical record.

5. Describe the best way to explain to a concerned parent why an immobilization device is a better alternative than having the parent hold the child.

6. Following radioiodine therapy for hyperthyroidism, what instructions should be given to a patient who is the mother of a 1-year-old child?

7. Describe how a technologist might reassure a patient who is apprehensive about the isolation required for radioiodine therapy.

8. A patient received 150 mCi of $^{131}$I. Immediately following dose administration, the dose rate at 3 meters from the patient was 90 mrem/hr. At what dose rate will the patient contain less than 33 mCi of radioactivity?

9. Explain how scintillation camera quality control relates to the ALARA concept and patient radiation safety.

10. Describe some techniques the technolo-

gist might use to ascertain that patients understand pre-examination instructions.

## Activities

1. Draw a floor plan of the nuclear medicine department and identify those areas to be surveyed on a daily basis. Determine the background level for each area with a survey meter and record it on an appropriate form.

2. After completing activity 1, review all radiation signs posted in the nuclear medicine department. Are restricted and unrestricted areas posted correctly based on the radiation levels recorded for those areas?

3. Review your monthly radiation dosimetry reports for the past few months. Are the exposures similar from month to month? If not, can you identify reasons why exposures were greater in certain months? Propose some changes in your work habits to reduce your exposure.

4. Observe graduate nuclear medicine technologists in the clinical setting. Which radiation safety practices are most frequently ignored? If you were the nuclear medicine supervisor, how could you encourage these technologists to follow the ALARA philosophy?

5. Using a survey meter, measure the radiation dose rate from patients receiving various diagnostic procedures in nuclear medicine. Use the same counting geometry for each patient. Tabulate your results and summarize your findings.

6. Develop an in-service session to help housekeeping personnel work more safely in restricted areas. List the information that this group should have regarding radiation areas.

7. Develop a justification to be presented to the assistant hospital administrator for the purchase of a new xenon administration and trapping device. Base the justification on radiation safety considerations.

## Answers

### Questions

| | |
|---|---|
| 1. a | 6. a |
| 2. d | 7. c |
| 3. c | 8. d |
| 4. c | 9. d |
| 5. d | 10. b |

### Exercises

1. Key elements for any ALARA program include effective use of time, distance, and shielding. In the hot lab, these methods can be employed in the following ways:

*Shielding*

- Shield all vials and syringes containing radioactivity.
- Work behind an L-block.
- Shield radioactive waste containers.
- Store all radioactive materials behind lead bricks.
- Add additional shielding around radionuclide generator.

*Distance and Time*

- Keep radioactive materials at arm's length or use tongs if practical.
- Gather and organize supplies before manipulating radioactivity.
- Work quickly and efficiently.
- Store radioactive waste for decay in storage area away from hot lab.
- Perform routine paperwork and record-keeping outside of the hot lab.
- Rotate hot lab responsibilities among available staff.

*Miscellaneous*

- Purchase the smallest radionuclide generator needed to complete clinical schedule.
- Wipe test the lab daily to detect removable contamination.

2. To minimize radioactive contamination during the performance of lung ventilation studies, the technologist should:

a. ensure that the charcoal filter in the radioxenon trap is changed when it becomes saturated with radioxenon.

b. ensure that the tubing connections are firmly attached and that the hoses do not leak. Leakage may be determined by collecting air samples during the performance of a radioxenon study. Wipe tests following an aerosol study should be performed on the exhaust vent of the aerosol administration device and areas around the patient such as the floor.

c. activate the room ventilation system to maintain negative pressure within the imaging room to prevent escape of leaked radioxenon into other areas.

d. have the patient wear a nose clamp during a radioxenon study.

e. allow the patient to practice breathing on the administration system to familiarize the patient with the study routine and sensations of breathing into a closed system.

f. offer encouragement to the patient during the ventilation study to elicit cooperation.

g. ensure that adequate oxygen flow is being delivered to the closed breathing system.

3. Nursing personnel should be made aware of the routes by which radiopharmaceuticals are excreted from the body and that most excretion takes place through the urine. Therefore, if Standard Precautions are observed when handling patient excreta, the likelihood of radioactive contamination is very small. Nurses should also be informed that radioactive patient excreta can be disposed of into the sewer system.

   As for external radiation, most of the agents in nuclear medicine are tagged with Tc-99m, which has a very short half-life. The short half-life, in conjunction with the excretion of the radiopharmaceutical from the body, decreases the amount of radiation emitted from the patient over time. Several studies have shown that the amount of exposure a nurse would receive from providing care even to very ill patients is quite

small and below the regulatory exposure limit for the general public. However, whenever practical, nurses could minimize the amount of time spent in proximity to the patient as well as increasing their distance.

4. Review of the medical record and interviewing the patient are intended to ensure that the patient receives the maximum medical benefit from a nuclear medicine test and that this benefit outweighs the small risk associated with exposure to diagnostic radiation. Identification of certain information in the patient's medical history and medical record supports the medical need for the examination. This information should include:

   • verification of the referring physician's order for the nuclear medicine examination for a particular patient

   • confirmation of an appropriate clinical indication for the test to ensure that the test will supply the information the patient's physician is seeking

   • previous diagnostic tests (other imaging examinations, laboratory tests), therapies (i.e., radiation therapy, surgery), or medications that may affect the biodistribution of the tracer in the patient

   • for fertile female patients, date of last menstrual period to help ascertain pregnancy status

5. The technologist should assure the parent that completing a technical satisfactory examination is the goal, while demonstrating sensitivity to the feelings of the parent and the child. First, immobilization devices more effectively prevent patient movement than holding by another individual. Also, they are used in place of sedation, if possible. Second, movement affects the quality of the images and their accurate interpretation. Third, severe motion artifacts may require repetition of the examination, exposing the child to an additional dose of radioactivity. Last, holding the child would expose the parent to a small amount of radiation though an amount associated with very low risk to the parent. One alternative way may be to use

restraint devices on the child but place the parent in a location where the child can see him or her. The parent should also be reassured that there is no sensation associated with acquisition of the image itself and that the procedure is not physically painful.

6. It should be stressed that the intent of the precautions is to minimize radiation exposure to family members who will derive no direct medical benefit from it. To prevent external irradiation of family members, prolonged close contact should be avoided. Spouses should not sleep in the same bed, and children should not be held for extended periods, as for bottle-feeding. Internal transfer of radioiodine can be avoided by preventing the exchange of body fluids (saliva, perspiration, urine) to other family members. Therefore, kissing, sharing of eating and drinking utensils, and holding or caressing are activities between family members and the patient to be avoided. Also, a strict handwashing regimen, particularly before food preparation, should be observed by the patient. The patient should also be aware that bathroom fixtures are potential sources of contamination to others. If a separate bathroom is available, it should be designated for exclusive use by the patient. Breastfeeding, if still occurring, should be discontinued.

7. The technologist should first attempt to identify the source of the patient's apprehension. If this is the patient's first therapy, the term *isolation* may be interpreted by the patient to mean that there will be no communication between the patient and hospital staff or family members. The patient should be reassured that both nuclear medicine and nursing staff will communicate in person with the patient several times a day. Any emergency medical care, should it become necessary, will not be withheld because of the patient's isolation. Also, visitors will be permitted, although they will be required to stand outside the isolation room and to refrain from physical contact with the patient. If a

telephone is permitted inside the isolation room, the patient will be able to keep in contact with friends and family.

It should be stressed that restricting the patient to one room is the most practical method of protecting hospital staff and visitors from unnecessary exposure to radiation. Nuclear medicine personnel will monitor the patient daily to determine the earliest possible time that the patient can be released from isolation. Many hospitalized patients fail to drink sufficient fluids and become dehydrated. The technologist may suggest that the patient drink fluids liberally and void frequently to enhance clearance of the unbound iodine from the body. However, the technologist should be cautious about predicting the time of release from isolation. The patient should also be encouraged to bring some activities that will occupy the time. A television and radio should be provided in the isolation room, if possible.

8. $$\frac{\text{initial dose rate}}{\text{mCi administered}} = \frac{\text{subsequent dose rate}}{\text{mCi retained}}$$

$$\frac{90 \text{ mrem/hr}}{150 \text{ mCi}} = \frac{x}{30 \text{ mCi}}$$

$$x = \frac{30 \text{ mCi } (90 \text{ mrem/hr})}{150 \text{ mCi}}$$

$$x = 19.8 \text{ mrem/hr}$$

If 30 mCi yields a dose rate of 19.8 mrem/hr, any dose rate less than 19.8 mrem/hr indicates that the patient has retained less than 30 mCi.

9. The ALARA concept stresses that radiation exposure should be reduced to the lowest level possible through reasonable and cost-effective means. Performing scintillation camera quality control is one way that the technologist helps to ensure that the patient will derive the most medical value from a nuclear medicine examination with the least amount of radiation exposure. Properly functioning imaging equipment is key to providing the physician with the most accu-

rate diagnostic information. Artifacts caused by equipment malfunction and introduced into diagnostic data may adversely influence the patient's treatment, or require that an examination be repeated with an additional dose of radioactivity. Technically unsatisfactory images decrease or negate the benefit patients receive from being exposed to even a small amount of radiation. Routine monitoring of instrument performance is one way to minimize technically suboptimal studies.

10. To increase patient understanding of pre-examination instructions, the technologist should:

- discuss the requirements of the examination in a quiet, private area away from any distractions.
- explain the reasons behind the instructions and the consequences of not following them.

- avoid technical jargon and use terms the patient can understand. Some patients may be embarrassed to admit that certain words are unfamiliar. Also, patients' definitions may vary from those of health care personnel. For example, some patients may not consider over-the-counter medications or birth control pills to be medicine.
- discreetly test the patients' understanding by asking questions or by asking them to repeat the instructions.
- allow time for questions. Answer questions honestly; avoid belittling patients for asking questions with obvious answers or that you have already answered.
- ask open-ended questions that encourage patients to express their concerns or problems in carrying out the instructions. Offer practical advice to solve problems. Show respect for patients' concerns.

## CHAPTER 13

# Applying Radiobiology and Protection to Radiation Therapy

**Laurie Adams** • **Jan Carlisle**

## Chapter Outline

## Objectives

At the end of this chapter, the student should be able to:

1. Describe the role of radiation therapy in treating cancer.

2. Give advantages of using high-energy beams.

3. List the five factors that affect a tumor's response to ionizing radiation.

4. Differentiate between teletherapy and brachytherapy.

5. Describe the most commonly used teletherapy equipment.

6. List the rationale for various types of treatment, such as palliative and combination treatment.

7. Describe the goals and applications of treatment planning.

This chapter was adapted from the chapter in the first edition written by Steven B. Dowd and Stephanie Eatmon.

8. Describe the applications of the three cardinal principles of radiation protection to radiation therapy.

9. Describe the function of quality assurance programs in radiation therapy.

10. Describe the two methods of delivering therapy—brachytherapy and teletherapy.

<u>Important Terms</u>

abscopal
afterloader
alopecia
beta
brachytherapy
cancer
carcinoma
cerrobend
cobalt-60
critical structures
deep therapy
depth dose
fractionation
heavy ions

hyperthermia
$LD_{100}$
linear accelerator
megavoltage
neutrons
orthovoltage
palliation
penumbra
pions
protons
radiocurability
recovery
redistribution
reoxygenation
repopulation
sarcoma
shaping blocks
simulation
skin sparing
superficial therapy
teletherapy
tolerance dose
transmission target
treatment planning

## INTRODUCTION

This chapter is designed to be an overview of the use of radiation protection and the application of radiobiologic principles in radiation therapy, also called *radiation oncology*. First a brief description of radiation therapy will be presented. Then two applications of radiation protection in radiation therapy, higher energy beams and treatment planning, are discussed. The three cardinal principles of radiation protection—time, distance, and shielding—are described as they relate to teletherapy and brachytherapy. Finally, quality assurance, a means of improving patient care and reducing radiation dose in therapy, is reviewed.

## THE ART AND SCIENCE OF RADIATION THERAPY

For many years, radiation therapy has been shrouded in mystery. This is probably based on humankind's fear of cancer, as well as the negative connotations often associated with radiation. Abrahamson notes that:

[E]ven though the specialty [of radiation therapy] has existed for over 75 years, radiation therapy remains one of the most elusive, most mysterious, and most misunderstood specialties in medicine. The very word *radiation* conjures up in most patients and some physicians a myriad of old wives' tales and incantations: "I will surely die; if not, I'll certainly be burned over most of

Chemcial carcinogen → Ultimate carcinogen → Altered receptor expression →
Latent tumor cell (metabolic activity; DNA) growth and promotion →
Differentiated tumor progress → Undifferentiated cancer

**Figure 13–1** Model for most types of cancer. The first three steps are known as neoplastic conversion, the last three as neoplastic development and progression.

my body." "I'll be sterile." "I had a friend who had it—didn't die, but went crazy." "My hair will fall out."

Radiation therapists, the technologist members of the radiation oncology team, must function as part physicist, part radiobiologist, part diagnostic imager (in the performance of simulation), and part patient care specialist—a variety of roles that combine scientific knowledge with professional artistry. The basic goal of a radiation therapist, as described in Chapter 1, is to ensure that radiation is used in a manner that increases its therapeutic effectiveness while providing physical and emotional care to the patient.

All medical disciplines have an artistic side and a scientific side. Artistic does not mean lack of methodology or "free-spiritedness," it relates to special skills used by the practitioner. These skills are based on scientific knowledge. Thus, a radiation therapist uses knowledge gained in educational programs, in clinical settings, and in self-directed activities to provide effective patient care.

## Cancer and Cancer Treatment

About one in six Americans dies of cancer, a cause of death second only to heart disease. Thirteen hundred people die of cancer each day. Today the overall 5-year survival rate is 40% (4 in 10 patients), up from 33% in 1960 (1 in 3). Much of this increase in survival is due to better detection methods and improved treatment techniques.

There is probably no single cause for cancer. Today scientists still search for answers to the potential causes of cancer. It is accepted that cancer generation follows a series of steps beginning with metabolic activation. One of the

accepted models can be found in Figure 13–1. The text boxes on the next page show how exposure to the sun leads to skin cancer.

What makes cancer difficult to treat is that malignant cells from the primary tumor spread to other sites within the body and form secondary or metastatic tumors. Malignant cells can spread by means of lymphatic channels or through the blood, which is called *hematogenous spread*. Tumors that have not metastasized and that remain localized have the greatest chance of cure.

For many years, radiation was a second treatment for advanced tumors only. Many older people still regard radiation as a last resort. Today about half of patients with malignancies receive radiation therapy alone or in combination with another method of treatment such as surgery or chemotherapy. In fact, cancer today is diagnosed, as well as directed and treated, through a multidisciplinary approach.

The decision to use surgery, radiation therapy, chemotherapy, or experimental modalities depends on several factors, including the histology of the tumor, stage of the disease, location of the tumor, and physical condition of the patient. Histology provides information about the type and aggressiveness of the tumor, and stage gives an indication of the size, extension, or spread. Location of the tumor within the body is important for both radiation therapy and surgery. Tumors that are easily accessible are more likely candidates for surgery, whereas those that are difficult or impossible to excise are candidates for radiation therapy. Radiation therapy is further limited when a tumor is located close to a critical organ that is more radiosensitive than the tumor. The patient's physical condition must be amenable to treatment to withstand the acute side effects from each modality.

## How the Sun's Rays Can Lead to Skin Cancer

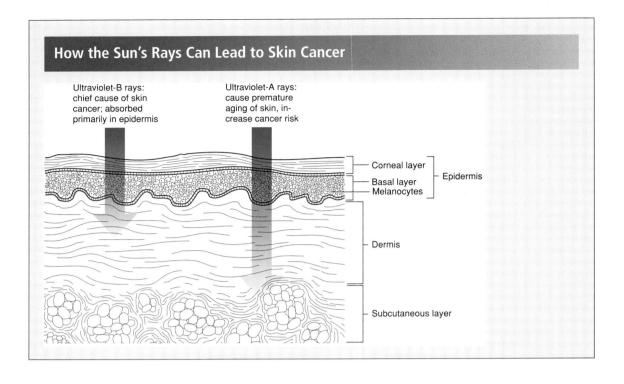

Ultraviolet-B rays: chief cause of skin cancer; absorbed primarily in epidermis

Ultraviolet-A rays: cause premature aging of skin, increase cancer risk

Corneal layer
Basal layer
Melanocytes
Epidermis

Dermis

Subcutaneous layer

## Suntan: The Skin's Attempt at Self Defense

1. Ultraviolet rays hit the epidermis; the melanocytes synthesize melanin pigment granules.

2. The granules travel through extensions of melanocytes into epidermal cells.

3. Melanin-rich cells move up to form the outer skin layer. They flatten and eventually slough off. The extra pigment gives the tan, and underlying skin cells are protected by extra absorption of ultraviolet rays.

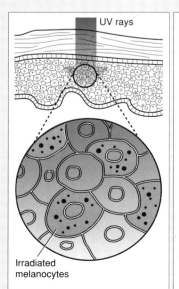

UV rays

Irradiated melanocytes

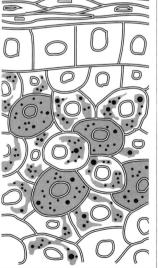

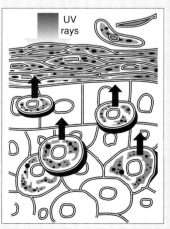

UV rays

## Skin Cancer: The Result of Sun Damage to Skin Cells' DNA

1. Intense or prolonged skin exposure alters the DNA as a result of excessive irradiation.

2. Cells with altered DNA then multiply.

3. Cancer results as abnormal cells undergo uncontrolled multiplication and disorganized growth. If untreated, the cancer cells can infiltrate and destroy adjacent tissue, eventually spreading to distant parts of the body.

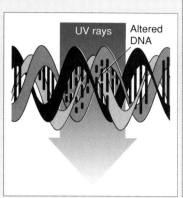

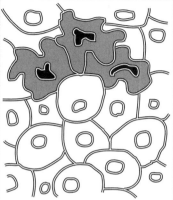

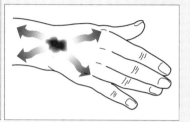

### Evaluating the Tumor for Treatment

Once a tumor has been positively diagnosed as malignant, the tumor is evaluated for treatment. When radiotherapy is selected as the treatment modality, either alone or in combination with other modalities, the tumor response to radiation is evaluated. Five factors affect the response of a tumor to ionizing radiation and must be considered:

1. The relationship between radiosensitivity, radiocurability, and the tolerance dose, all of which relate to the tumor's location to critical structures
2. The oxygen effect
3. Fractionation of dosage
4. Volume effect
5. Linear energy transfer of the radiation. (See Chapter 5 for more information on OER, fractionation, and LET.)

### Radiosensitivity, Radiocurability, and the Tolerance Dose

The goal of radiotherapy is to deliver a sufficiently high dose of radiation to sterilize tumor cells with minimal damage to surrounding normal tissues. Ideally, an $LD_{100}$ would be delivered—the dose needed to destroy 100% of cancer cells. The problem is that all tumors can theoretically be sterilized with radiation, but normal tissue will also be affected. The goal is to deliver the highest dose possible to the tumor while sparing surrounding normal tissue. In Chapter 1, this was called the *therapeutic efficacy;* it is also called the *therapeutic ratio* (Figure 13–2).

Radiosensitivity of a tumor is primarily a function of the primary tissue from which it arose (Table 13–1). It can be defined as the ability of radiation to change cells biologically that make up a tumor or other tissue, either by cell killing or by destruction of reproductive capability.

Radiation does not distinguish between normal tissue and tumor tissue; this is a random interaction. All normal tissue has a tolerance dose—the maximum dose that can be delivered to the tissue or critical structure. If exceeded, this maximum dose will show a large increase in the probability of occurrences of severe reactions. Tolerance is superior to radiosensitivity in clinical

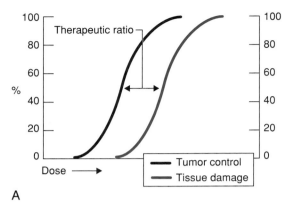

A

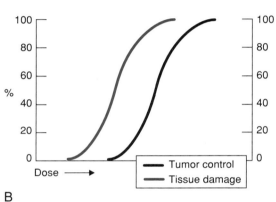

B

**Figure 13–2** (*A*) A good therapeutic ratio. Tumor control is achieved at a dose lower than one that would cause damage to surrounding tissue. (*B*) The opposite. Tumor control cannot be achieved without greater damage to surrounding tissue.

**Table 13–1  Radiosensitivity of Various Tumors and Tissues\***

| Radiosensitivity | Tumors | Potential Tissue of Origin |
| --- | --- | --- |
| High | Lymphoma | Lymphoid |
| | Leukemia | Hematopoietic |
| | Seminoma | Spermatogenic epithelium |
| Fairly high | Squamous cell cancers | |
| | Oropharynx | Oropharyngeal stratified epithelium |
| | Bladder | Urinary bladder epithelium |
| | Adenocarcinoma of alimentary tract | Colon epithelium |
| Medium | Vascular and connective tissue elements of all tumors | Interstitial tissue |
| Fairly low | Salivary gland tumors | Salivary gland epithelium |
| | Renal cancer | Renal epithelium |
| | Osteogenic sarcoma | Osteocytes |
| Low | Rhabdomyosarcoma | Muscle tissue |
| | Leiomyosarcoma | Muscle tissue |
| | Ganglioneurofibrosarcoma | Neuronal tissue |

\*Not a totally representative list of all tumors and all possible tissue origins.

Modified from Rubin P (ed): Clinical Oncology for Physicians and Students: A Multidisciplinary Approach, 7th ed. Philadelphia, WB Saunders, 1993, p. 75.

applications. It takes into account the inherent radiosensitivity of stroma and parenchyma, capabilities for repair, the need for preservation of functional integrity, and the organ's importance to life (Travis, 1989). Most tolerance doses are expressed in terms of the $TD_{5/5}$—the dose given to a population of patients that will result in 5% of complications in 5 years. In some cases, however, as low as 1% or as high as 50% may be an acceptable complication rate, depending on circumstances. Tolerance doses depend on the volume of tissue treated, the total dose, and the dose per fraction.

Strandqvist (1944) conducted a now classic study that related the time and dosage of treatment of skin and lip cancers to clinical results. These results included early and late complications and cure. He found that some time–dose relationships (fractionations) cured the cancer but produced a variety of severe late complications. From this, the concept of tolerance was developed.

Tolerance must be balanced with the curative dose for the tumor (radiocurability). The curative dose is the dose that will sterilize the tumor (Table 13–2) and is based on radiosensitivity. Some critical structures have such a low tolerance dose that tumors located in these areas cannot be given a tumorcidal dose. Tumors usually considered curable include the childhood tumors of neuroblastoma, retinoblastoma, and Wilms' tumor; squamous cell lesions of skin, oral cavity, pharynx, larynx, and cervix; lymphomas; testicular tumors; nasopharyngeal cancer; adenocarcinoma of the prostate; and pituitary tumors. Strandqvist's research into time–dose relationships has also been extended, now making it possible to deliver tumoricidal doses to areas such as the pancreas and stomach that previously could not be treated because of a low tolerance by critical structures.

## Oxygen Effect

The oxygen effect, described in Chapter 5, can enhance or limit the effectiveness of radiation therapy. Recall that oxygen enhances the free radical effect. Larger doses of radiation are needed to treat a tumor containing hypoxic cells. Fully oxygenated cells can have a radiosensitivity 2.5 to 3 times that of anoxic or hypoxic cells.

**Table 13–2  Tumor Type and Radiocurability Levels**

| Dose Needed for Cure (rad) | Tumor Type |
| --- | --- |
| 2000–3000 | Seminoma<br>Central nervous system cancer<br>Acute lymphocytic leukemia |
| 3000–4000 | Seminoma<br>Wilms' tumor<br>Neuroblastoma |
| 4000–5000 | Hodgkin's disease<br>Lymphosarcoma<br>Histiocytic cell carcinoma<br>Basal and squamous skin cancer |
| 5000–6000 | Metastatic lymph nodes<br>Squamous cell carcinoma<br>Cervical cancer<br>Head and neck cancer<br>Embryonal cancer<br>Breast cancer<br>Medulloblastoma<br>Ewing's tumor<br>Dysgerminoma |
| 6000–6500 | Larynx (<1 cm)<br>Breast cancer, lumpectomy |
| 7000–7500 | Oral cavity (<2–4 cm)<br>Oronasolaryngopharyngeal cancers<br>Bladder cancers<br>Uterine fundal cancer<br>Ovarian cancer<br>Metastatic lymph nodes (1–3 cm)<br>Lung cancer (<3 cm) |
| 8000 | Head and neck cancer (>4 cm)<br>Breast cancer (>5 cm)<br>Gliomas<br>Osteogenic sarcomas<br>Melanomas<br>Soft tissue carcinomas<br>Thyroid cancer<br>Metastatic lymph nodes (>6 cm) |

Modified from Rubin P (ed): Clinical Oncology for Physicians and Students: A Multidisciplinary Approach, 7th ed. Philadelphia, WB Saunders, 1993, p. 72.

Hypoxic cells in tumors are known to reoxygenate. This occurs after the well-oxygenated cells within a tumor have been destroyed with initial doses of radiation. The cells that were previously resistant to radiation will now be

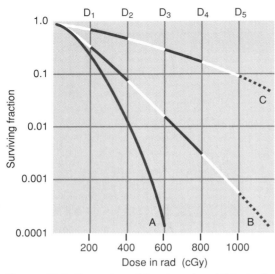

**Figure 13–3** Illustration of fractionation. (*A*) is single dose; (*B*) is fractionated dose; (*C*) is very fractionated dose.

more sensitive. This improves the therapeutic ratio and is one basis for the fractionation of doses.

### Fractionation of Dose

Dose fractionation is the division of large doses of radiation needed for treatment into smaller, usually daily, increments (also described in Chapter 5). Recall that the ram testes were sterilized in the French study without injuring surrounding tissue by dividing the dose needed to sterilize the testes into smaller fractions. This model works for tumor growth as well. Figure 13–3 illustrates the use of fractionation in therapy. The sidebar also describes the "four R's" of fractionated radiotherapy.

### Volume Effect

The volume effect relates to the need to irradiate surrounding tissue as well as the tumor site. As tumor size increases, a larger volume must be irradiated. This limits the tolerance as a result of a greater involvement of normal tissues. For instance, a 10 cm$^2$ volume of spinal cord has an approximate tolerance of 4500 cGy. When a larger volume of tissue is treated, the tolerance decreases. Thus, the dose must be decreased. Conversely, when the volume treated decreases in size, the dose may be safely increased.

### Linear Energy Transfer

As linear energy transfer (LET) increases, so does the chance of causing irreversible cellular damage to the tumor. Because x-radiation and gamma radiation are low-LET radiations, they are not as efficient at causing damage to a tumor as some other forms of radiation. This had led to increased research in the use of "heavy ions" that have a higher LET than x-radiation or gamma radiation.

### Combination Treatment

Radiation therapy may be used alone or in unison with surgery, chemotherapy, or immunotherapy. The determination to use a certain modality is based on histology, staging, site, patient characteristics, available resources, and physician preference. Radiation therapy and surgery are local or regional rather than systemic. That is, they treat a specific cancer site rather than an entire system. Chemotherapy is systemic treatment.

One example of combination treatment involves giving a single large dose of radiation 24 hours after colorectal cancer surgery to prevent seeding of tumor cells during surgery. Radiation is also given preoperatively for three reasons:

1. It can make surgery easier.
2. It can, as described previously, sterilize tumor cells on the surface, which decreases the possibility of seeding.
3. It can alter the surrounding normal tissue, decreasing the possibility that tumor cells will be "taken" in normal tissue.

In soft tissue sarcomas of extremities, a wide excision can be made that spares the limb, and then a full course of radiation to the surgical site is delivered.

A common mistake is to assume that alopecia (loss of hair) to lung patients is caused by

## The Four R's of Fractionated Radiotherapy

Early radiotherapy did not always make use of fractionated doses or make use of them in a scientific manner. Not until animal experiments indicated that certain effects could be achieved, and others avoided, by using fractionation was it practiced. These experiments indicated four primary biologic factors named the "four R's" that have been discussed here and in previous chapters:

1. Mammalian cells show a tendency to *recover* from the effects of radiation damage.
2. Some cell types (e.g., the epithelium of the gastrointestinal tract) are capable of rapid *repopulation* while receiving fractionated doses of radiation. This would not be possible with large single doses of radiation (recall the gastrointestinal syndrome described in Chapter 7).
3. The rate of *reoxygenation* of the tumor is important. A typical tumor receives a dose of 200 cGy (rad) per fractionation. This destroys the well-oxygenated tumor cells, and the time interval to the next fraction allows the cells of the tumor that were hypoxic to take in additional oxygen that will increase their radiosensitivity. This can necessitate the use of different fractionation intervals for some tumors and, in some cases, the use of hyperbaric oxygen.
4. The radiosensitivity of cells varies throughout the cycle. The clinical effect of radiotherapy depends on both the dose delivered and in some cases the interval between treatment fractions (the *redistribution* of cells in the cycle). Radiation causes a delay in the progression of the cell cycle (previously called *division delay*) and causes a surviving population of cells to become synchronized (putting all or most cells in the same phase of the cell cycle. This holds true for tumor cells and acutely responding cells (described in Chapter 5) only, and its clinical value remains largely unclear.

radiation. The short-term side effects of radiation are localized rather than systemic. The alopecia is from the chemotherapy portion of a combination treatment of chemotherapy and radiation therapy. The loss of hair seen in the early x-ray pioneers was due to the fact that they allowed their heads to be exposed to large amounts of radiation. Recall that the epilation described in Chapter 5 was from testing fluoroscopic equipment by observing the shadow of a watch through the operator's skull.

Side effects can occur as a result of radiation therapy. Since effects are localized, esophagitis, for example, may occur as a result of mediastinal irradiation; pelvic treatments can cause diarrhea. These effects are usually minor and transient.

It is not possible to cure all tumors, but patients can be given relief of symptoms through shrinkage of tumors. Palliation means to relieve pain or obstruction by shrinking the tumor. Palliative therapy is also used for large bulky tumors that are a social and aesthetic problem. For example, treatment may be delivered to a metastatic bone tumor of the femur for pain and impending fracture that would interfere with mobility. Seizures, paresthesias, and visual disturbances all can be relieved with brain irradiation. Palliative therapy is also given in emergency situations such as spinal cord compression.

Abramson notes that symptoms and signs such as bone pain, cough, hemoptysis, shortness of breath, neurologic symptoms, obstruction, hemorrhage, ulcerations, and jaundice can be relieved through radiation. Some authorities call this the "four B's"—bone, brain, bleeding, and blockage—in reference to the symptoms treatable by palliative therapy. Recall from Chapter 5 the concept of telangiectasis, a dilation of small blood vessels that leads to impaired blood flow. This normally negative outcome can be used positively to minimize internal bleeding.

## Teletherapy Equipment

Cobalt-60 (Co-60) is highly efficient, although some authors (e.g., Stanton and colleagues, 1992) believe it is inefficient compared with the linear accelerator. However, it is still recognized as a viable treatment option in many facilities, including leading centers such as M.D. Anderson in Texas. It is very effective when used for head and neck cancers.

Two disadvantages of Co-60 are penumbra and low percentage depth dose (%DD). Co-60 is unstable and undergoes continuous decay, emitting gamma radiation. Its sources continually lose energy and thus must be replaced. As a radioisotope, Co-60 has a certain half-life, or amount of time it takes the radioisotope to decay to 50% of original activity. Co-60's half-life is approximately 5.3 years. As the source decays, the exposure times must be increased, lengthening treatment times.

Linear accelerators (linacs) produce radiation by accelerating electrons at a target, producing high-energy photons or x-rays. Electrons are used when the lesion is on the body surface or extends only a few centimeters into the skin. Linacs use a transmission target that generates an x-ray beam along the same line of path as the accelerated electrons. If the target is removed, the beam consists solely of electrons. This spares normal tissue under the tumor since electrons do not penetrate deeply. However, skin reactions may be more pronounced.

Other forms of equipment and radiation include neutrons, protons, heavy ions, pions, and hyperthermia (the use of heat to treat tumors). Most of the interest in other forms of radiation is due to their physical (LET) or radiobiologic properties. Facilities using these types of radiation are rare, but the beam characteristics allow greater tumor dose with less normal tissue destruction. The Bragg peak is an interesting aspect of heavy ions and protons: cell killing is independent of oxygen, there is a high relative biologic effect (RBE), and there is a sparsely ionizing path that has a very high peak LET that then rapidly drops to zero.

## Brachytherapy

Brachytherapy is the use of sealed radioactive isotopes inserted temporarily or permanently into hollow cavities, within tissues, or on the surface of the body. Alexander Graham Bell is credited with first describing the possibility of internal radiation therapy in 1903. External (*tele-*) therapy delivers a fractionated dose of radiation, generally 5 days a week for up to 7 or 8 weeks. Internal sources of radiation deliver radiation continuously over hours or days. This radiation is delivered in a more concentrated fashion to a tumor site. Brachytherapy is contraindicated when a tumor infiltrates bone, when there is an active infection in the tissue to be treated, or when the boundaries of the tumor are not clearly identifiable.

A radioisotope such as gold (Au-198) has a half-life of 2.7 days and can be inserted and left permanently in place. Radioisotopes such as radium, with a half-life of 1600 years, must be removed from the body after a certain period. For this reason, radium is no longer commonly used for brachytherapy. A commonly used isotope is iridium-192 (Ir-192). It is easily shaped into wires and other forms, can be prepared in different strengths, and requires only 2 cm of lead for adequate shielding (as opposed to 10 cm for radium).

The two basic types of radioisotopic implants used are intracavitary, which is inserted ("afterloaded"; see the text box) by a physician into a body cavity such as the vagina, and interstitial, which is placed in the form of catheters, seeds, wires, and needles in body tissues (Figures 13–4 and 13–5).

## The Afterloader Controversy

Early in 1993, one company lost its license to perform high-dose-rate (HDR) brachytherapy because of the death of a patient from what was described as "acute radiation exposure and consequences thereof." *Afterloading* refers to techniques in which applicators are positioned in a patient and the radioactive sources are introduced at a later stage (Godden, 1988). Manual afterloading reduces dosage to the staff doing the insertion but not to the nursing staff or visitors, as the source remains inserted. High-dose-rate afterloading is a type of remote afterloading in which sources are removed. The source can also be removed if a radiation worker has to enter the room. The treatment is fractionated over days, which necessitates multiple visits by the patients. Treatment times are a matter of minutes or hours, as compared with days in low-dose-rate afterloading.

In the HDR controversy, the source remained in the patient, which exposed the patient, staff, and visitors to radiation without their knowing that exposure was taking place. This mistake occurred because of what appeared to be a combination of human and machinery errors. Evidently, alarms were disabled as it was thought that they were malfunctioning; additionally, staff

were not appropriately trained in radiation safety but were allowed to operate the machine. The NRC found that a total of 94 people were exposed, including nursing home staff who, unaware of its radioactivity, found the catheter and stored it in a biomedical hazards bag.

What is the positive outcome of such a tragic event? As many program directors noted after the incident, students can learn from such a negative experience the value of proper radiation safety practices. The following comments were published in the March 8, 1993, issue of *ADVANCE for Radiologic Science Professionals* in an interview with Dennis Leaver, M.S., R.T.(T.), radiation therapy program director at Southern-Maine Technical College: "Educators can use these examples to reinforce the seriousness of the radiation therapy profession. I take every opportunity I can to discuss this with students and give them copies of articles to help them understand what occurred and what their responsibility would have been if they were in that situation." What will serve students best, he later notes, are good problem-solving skills and observational techniques, to prevent these incidents from occurring to them as graduates.

## USING HIGHER ENERGY BEAMS

Before the development of high-energy machines capable of megavoltage (millions of electron volts; MeV), most machines could deliver only orthovoltage (maximum energy of 500 kVp). Now machines are capable of megavoltage therapy. Both cobalt and linear accelerators (linacs) are capable of generating megavoltage beams, although cobalt units are being slowly replaced by linacs in many facilities. There are three major advantages to using

megavoltage beams rather than orthovoltage beams for the treatment of deep lesions:

1. Megavoltage beams provide greater beam penetration (depth dose). Simply, this refers to the relative dose of radiation at any depth.
2. Greater penetration translates also into a lower skin dose. This is known as skin sparing. This is illustrated in Table 13–3.
3. Megavoltage beams provide less penumbra. Whereas in diagnostic imaging

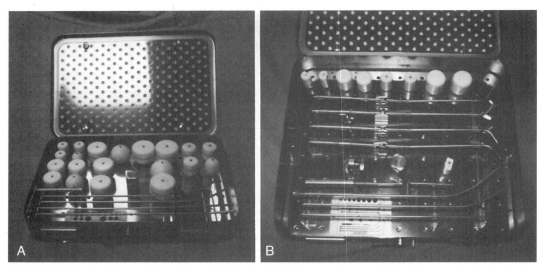

**Figure 13–4** Intracavitary devices for brachytherapy. (*A*) Instrument: vaginal mold; cancer treated: vaginal. (*B*) Instrument: Fletcher; cancer treated: cervical.

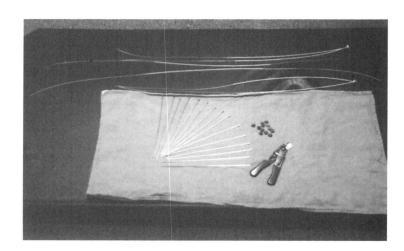

**Figure 13–5** Intrastitial devices for brachytherapy. Syed needles are placed directly into the tumor. Cancers treated by this method include cervical, endometrial, ovarian, head and neck, and prostate cancers and sarcomas.

penumbra refers to a loss of sharpness at the edge of the radiograph, in therapy it also refers to an area of dose gradient at the edge of a beam. With a large penumbra, a larger field size must be used to deliver a uniform dose to the tumor. This also increases dose to surrounding healthy tissue.

## TREATMENT PLANNING

Several professionals work as a team in providing the course of treatment to a patient in radiation therapy. The radiation oncologist (a physician), physicist, dosimetrist, and radiation therapist are the primary professionals that determine the patient's course of treatment.

Table 13–3 Variations in Depth Dose with Higher Beam Energies*

| Linear Accelerator Energy (MeV) | Depth Dose* (%) |
| --- | --- |
| 4 | 62.7 |
| 6 | 67.7 |
| 8 | 71.0 |
| 10 | 75.3 |

*Assumes 100-cm source-to-skin distance.

Modified from Stanton R, Stinson D: An Introduction to Radiation Oncology Physics. Madison, WI, Medical Physics Publishing, 1992, p 109.

The primary objective of treatment planning is to increase the therapeutic efficacy of radiation therapy by ensuring that the tumor receives a uniform and effective amount of radiation while sparing normal tissue as much as possible from the effects of radiation.

There are four basic aspects to treatment planning:

*Localization* is the determination of the location and extent of the tumor as related to surrounding anatomic landmarks. All types of diagnostic examination, including palpation, x-ray examination, and scopic study are used to localize the tumor (Figure 13–6). From this information, treatment fields and techniques are selected.

*Simulation* uses a radiographic imaging unit called a *simulator* that simulates (mimics) movements of the treatment unit and other aspects such as geometry (Figure 13–7). During simulation, treatment fields are transferred from the treatment plan to the patient.

*Field selection and placement*

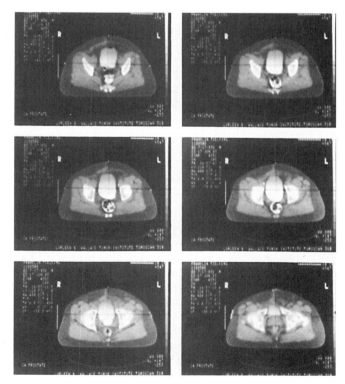

**Figure 13–6** CT treatment planning film used to localize the tumor and determine spinal cord depth. This ensures that a dose of less than 45 Gy will be delivered to the spinal cord; otherwise, myolitis may result in about 5 months.

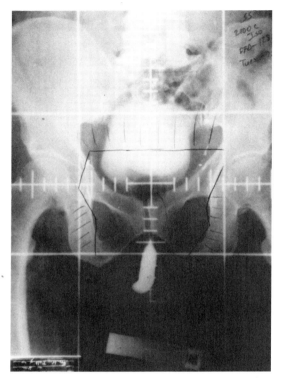

**Figure 13–7** Simulator film of the prostate, approximate field size of 12 cm by 12 cm. Hypaque is placed within the bladder and barium into the rectum to pinpoint the exact location of the prostate, as well as critical structures in case blocks are needed. At the bottom, a silver clamp is on the penis to hold the Hypaque in the bladder.

*Verification* ensures that the areas selected for treatment are actually being treated. This includes the use of port films taken on the treatment machine.

Patients must be positioned exactly the same way with each treatment. Devices that ensure accurate alignment of the beam to the patient include field lights, protractor or gantry angle indicator, lasers, and back pointers. Patient-positioning aids include custom mouthpieces known as *bite blocks* for the head and neck, face masks using plastic material, and cast styrofoam materials for the thorax.

Shaping blocks made of cerrobend (an alloy of lead, tin, bismuth, and cadmium) are used to "shape" the beam. These blocks are placed onto a tray attached to the head of the treatment unit. The usual thickness of a cerrobend block is five half-value layers (HVLs). This reduces intensity to about 3% of original value. Another means of beam shaping is the use of multileaf collimators.

Additional skin sparing is often achieved through the use of compensating filters. As with x-ray compensating filters, the material of choice is often aluminum, although a variety of materials, such as brass, can be used. Equipment is now available that allows the use of cerrobend for construction of a compensating filter. A compensating filter must be inserted a sufficient distance (at least 15 cm) from the patient to ensure that electrons generated by the interaction of the megavoltage beam with the filter do not strike the patient.

## CARDINAL PRINCIPLES OF RADIATION PROTECTION

The three cardinal or basic principles of radiation protection are:

- Minimize time of exposure.
- Maximize distance from the source of radiation.
- Maximize amount of shielding.

In almost all situations, distance is the superior single method of radiation protection; it is always desirable to use a combination of the above three methods. For example, using lead shielding of 1 HVL will reduce intensity by half. Doubling distance from a point source will reduce intensity by one fourth. Together these methods will reduce intensity by one eighth. Thus, an intensity that was 100 mR/hr becomes 50 mR/hr after the shielding. Doubling distance alone reduces an intensity of 100 mR/hr to 25 mR/hr. Using both reduces intensity to 12.5 mR/hr.

The radiologic technologist must often function as an educator for other health professionals, patients, and the general public regarding the safe uses of ionizing radiation (Chapter 1 discussed this in some detail). For example, the myth persists among a small minority of health care workers that patients receiving teletherapy treatments become radioactive and thus are a source of exposure to the worker. This belief will compromise patient care.

Often, "teachable moments" arrive in which the radiologic technologist is called on to educate patients, visitors, or other workers about the safe uses of ionizing radiation. Effective education of others contributes to better patient care and elevates the status of our profession in the eyes of outsiders. It is extremely important that radiologic technologists take their role as educator seriously.

## Time

### Teletherapy

Since a cobalt source continually emits radiation, radiation levels in treatment rooms with a Co-60 unit will be higher than normal background radiation and thus a potential source of occupational dose to the operator. Also, the source may stick in the "on" position, which can lead to increased levels of radiation to the operator. This is rare, but a therapist working with a cobalt source must know the departmental routine for shutting down the machine and evacuating the patient.

### Brachytherapy

A direct relationship exists between time of exposure and dose received. Thus, if time of exposure can be cut in half, dose is also cut in half for sources with a long half-life. At one time, radiographers may have been responsible for taking a localization film for brachytherapy patients; however, most sources are now afterloaded, leading to no exposure at this time. Afterloading means that the radioactive sources are placed in the implant devices after radiographs have been taken following surgery. Sources or seeds seen on the radiograph are dummy sources placed in the implant applicators for purposes of treatment planning. Information from these radiographs will help determine the dose distribution and doses to normal tissues and organs. Radioactive sources are placed when the patient is in the hospital room.

Nurses should be encouraged to minimize their time of exposure. It is generally wise to recommend that each provider limit the time of exposure to 30 minutes while the source is in place, although this is a broad recommendation that will vary based on circumstances. See the sidebar for additional general guidelines for nursing and other staff.

## Distance

### Brachytherapy

For point sources of radiation, intensity of radiation varies by the inverse of the square of the distance from the source. In all cases, individuals caring for the patient should stay as far as possible from the radiation source. If possible, caregivers should be encouraged to stand at either the head or foot of the bed, depending on the site, for intracavitary implants, as well as behind lead shields as much as possible. For head and neck implants, the caregiver should stand at the side of the bed farthest from the implant.

When possible, communication with the patient should be performed at a distance. However, it is also important *not* to treat these patients as if they had some sort of highly contagious fatal disease. Patient care must be balanced with radiation protection.

## Shielding

### Teletherapy

In teletherapy using linacs, there is little chance of a therapist receiving radiation exposure, although these machines do produce a variety of sources of radiation that require shielding. Scatter is produced when the primary beam interacts with the patient. Additionally, all x-ray-producing machines generate radiation that travels in all directions, not just as desired in a forward direction. This is known as *leakage radiation*. Because the radiation therapist is outside the room when the exposure is delivered, there is no exposure.

A wall that can be exposed to the primary beam requires a primary barrier. Walls that can be exposed only to leakage and scatter require secondary barriers. Barriers in therapy are

## Additional Guidelines for Caring for Brachytherapy Patients

Certainly, radiation therapists will be called on to provide guidelines for caring for the patient undergoing brachytherapy. Other radiation workers, such as radiographers working the evening shift, may also be called on for advice. As described in previous chapters, these individuals should seek to know as much as possible about radiation but provide only advice they are qualified to give. Guidelines for patient care should be contained within the patient's chart, based on prescriptions of the radiation oncologist and radiation safety officer. In most cases, it is best to contact the radiation oncologist, radiation safety officer, or the radiation therapist on call for specific advice. The following guidelines for nurses are based on those developed by Hassey (1988):

- The patient should be assigned to a private room with private bath.
- A "Caution: Radioactive Material" sign is placed on the patient's door.
- Nurses caring for brachytherapy patients should wear dosimeters. They should not share monitoring devices unless a pocket dosimeter is used.

- Pregnant women and children under 16 years should not enter the room.
- Visitors should stand at 6 feet and limit their visits to 30 minutes per day.
- A dislodged source should be picked up with long-handled tongs and deposited in a shielded container in the patient's room. If the source sometimes cannot be found, a "No Visitors" sign should be hung on the patient's door until technical staff locate it.
- Dressings and bed linens should be retained until the source is removed then disposed of as usual. Since the source is sealed (unlike radionuclide therapy), the source should not be excreted in urine, feces, or other body fluids.

If these guidelines are given to other health care workers, it must be noted that these are general guidelines based on sound practice, but are *not* the specific guidelines of those responsible for radiation safety (e.g. the oncologist and the radiation safety officer).

designed in a manner similar to those in diagnostic radiology (see Chapter 9), but of course are much thicker because of the greater energy of the beam. These walls are commonly in excess of 3 feet thick. Concrete is often used instead of lead, which reduces the shielding costs.

Walls and other objects in the treatment room exposed to megavoltage sources of radiation become radioactive for short periods of time. This depends on several factors, and not all authorities think that this is a significant source of exposure. Stanton and colleagues (1992), on the other hand, indicate that therapists can receive a whole-body equivalent of about 20 mrem per month and as much as 150 mrem to the extremities from these sources.

They recommend that therapists wear a ring dosimeter as well as the regular film badge to monitor this exposure.

### Brachytherapy

If properly used, lead shielding can sometimes provide additional safety from radiation exposure from brachytherapy patients. In most cases, however, shielding such as lead aprons is not of value, and nurses caring for a brachytherapy patient should instead be counseled to limit their time of exposure. There are rolling lead shields, similar to those used in angiography, that can be placed beside the patient's bed to reduce exposure to caregivers and fam-

Table 13–4  Quality Assurance Tests Performed by Physicists and Therapists

| Test | Range of Acceptance |
|------|--------------------|
| **Daily tests** | |
| Interlocks, lamp | Working |
| Patient audiovisual | Working |
| Output constancy of arc | ±3% |
| Radiation monitor | ±3% |
| Radiation warning lights | Working |
| Laser localization lights | ±3 mm |
| Optical distance indicator | ±3 mm |
| **Weekly and monthly tests** | |
| Congruence of radiation and light field | ±3 mm |
| Cross-hair alignment | ±2 mm |
| Radiation output | ±3% |
| Beam energy | ±1% TMR |
| Mechanical inspection | Shows no loose wires, covers, screws, or other items |
| Emergency off switches | Working |
| **Annual tests** | |
| Mechanical and digital indicators | ±2 mm or 1 degree |
| Machine isocenter | ±1 mm |
| Isocentricity of couch and sag | ±3 mm |
| Radiation beam symmetry | ±2% |
| Radiation beam flatness | ±3% |
| Monitor chamber linearity and end effect | ±1% |
| Beam stability at gantry angles of 0, 90, 180, and 270 degrees | ±1% |

Modifed from Stanton R, Stinson D: An Introduction to Radiation Oncology Physics. Madison, WI, Radiation Physics Publishing, 1992, p 135.

ily members. A general guideline was given earlier; the recommended guidelines for specific patients should be contained within the patient's chart. Counseling nurses and other health care professionals is sometimes difficult since those inexperienced in the care of brachytherapy patients often believe that lead and lead aprons are some form of absolute protection against radiation exposure. This is a myth that is perpetuated by their use in other areas (e.g., fluoroscopy and portable radiography) as well as television and movies that inaccurately portray radiation and its effects.

## QUALITY ASSURANCE PROGRAMS

Standards for quality assurance programs are set forth in the American College of Radiology Quality Assurance Manual. Quality assurance programs are usually administered by a radiation physicist, but it is important that all employees participate in the quality assurance program. Some tests can be performed only by a physicist, but many tests are also performed by therapists on a daily basis (Table 13–4).

The goal of a quality assurance program is to ensure that the radiation dose delivered is as low as is reasonably achievable while increasing the therapeutic efficacy of procedures. This requires the input of all employees, including therapists, and it extends beyond simple checks of equipment.

## SUMMARY

Cancer is a common disease that is feared by the general public. Today about half of patients with cancer receive radiation therapy as the sole treatment or in conjunction with another treatment method such as chemotherapy. Radiation therapists are the technologist members of the team responsible for ensuring that radiation is used effectively to destroy cancer tissue while sparing normal tissue.

Five factors affect the response of a tumor to radiation: (1) the relationship between radiosensitivity, radiocurability, and the tolerance dose; (2) the oxygen effect; (3) fractionation of dosage; (4) the volume effect; and (5) linear energy transfer. Radiation therapy cannot always produce a cure; many treatments are given for the relief of pain (palliation). The two major forms of treatment are teletherapy (at a distance) through cobalt-60 and linear accelerators capable of megavoltage beams, and brachytherapy, which involves insertion of radioisotopes into body cavities (intracavitary) and into tissue (interstitial).

Means of radiation protection include the use of higher energy beams and the effective use of treatment planning. Treatment planning uses localization, simulation, field selection and placement, and verification. The beam is often shaped by the use of cerrobend filters and multileaf collimators; compensating filters are also used to further spare the skin. Additionally, for treatments to be effective, patients must be in the same position for each treatment.

The three cardinal principles of radiation protection are (1) minimize time; (2) maximize distance; and (3) maximize shielding. Each of these can be practiced during both teletherapy and brachytherapy to minimize exposure to operators, other health care workers, and patients. One additional means of improving patient care and minimizing radiation dose is through the use of quality assurance programs.

## Questions

1. The maximum dose that can be delivered to a critical structure is known as the:

   a. tolerance dose.      b. curability dose.
   c. depth dose.          d. LD50.

2. The determination of the location and extent of the tumor as related to surrounding anatomic landmarks is known as:

   a. simulation.          b. localization.
   c. field selection.     d. verification.

3. Electron beam treatments are used when:

   a. the tumor is deep-seated.
   b. the tumor is superficial.
   c. skin reactions could be a problem.
   d. a high oxygen enhancement ratio (OER) is desired.

4. Which of the following are advantages of high-energy beams?

   I. greater depth dose
   II. lower skin dose
   III. greater penumbra

   a. I and II only        b. I and III only
   c. II and III only      d. I, II, and III

5. About how many Americans die of cancer?

   a. one in two           b. one in four
   c. one in six           d. one in eight

6. When specific guidelines are not available for brachytherapy patients, caregivers should be encouraged to limit their time of exposure to:

   a. 10 minutes.          b. 20 minutes.
   c. 30 minutes.          d. 45 minutes.

7. At what distance must a compensating filter be placed to avoid having electrons generated by the beam strike the patient?

   a. 5 cm                 b. 10 cm
   c. 15 cm                d. 20 cm

8. Beam-modifying blocks are most often made of:

   a. lead.                b. aluminum.
   c. cerrobend.           d. cobalt.

9. Which of the following are types of implants used in brachytherapy?

   I. interarticular
   II. interstitial
   III. intracavitary

   a. I and II only        b. I and III only
   c. II and III only      d. I, II, and III

10. How does a linear accelerator target differ from a diagnostic x-ray target?

I. A linac target produces x-radiation along the same path of travel as electrons.
II. A linac target can generate gamma radiation as well as x-radiation.
III. A linac target can be removed to generate an electron beam.

a. I and II only
b. I and III only
c. II and III only
d. I, II, and III

## Exercises

1. Why is the treatment of a tumor more than simply the determination of the curative dose?

2. How should nurses be counseled about the use of shielding during care of a brachytherapy patient?

3. What is treatment planning, and what are its basic aspects?

4. What are the similarities and differences between cobalt-60 and linear accelerators?

5. How is beam shaping and skin sparing achieved in therapy?

## Answers

Questions

| | |
|---|---|
| 1. a | 6. c |
| 2. b | 7. c |
| 3. b | 8. c |
| 4. a | 9. c |
| 5. c | 10. b |

Exercises

1. The curative dose is the dose needed to sterilize a tumor and is a reflection of tissue radiosensitivity. This must be balanced with the tolerance dose of the organ or area that will be treated. The goal of radiotherapy is to destroy cancer cells while sparing normal tissue.

2. Nurses, especially those inexperienced in the care of brachytherapy patients, often do not understand that shielding can be of little value in caring for patients with radioactive implants. It is necessary to inform them of the three cardinal principles of radiation protection—time, distance, and shielding—and of how the effective use of time and distance from the source can be superior to shielding. Shielding can actually slow a worker down to the point that dosage is increased rather than decreased. Nurses should attend continuing education inservices that discuss radiation protection and care of the patient receiving brachytherapy treatments.

3. Treatment planning increases the therapeutic efficacy of radiation therapy by ensuring that the tumor receives a uniform and effective amount of radiation while sparing normal tissue as much as possible from the effects of radiation. The basic aspects of treatment planning are (1) localization or the determination of location and extent of the tumor as related to surrounding anatomic landmarks; (2) simulation, which uses a radiographic imaging unit called a simulator that simulates (mimics) movements of the treatment unit and other aspects such as geometry; (3) field selection and placement; and (4) verification.

4. Both cobalt-60 and teletherapy equipment are teletherapy units and are capable of providing radiation in the megavoltage range. Co-60 units use a radioisotope of cobalt to produce gamma radiation. Linear accelerators function like x-ray generators with the exception that they use a transmission target and can also generate an electron beam.

5. Higher voltage beams, since they transmit a higher energy of radiation, lower skin dose. Also, compensating filters made of aluminum are used to lower skin dose. The beam is shaped through the use of cerrobend blocks and multileaf collimators.

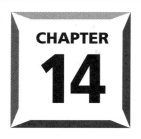

# CHAPTER 14

# Patient Education

### Steven B. Dowd • Elwin R. Tilson

## Chapter Outline

## Chapter Objectives

At the end of this chapter, the student should be able to:

1. List reasons why patient education is important in the modern practice of the radiologic sciences.

2. Using mammography as an example, discuss some of the issues involved in explaining risks and benefits to the patient.

3. Describe the commonalities of good teaching.

4. Explain the difficulties in using numerical expressions of radiation dosage and radiation risk.

5. Compare the relative utility of different risk comparisons and explanations.

## Important Terms

brief encounter
commonplaces
expert
hider
informed relationship
involuntary risk
numeracy
revealer
risk
therapeutic relationship
trust
voluntary risk

## PATIENT EDUCATION AND RADIATION PROTECTION

There are a number of reasons why patient education is more important today than ever before. One of the most important is the growing awareness that patients are not passive objects to be poked, prodded, or radiographed, but are active participants in a process designed to improve their health. If nothing else, this is consistent with good customer service. A patient who feels that his or her concerns have been dealt with is likely to return to that department. However, patient education also makes better use of a shrinking health care dollar. For example, a patient who understands the tests that he or she has undergone will be better able to interact with his or her physicians when it comes time to have "more tests." Are those tests really necessary? Didn't we just collect that information six months ago? Good patient education makes the patient more of a participant in the process and makes better use of the health care dollar.

How does this relate to radiation protection and radiobiology? Radiation exposure involves a risk. That risk may be very small or it may be very large, depending on the dose of the examination. Research clearly shows that patients more readily undertake voluntary risks than involuntary risks (Dowd and Steves, 1997). Thus, a patient who feels fully informed will readily undergo an examination, cooperate to the best or his or her ability, and return to that facility. It is regretful that in imaging, as in many other medical disciplines, we tend to think of the informed relationship only in terms of signing forms for informed consent (Dowd, 1994). In reality, all patient care procedures require an informed relationship—the patient, unless somehow unable, must be able to agree to a procedure based on a full understanding of that procedure.

Being able to educate patients about radiation exposure is also important due to the complexity of the information. As you have seen in previous chapters, there are few right or wrong answers, especially in the low-dose regions. "Can radiation cause cancer?" is directly answered with "Yes, but. . . ." However, as we will see, this direct answer may not be the most therapeutic response for a patient.

### The Example of Mammography

To see the need for patient education in its proper context, consider the example of mammography. The guidelines about when to have mammography vary among experts, and in any case, the decision is a personal one made by the patient. However, mammographers (technologists who perform mammography) take their patient education responsibilities very seriously. Mammograms are often painful due to compression and thus are easy to avoid. Women may also fear developing cancer from the radiation used. The media tend to overdramatize (often in both directions), so women are unsure whom they can trust. Therefore, a mammographer wants to be sure that the patient understands the procedure and risks of the procedure as well as its potential benefits. It is extremely important that the patient make an informed decision.

Studies have shown that women have a number of faulty assumptions about the risks of breast cancer and the value of mammography as a screening tool (this is consistent with studies of other disease processes of both male and female subjects). Studies have found that educated women tend to overestimate their risk of dying of breast cancer and also overestimate the value of mammography; however less educated and older women tend to underestimate their risk of breast cancer (Black et al., 1995; Costanza et al., 1992).

The "best" means of telling patients about risks and benefits has not been determined and may not ever be. However, it is important that women be both informed and told how the communicator (e.g. the technologist) has come to this conclusion (Rimer, 1995). It is important that, in patient education, we are not seen as simple apologists for the use of ionizing radiation—that is, that we recommend mammography because we truly believe it is the best method of diagnosing cancer. To do this will require the establishment of the technologist as a competent professional *and* the formation of a bond between the patient and technologist that is based on trust.

## WHAT IS EFFECTIVE TEACHING?

All health professionals have a teaching role. Although teaching in the classroom and clinic are not identical to patient education, consider what makes or made your teachers effective in your radiologic technology education. All teaching involves four commonplaces (Dowd, 1996):

- *someone* (a teacher) teaches
- *someone else* (a learner) about
- *something* (a curriculum or information)
- *someplace* (in the case of patient education in the radiology department, a radiology room)

Good teachers also take the time and effort to evaluate the learning needs and readiness of their learners. For example, you probably were taught the basics of radiation safety in a course called Introduction to Radiologic Technology. At that point, you probably knew the rudiments of safety such as time, distance, and shielding but didn't really understand it well. Later you took Radiologic Physics and courses in Radiation Protection and Biology (as well as your associated clinical experiences), and now you probably know a lot about radiation safety and protection, and are ready to apply it to patient education—which you could not have done earlier.

It is similar with patients, although they are a much more diverse group—some are not very literate, some are very young, some are very old, and so on (Table 14–1 lists some of these factors). Each has a right to be educated, but the level and amount of information presented will vary.

The patient encounter that technologists typically have with patients has been called the *brief encounter*—a term borrowed from communications theory. In the course of a few minutes, a technologist must assess the patient, take a patient history, provide the patient with the information he or she needs for successful completion of the examination and follow-up (patient education), and perform an examination. This is a difficult balancing act. In some cases, staff technologists are so skilled at this

process that they have integrated it to the point that it is difficult to separate out the parts of the process! Thus, it is difficult or even impossible to provide you with a lock-step description of the process.

One of the best ways to learn how to teach patients is to observe technologists whom you have separated into two categories—one that you feel is very adept at patient care and education, and another that you feel is not. Observe and then reflect on the attributes that make each good or bad at the process. How can you emulate the good behaviors and avoid the bad ones?

### The Role of Trust

Good teachers in any setting try to establish a connection with their learners; that connection is based on trust. According to van Servellen (1997), trust "is felt to be the single most influential factor behind the patient's acceptance of provider opinion and his or her willingness to engage in positive health-related behaviors."

Trust is a facilitator to any therapeutic relationship; lack of trust is a barrier. Trust is established through a communication of respect and genuineness; it is lost when excessive professional distance is created through disinterest and lack of concern.

Van Servellen (1997) believes that there are three phases in the establishment of trust: an initiation phase, an implementation phase, and a termination phase. In the relationship that radiographers and other imaging professionals have with patients, these correlate with the introduction of patient and practitioner; the performance of the examination; and the termination of the examination.

When the patient is introduced to the technologist, there is often an initial attempt at communication in the form of small talk and the taking of the patient history. It is most likely during this phase that questions about radiation exposure will occur. We have had practitioners exclaim to us, sometimes incredulously and sometimes proudly, "My patients have *never* asked questions about radiation exposure!" Others have indicated that this is a common process and that they have at least one patient per day ask

**Table 14–1** Items to Assess for Effective Patient Education

| Factor | Considerations |
|---|---|
| Health beliefs determine the patient's response to illness | Patient needs to feel like a partner and that his or her actions will influence the outcome. |
| Sociocultural background | Some cultures expect to be told what to do; some react stoically, etc.* |
| | A Japanese patient from Hiroshima or a patient from the Utah Testing Grounds may have a quite different view of radiation than the "average" patient. |
| Physical illness | Changes individual's view of self; even threatened disease (undiagnosed symptoms) may cause a patient to react differently than "normal." |
| | Many times disease threatens factors seen as peripheral to the exam, such as socioeconomic status. Patients who feel their illness may "bankrupt" them may react irrationally to treatment. |
| Mental illness | All mental illnesses are not the same; some patients may be able to understand; as humans, they deserve the right to participate to the best of their ability. |
| Age (youth) | Younger patients not able to understand; thus, parents may receive most education. However, adolescents are a mix of child and adult, making education of parent and child extremely important. |
| Age (old age) | Many old people are stereotyped as "senile"; in reality most have small changes that only slightly change their ability to learn and most can adapt to those small changes. |
| Preferred learning style | Some like to learn by seeing or reading (visual); some by listening; some by doing (tactile/psychomotor). Many people are combinations of these; for example, many radiography students like to learn by seeing and doing. |
| Environment | Many environments are not conducive to learning; a good example is the often cold and dark radiology room. Mammography rooms are often designed in the opposite form: open, bright, comfortable—conducive to learning. |
| Literacy | Often overlooked; a patient may read a consent form, for example, and sign it, but not really understand the information. Most people who are marginally literate or illiterate will state they do understand, even when they don't due to a fear of appearing "stupid."† |

*For a review of sociocultural considerations and how these relate to patient care, see Davidhizar RE, Dowd SB, Giger J: Model for cultural diversity in the radiology department, Radiol Technol 68:3, 233–238, 1997.

†For a review of patient literacy and how that relates to patient education, see Brownson K, Dowd SB: Informed consent: does the patient really understand? Images, Spring, 1997.

them about radiation exposure. We wonder if the establishment of trust might not have something to do with this—if patients see you as competent, yet cold and impersonal, they will not have sufficient trust to ask you a potentially hard question. In the case of the mammographic patient cited earlier, avoiding future mammograms will be easy because radiographers seem to cause pain and not even apologize for it!

The building of trust takes time, probably more time than we think we have. But to quote van Servellen (1997) again:

> Providers may argue that there are too many demands on their time to build trust in their relationships with patients. While the building of trust does take time, it is a task that cannot be neglected even in this era of fleeting episodic encounters with patients. It is not that we cannot afford the time to build trust; rather, we cannot afford not to build trust.

### Building Trust and Educating the Patient— "Give 'Em an Apron!"

One of the best ways to establish trust for a radiographer, beyond efficient and compassionate patient care, is to provide patients (when appropriate, see Chapter 11) with a lead apron or other forms of shielding. This lets the patient know that you care about his or her welfare. A simple explanation, such as "I am putting this here for your protection," is typically sufficient.

It also encourages patients in the future, to ask for an apron, "Hey, where's my apron?" Thus, giving an apron to one patient can have a domino effect that may encourage more radiation protection of all patients, and may encourage those "sloppy" technologists to do the right thing.

## SHOULD TECHNOLOGISTS TELL EVERYTHING THEY KNOW?

One of the dilemmas of any allied health professional or nurse is the need to provide only what is relevant and to be careful that one is not providing so much information that one is practicing medicine or increasing, rather than reducing, patient anxiety about the procedure. There are four basic considerations that should be made, for example, before answering any question a patient poses (Carson and Arnold, 1996):

1. What are the motivations for this question?
2. What effect will answering the question have?
3. Who is the proper person to answer the question?
4. How much information is appropriate?

For example, many patients come to the radiology department with undiagnosed symptoms (Davidhizar and Dowd, 1996). These patients are naturally anxious and may ask a slew of questions. Are they asking these questions because they want information or because they want to be reassured? In many cases, it is the latter rather than the former. Proper assessment is the key. A biology professor or a college student may be asking a lot of questions about radiation exposure out of natural curiosity. An adolescent, on the other hand, may have, buried beneath the surface questions, an unstated one, "Will this make me sterile?" The adolescent is in a life stage in which sexuality is important, and there is much confusion about sexuality—he may not know the difference between "sterility" and "impotence," for example. The adolescent may be looking for reassurance that having an x-ray will not compromise his sexuality. This may seem very silly to us, but it is a real concern to the patient, and thus, important.

A patient who asks questions about radiation exposure may have other hidden agendas. For example, not all patients understand the difference between radiography and nuclear medicine for diagnosis and radiation therapy for the treatment of disease. Many patients know that certain disease processes take higher doses for treatment. They may associate those doses with more virulent forms of the disease. A logical extrapolation to them is that radiographic examinations with a lower dose of radiation are done for more benign diseases—we know this is not logical, but the patient does not. Thus, they may be relieved when they hear that the dose from a particular examination is low, "Great! I can't have anything that bad."

Another mistake in logic that patients make is assuming that examinations without radiation are "risk-free" and that all examinations provide the same level of information. Thus, patients who have an x-ray and then an MRI or ultrasound think that their physician or the hospital must be "double-dipping" and ordering unnecessary examinations. They will find the x-ray particularly galling as they associate that examination with a risk. They need to know that all examinations are not equal and that there is a logical reason for having two (or three or more) examinations of the same region using different modalities. However, as the case study shows, this information exchange must often be presented with caution and skill.

When patients ask questions such as, "What will this test show?" very often what they *really* want to know is whether the test will be painful, stressful, and whether the technologist is really competent to do that test (Lewis, 1986). Radiographers are also "convenient targets"—the patient may just have left the physician's office, for example, but the doctor seemed so *rushed*— "I'll just ask the technologist," they think. However, the technologist may not be the best individual to provide this information.

## CASE STUDY

Sam Smith is a radiography student in the second year of his education. When a patient presents for a skull radiograph, she asks whether this examination will show a brain tumor. She has had a bump on the back of her head for about 2 weeks, not painful, but obvious. He answers, "No. This test is designed to show the bony anatomy of the skull and perhaps the surrounding soft tissue. We normally do CT scans for brain tumors."

The next day, her physician storms into the department asking, "Who is the moron who told my patient she needed to have a CT scan?" When he finds out it is Sam, he calls up his program director and seeks to have him removed from the program for "practicing medicine without a license."

1. Do you think Sam did the right thing?
2. If not, what should he have done?
3. Ask two technologists separately how they would have handled this situation. Did they agree?
4. What could be done to avoid this situation in the future?

Don't take these admonitions as an excuse to not provide information and think that all patients need are pats on the head, "There, there, Mr. Jones, it will be alright." As we noted earlier, patients both need and now are beginning to demand more information about their care, but remember that the proper administration of information is no easier than the proper administration of medication or radiation. Both too much and too little serve no useful purpose, and can actually pose a danger to the patient.

### Hiders, Revealers, and Experts

Davidhizar and Dowd (1997) postulate that there are three types of individuals when it comes to revealing information to patients. The first are *revealers*. These individuals tell everything they know. These individuals are often new technologists who want to reduce patient anxiety and have a need to be seen as experts. They have not often dealt with patient anxiety and have a need to reduce it as quickly as possible.

The second group are *hiders*. These are often technologists with some clinical experience who have been "burned" when it comes to providing (probably too much) information. They may also be from the "old school" when technologists were told specifically to tell the patient nothing—after all, they were "only technicians." In some cases, hiders give information that is false, or that has only a "grain of truth" to it ("Having an x-ray is like spending a day in the sun"). They also seek to alleviate anxiety quickly, often by deceptive or close to deceptive means ("After all, it's easier on the patient that way," they rationalize). Many of these individuals are skeptical that patient education is a role of the technologist and believe that it is a function better reserved for doctors or nurses. Taking x-rays is their job; everything else isn't.

The final group are the *experts*. An expert knows just how much information it is appropriate for a technologist to reveal—that is, knows the scope of practice of a technologist. An expert is able to evaluate what the patient needs to know and knows how to respond with simple comments at first that begin the assessment process and gradually unfold into what needs to be revealed. Experts also know that each case is situational and must be evaluated on its own merits. No one method works well all the time or in all situations. A contrasting of the three types can be found in Table 14–2.

### NUMERACY

Numeracy refers to an individual's ability to understand numbers and their meaning. Numbers are abstract representations of concrete things. A classic article by Miller (1956) indicated that most people can comprehend up to the number seven in concrete terms, beyond which numbers become an abstraction. Although education and experience with numbers increase one's ability to deal with them, the unfamiliar nature of radiation exposure risks may make numerical comparisons more confusing than illuminating.

Many radiation risks are expressed in terms

Table 14–2  Revealers, Hiders, and Experts

| Question | What the *Hider* Would Say | What the *Revealer* Would Say | What the *Expert* Would Say |
|---|---|---|---|
| Does this test show if I have cancer? | Ma'am, I don't know; I'm just the technician. | Yes, Ma'am! We had such a case just last week! | Do you think you have cancer, Ma'am? *or* Most tests are performed to rule out disease rather than rule it in, Ma'am. |
| Will this x-ray hurt me? | No. It's just like a day in the sun. | Well, it depends on whether you are talking about stochastic or nonstochastic effects. In school, we learned that . . . (long monologue) | Sir, your physician ordered an x-ray because he sees it as necessary to your care. What do you mean by "hurt" you? |
| Has anyone ever died from having one of these barium enemas? | No. | Well, yes. There is a rare possibility that your colon could be perforated, and barium could leak into your peritoneum . . . | Are you worried about this test? (and if yes): We are all very qualified to do this exam, but no examination is risk-free. Would you like to speak with Dr. Jones, our radiologist, before the examination? |

Note how the *Hider* tries to terminate the question abruptly and "move on," while the *Revealer* seems compelled to provide every bit of information known to medical science. The *Expert* asks a simple reflective question or makes a statement that allows further response. The dialogue between an *Expert* and a *Patient* may take as long as the monologue delivered by a *Revealer,* but it will be an *exchange* of information that benefits the patient.

Adapted from Davidhizar and Dowd (1997). Used with permission.

of numbers. For example, radiation exposure might be compared to a certain number of days of sunbathing or number of days of life lost, or a "one in a million risk." Although it has been repeatedly affirmed that statistical abstractions such as a "one in a million risk" have little meaning to most individuals, they are still often used. One study showed that even trained health physicists had difficulty with the abstractions used in quantifying risk (Watson and Walsh, 1980). There exists the potential for even well-educated professionals to misuse these numbers. For example, the authors are familiar with a case in which a mammographer informed a patient that the radiation exposure from a mammogram was the same as from a cross-country plane flight. This is wholly incorrect. The *calculated risk of death* from a mammogram is the same as a cross-country air flight. The radiation exposure from a cross-country air

flight is much less than that of a mammogram. In this case, the mammographer made a classic "apples and oranges" comparison and gave the patient incorrect information.

There are certainly cases in which numerical information about radiation and radiation risk can be helpful; they are relatively rare. Certainly technologists should "know the numbers," but they should use them sparingly in dealing with patients.

## WAYS TO EXPLAIN RADIATION EXPOSURE TO PATIENTS

If patients ask directly and if, upon further probing, it seems that they really want to know how many "mrem" a procedure provides, it is probably best to provide that information. A technologist who does not know representative exposures from common exams (see Chapter 11) does not know much about his or her profession. However, one way to provide patients with information about radiation exposure is to compare that exposure with something else (see Chapter 1 for some examples). What do you think about the following approaches?

1. A technologist who compares radiation exposure to exposure from the sun or natural background radiation (probably the most common approach).
2. A technologist who compares radiation exposure to flying in an airplane.
3. A technologist who compares radiation exposure to smoking.
4. A nuclear medicine technologist who compares the exposure from nuclear medicine examinations to chest x-rays (saying, for example, that the exposure from a hepatobiliary study is the same as a chest x-ray).

Each of these has pluses and minuses. We recall that individuals accept voluntary risks much more so than involuntary risks; thus approach 1 might have more merit than approaches 2 or 3 to individuals who do not smoke or who do not fly in airplanes. In fact, with all the negative press cigarettes have received, such an approach might not even work with a smoker, who might be a smoker only because he or she can't give up the habit. It might be easier not to have that x-ray.

Approach 4 is a statement that is both true and false. There are some valid comparisons in terms of overall dose; however, the radiation from a nuclear medicine scan is delivered in a much different manner. In teaching, there often is a fine line between "misleading" and "bringing it to the level of the student," as you probably know. Radiologic physics instructors are often faced with this dilemma since making a complicated physics principle *too* simple also will make it *wrong* in many cases. However, it is important to realize that this line should not be crossed.

## SUMMARY

Patient education has become more important than ever before. Technologists are responsible for informing patients about the proce-

dures they are about to undergo; they are also responsible for providing radiation protection and informing patients who want to know about the radiation exposure and risks of the procedure as regards radiation exposure.

All health care professionals have a teaching role, and good teaching involves someone teaching someone else about something in a place. In radiography, teaching typically happens within a brief encounter—a short period of time, which means that technologists must be really sharp with their teaching skills to be effective. Building trust is extremely important and, in radiology, means showing compassion, answering questions as honestly as possible within the confines of acceptable practice, and providing patients with radiation protection.

Technologists should realize the fears and misconceptions that people have about ionizing radiation. They also have to realize that it is improper for a technologist to tell a patient nothing or to "tell everything they know"—the proper administration of information is no easier than the proper administration of medication or radiation. It is useful to think of three types of technologists—hiders, who give no information, revealers, who tell all, and experts, who know how much information to give at the right time.

There are many ways to analogize radiation exposure, and no one right way to do so. Technologists need to be certain, however, that the method they use is both accurate and understandable to the patient. They also need to be aware of some of the potential issues behind the actual questions asked in order to deal with the real concerns of the patient. Sometimes, questions about radiation exposure are actually a concern over the technologist's ability to provide empathetic care, which should always be answered affirmatively.

## Questions

1. Research clearly shows that individuals more readily take on voluntary risks than involuntary risks.

   a. true
   b. false

2. Studies have found that less-educated and older women tend to underestimate their risk of breast cancer.

   a. true
   b. false

3. One of the most important factors in communicating risk is that the communicator tell how he or she has come to that assessment of risk.

   a. true
   b. false

4. Which of the following should be considered before answering any patient questions?

   a. What are the motivations for this question?
   b. What effect will answering the question have?
   c. Who is the proper person to answer the question?
   d. How much information is appropriate?
   e. All of the above

5. Which of the following answers would a hider probably give in response to the question, "how much radiation will this examination give me?"

   a. "One hundred millirems"
   b. "Less than you might think"
   c. "Well, it depends on whether you are talking about skin dose, internal dose, organ dose, or exit dose"
   d. None of the above

6. Research has shown that people can understand and use in concrete terms numbers up to _____, plus or minus 2.

   a. 3              b. 7
   c. 30             d. 70

7. Comparing radiation risk to the risk of flying would be a bad idea:

   a. in all cases.
   b. if your patient had a fear of flying.
   c. the day after an airplane crash hit the news.
   d. Two of the above

8. Comparing a nuclear medicine scan to an x-ray has value because:

   a. all x-rays have low exposure.
   b. people are familiar with x-rays, for the most part.
   c. nuclear medicine uses a different form of administration than x-ray.
   d. None of the above

9. Comparing a nuclear medicine scan to an x-ray might not be good because:

   a. all x-rays have low exposure.
   b. people are familiar with x-rays, for the most part.
   c. nuclear medicine uses a different form of administration than x-ray.
   d. None of the above

10. Which of the following is probably the most common approach to informing patients about radiation risk?

    a. comparing radiation exposure to exposure from the sun or natural background radiation
    b. comparing radiation exposure to flying in an airplane
    c. comparing radiation exposure to smoking
    d. comparing radiation to eating common foods

## Exercises

1. What hidden agenda might each of the following individuals have in asking about radiation exposure?

   a. an adolescent
   b. an individual who wants to be assured that the dose is low

2. What usually causes people to fall into the categories of "hiders" or "revealers"?

3. How does providing patients with an apron or other forms of shielding establish trust?

4. What is one of the main problems with using numerical risk comparisons?

5. What does the expression "technologists are convenient targets" mean in this chapter?

## Answers

Questions

| | | | |
|---|---|---|---|
| 1. a | | 6. b | |
| 2. a | | 7. d | |
| 3. a | | 8. b | |
| 4. e | | 9. c | |
| 5. c | | 10. a | |

## Exercises

1. Adolescents may have concerns about sexuality and may worry that radiation exposure could make them "sterile"—which they may not have sufficient knowledge to differentiate from "impotent." Individuals who want to be assured that the dose is low may feel that low doses mean that the disease process they potentially have must then be relatively benign.

2. Revealers tell everything they know, even when they should not. Often new technologists who want to reduce patient anxiety and have a need to be seen as experts are revealers. They have not often dealt with patient anxiety and have a need to reduce it as quickly as possible.

   Hiders think that their job is only taking x-rays or other radiologic science duties. They may be from the old school or have been burned when providing (often too much) information. They also want to alleviate anxiety, but do so almost deceptively.

3. Providing shielding lets patients know that you care first and foremost about their welfare. It also establishes a professional baseline for good practice and might encourage the patient to ask the next radiographer, "Hey, where is my apron?"

4. Numerical risk comparisons are difficult to understand, even by trained professionals such as physicians or technologists. Thus, there is a danger that the professional may use them incorrectly or that the patient may misunderstand them.

5. Technologists are convenient targets to ask questions of, as they are knowledgeable health professionals who are not seen in the same light as "the doctor" and thus more easily approachable. However, this is a dilemma in that the technologist may not be the best person to answer the question.

## Further Discussion Questions

1. Without naming names, discuss some of the behaviors you have seen in clinic of hiders, revealers, and experts. What aspects of the expert's behavior can you emulate so that you can become an expert?

2. What are your views on providing shielding? If there are cases in which you would *not* provide a patient with a shield, what kind of explanation would you provide them for this decision?

3. Discuss the relative merits of the different types of risk comparisons. Which method would you or do you use?

4. Discuss how establishing trust is so important, and some possible negative outcomes that can result if a patient loses trust in you.

5. The assertion is made in this chapter that all health care professionals have a teaching role. Do you agree or disagree with this statement? If you disagree, why? If you agree, describe some of the ways in which technologists function as teachers that were not mentioned in the book.

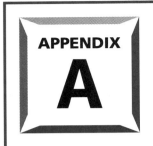

# Commonly Used Formulas

This section of the text covers some of the problems given in earlier chapters. We have selected these because we believe they have clinical utility and are commonly seen on certification examinations. This does not mean that other problems presented in this text are not important. It simply means that, in our experience, they are of limited use in the clinic or are not commonly asked on certification examinations. As with any selection of material, it reflects our experience as educators, and also our biases.

One good use of this section would be immediately before the certification examination. As the date of the examination draws near, students should progressively limit the amount of material they study. The rationale for this is that concepts were learned or not learned over a 2-year or greater course of study; 1 month before the examination is not the time to plunge into material in depth.

Most students learn the formulas used in the radiologic sciences by memorization. This is just the first step. As we have said in a previous section, the most important aspect of learning problem-solving is learning how to use the material in clinical practice. This involves attention to logical problem-solving, which we have also attempted to show here.

On many certification examinations, the correct answer can be ascertained or at least two choices eliminated by using logical decision-making. This is listed here as the presolving step for problems. In some cases, this may seem obvious, but the intent is to help all students with problem solving.

## CONVERTING UNITS

The following method for converting traditional units to SI units was given in Chapter 3:

$$1 \text{ R} \times (2.58 \times 10^{-4}) = \text{coulombs per kilogram (C/kg)}$$

$$1 \text{ rad} \times 0.01 = \text{gray (Gy)}*$$

$$1 \text{ rem} \times 0.01 = \text{sievert (Sv)}*$$

$$1 \text{ Ci} \times (3.7 \times 10^{10}) = \text{becquerel (Bq)}*$$

This works in reverse as follows:

$$1 \text{ C/kg} \div (2.58 \times 10^{-4}) = \text{roentgen (R)}$$

$$1 \text{ Gy} \div 0.01 = \text{rad}$$

$$1 \text{ Sv} \div 0.01 = \text{rem}$$

$$1 \text{ Bq} \div (3.7 \times 10^{10}) = \text{curie (Ci)}$$

*According to the ARRT (Conventions Specific to the Radiography Examination, May 1993), "Sieverts, greys, becquerels are not used on the radiography examination."

If the student is having trouble with problem-solving, an excellent resource is Dennis CA, Eisenberg RL: Applied Radiographic Calculations. Philadelphia, WB Saunders, 1993.

Recall that when converting from milliroentgens, millirads, and millirems to the whole units of coulombs per kilogram, grays, and sieverts, these units must first be converted to their whole unit by dividing the unit by 1000. Alternately, milliroentgens can be multiplied by $2.58 \times 10^{-7}$ to convert to coulombs per kilogram; millirads can be multiplied by 0.00001 to convert to grays; and millirems can be multiplied by 0.00001 to convert to sieverts. In algebra, to work the problem the opposite way (e.g. to convert sieverts to millirems), remember to use the opposite function (in this case, divide instead of multiply).

## Exposure

| | |
|---|---|
| *Sample problem 1:* | 10 R is how many coulombs per kilogram? |
| PRESOLVING STEP: | Since 1 R is $2.58 \times 10^{-4}$ C/kg, 10 R will be a larger number. |
| ADDITIONAL LOGIC STEP: | Remember that increasing a power of 10, when negative, *decreases* the superscript number. |
| FORMULA USED: | $10 \times (2.58 \times 10^{-4})$ C/kg<br>10 R = $2.58 \times 10^{-3}$ C/kg |
| *Sample problem 2:* | 10 mR is how many coulombs per kilogram? |
| PRESOLVING STEP: | Since 1 mR is $2.58 \times 10^{-7}$ C/kg, 10 mR will be a greater number. |
| ADDITIONAL LOGIC STEP: | Remember that increasing a power of 10, when negative, *decreases* the superscript number. |
| FORMULA USED: | $10 \times (2.58 \times 10^{-7})$ C/kg<br>10 mR = $2.58 \times 10^{-6}$ C/kg |
| *Sample problem 3:* | 1 C/kg is how many roentgens? |
| PRESOLVING STEP: | Since 1 R is $2.58 \times 10^{-4}$ C/kg, 1 C/kg will be many roentgens. |
| FORMULA USED: | Since we multiply in the first example, we must divide here. |

$1 \div 2.58 \times 10^{-4}$ C/kg (0.000258) = 3875.96

1 C/kg = 3875.96 R

| | |
|---|---|
| *Sample problem 4:* | 1 C/kg is how many milliroentgens? |
| PRESOLVING STEP: | Since 1 mR is $2.58 \times 10^{-7}$ C/kg, 1 C/kg will be many milliroentgens. Also, this number must be greater than the third sample problem. |
| FORMULA USED: | We must also divide here. |

$1 \div 2.58 \times 10^{-7}$ C/kg (0.000000258) = 3875000.96

1 C/kg = 3875000.96 mR

## Absorbed Dose

| | |
|---|---|
| *Sample problem 1:* | 100 rad is how many grays? |
| PRESOLVING STEP: | Since 1 rad is 0.01 (1/100) Gy, we can look at this problem and expect that 100 rad is 1 Gy. |
| FORMULA USED: | $100 \times 0.01 = 1$<br>100 rad is 1 Gy. |
| *Sample problem 2:* | 10 Gy is how many rad? |
| PRESOLVING STEP: | Since the gray is larger than rad, the answer must be greater than 10. |
| FORMULA USED: | $10 \div 0.01 = 1000$<br>10 Gy is 1000 rad. |
| *Sample problem 3:* | 100 mrad is how many grays? |
| PRESOLVING STEP: | This will have to be a very small number since the millirad is smaller than the rad, and the rad is smaller than the gray. |
| FORMULA USED: | $100 \times 0.00001 = 0.001$<br>100 mrad is 0.001 Gy.<br>100 mrad is 1 mGy. |

## Occupational Dose

*Sample problem 1:* If a radiographer receives 30 rem over her lifetime, what is her lifetime dose in sieverts?

PRESOLVING STEP: Since the rem is smaller than the sievert, the solution will be smaller than 30.

FORMULA USED: $30 \times 0.01 = 0.3$

30 rem is 0.3 Sv or 300 mSv.

*Sample problem 2:* The recommended lifetime dose is now 0.01 Sv for each year of age. How many rem can a radiographer accumulate per year of age?

PRESOLVING STEP: Since the sievert is a larger unit than the rem, the answer will be larger than 0.01.

FORMULA USED: $0.01 \div 0.01 = 1$

Radiographers can accumulate up to their age in rem (1 rem per year of age).

*Sample problem 3:* How many rem is 100 mSv?

PRESOLVING STEP: 1 mSv is 1/10 (0.1) of a rem.

FORMULA USED: Step 1: $100 \div 1000 = 0.1$

100 mSv is 0.1 Sv.

Step 2: $0.1 \div 0.01 = 10$.

100 mSv is 10 rem.

## RADIOACTIVITY

*Sample problem 1:* 10 Ci is how many becquerels?

PRESOLVING STEP: The curie is a much larger unit than the becquerel.

FORMULA USED: $10 \times (3.7 \times 10^{10})$

$3.7 \times 10^{11}$ Bq

*Sample problem 2:* 1000 Bq is how many curies?

PRESOLVING STEP: Since the becquerel is a very small unit, this will be a very small answer.

FORMULA USED: $1000 \div (3.7 \times 10^{10}) = 2.7 \times 10^{-8}$ Ci

## RELATIVE BIOLOGIC EFFECT

Relative biologic effect (RBE) is a ratio that compares a test radiation to 250 kVp of x-ray. A higher number indicates that the test radiation is *more effective* than the 250-kVp x-ray. Therefore:

An RBE of 2 indicates that the test radiation is twice as effective.

An RBE of 1/2 or 0.5 indicates that the test radiation is half as effective.

An RBE of 3 indicates that the test radiation is three times as effective.

An RBE of 1/3 indicate that the test radiation is one third as effective.

The formula for RBE is as follows:

$$\frac{\text{dose of 250-keV x-ray to produce the same effect}}{\text{dose of test radiation to produce an effect}}$$

*Sample problem 1:* If it takes 3 rad of test radiation to produce the same effect as 1 rad of 250-kVp x-ray, what is the RBE of the test radiation?

PRESOLVING STEP: Since it takes more test radiation to produce an effect than the 250-kVp x-ray, the RBE will be less than 1.

FORMULA USED: $\dfrac{1}{3}$

$\text{RBE} = \dfrac{1}{3}$ The test radiation is 1/3 as effective as the 250-kVp x-ray.

*Sample problem 2:* If it takes 1 rad of test radiation to produce the same effect as 10 rad of

250-kVp x-ray, what is the RBE of the test radiation?

PRESOLVING STEP: Since it takes less test radiation to produce an effect than the 250-kVp x-ray, the RBE will be more than 1.

FORMULA USED: $\frac{1}{10}$

RBE = 10

## mAs AND RADIATION INTENSITY

Since mAs directly controls the amount of radiation produced, changes in mAs, holding other factors equal, should produce equivalent changes in radiation intensity. Thus, as the mAs is doubled, exposure (entrance skin exposure) should also double. This relationship also holds for changing mAs or time as long as the other factor is held constant; doubling mAs doubles intensity so long as time and other factors are held constant.

Remember throughout that intensity and dose are related but not identical terms. If we are talking about entrance skin exposure, we can use the terms interchangeably. The formula for mAs and intensity is:

$$\frac{mAs_1}{mAs_2} = \frac{I_1}{I_2}$$

*Sample problem 1:* If the original intensity was 100 mR, and mAs is increased from 25 to 50 mAs, what will happen to intensity?

PRESOLVING STEP: Since mAs is increasing, intensity should also increase. Since mAs is doubling, intensity should double.

FORMULA USED: $\frac{25}{50} = \frac{100}{x}$

25x = 5000

x = 200

*Sample problem 2:* If the original intensity was 200 mR, and mAs is

decreased from 60 to 40 mAs, what will happen to intensity?

PRESOLVING STEP: Since mAs is decreasing, intensity should decrease.

FORMULA USED: $\frac{60}{40} = \frac{200}{x}$

60x = 8000

x = 133

*Sample problem 3:* A radiographer increases technical factors from 400 mAs and 0.1 second to 400 mAs and 0.15 second to increase density on a radiograph. What would the increase be to intensity?

PRESOLVING STEP: Calculate the mAs for each exposure. The first mAs is 40, the second is 60.

Since mAs is increasing, intensity should also increase.

ADDITIONAL LOGIC STEP REQUIRED: No first intensity or second intensity is given. Thus, the change in intensity must be a radio of the mAs change. The formula must be modified as follows:

FORMULA USED: $\frac{mAs_2}{mAs_1} = \frac{I_2}{I_1}$

$$\frac{60}{40} = \frac{I_2}{I_1}$$

$$\frac{1.5}{1} = \frac{I_2}{I_1}$$

Thus, the second intensity is 1.5 times the first.

## kVp AND RADIATION INTENSITY

kVp affects radiation intensity by a ratio of the kVps. The formula is as follows:

$$\left(\frac{kVp_1}{kVp_2}\right)^2 = \frac{I_1}{I_2}$$

*Sample problem 1:* If 75 kVp produces an intensity of 400 mR, what intensity will 80 kVp produce if all other technical factors are held constant?

PRESOLVING STEP: kVp is increasing with all other factors remaining constant. Intensity must increase.

FORMULA USED:

$$\left(\frac{75}{80}\right)^2 = \frac{400}{x}$$

$$\frac{5625}{6400} = \frac{400}{x}$$

$$5625x = 2,560,000$$

$$x = 455$$

80 kVp will provide 455 mR.

*Sample problem 2:* If a technique using 60 kVp provides 50 mR of intensity, what will switching to 70 kVp provide if all other factors are held equal?

PRESOLVING STEP: kVp is increasing with all other factors held constant. Intensity should increase. Knowledge of the general rule (see below) that increasing kVp by 10 at 60 will increase intensity by 36% will help solve the problem.

FORMULA USED:

$$\left(\frac{60}{70}\right)^2 = \frac{50}{x}$$

$$\frac{3600}{4900} = \frac{50}{x}$$

$$3600x = 245,000$$

$$x = 68 \text{ mR}$$

To check: 18 (intensity increased by 18 from 50 to 68) is 36% of 50 (0.36 × 50 = 18).

Note also the following general guidelines for kVp and intensity that will work well in clinical practice:

Increasing kVp by 10 at 60 kVp would increase intensity by 36%, increasing film density.

Increasing kVp by 10 at 60 kVp *and* decreasing mAs to compensate will *decrease* intensity by 14%, while maintaining overall film density.

Increasing kVp by 10 at 70 kVp would increase intensity by 30%, increasing film density.

Increasing kVp by 10 at 70 kVp and decreasing mAs to compensate will *decrease* intensity by 20%, while maintaining overall film density.

Increasing kVp by 10 at 80 kVp would increase intensity by 26%, increasing film density.

Increasing kVp by 10 at 80 kVp and decreasing mAs to compensate will *decrease* intensity by 24%, maintaining overall film density.

## INVERSE SQUARE LAW AND DISTANCE

For point sources of radiation, intensity varies by the inverse of the square of the distance. For extended sources such as the patient and other scattering objects, intensity decreases by 1/1000 at 1 meter; after that, the increase square law applies.

The inverse square law is:

$$\frac{I_1}{I_2} = \left(\frac{D_2}{D_1}\right)^2$$

*Sample problem 1:* If the intensity is 50 mR at 1 meter, what is intensity at 2 meters?

PRESOLVING STEP: Distance is increasing; intensity must decrease (by the inverse of the square).

FORMULA USED:

$$\frac{50}{x} = \left(\frac{2}{1}\right)^2$$

$$4x = 50$$

$$x = 12.5$$

ADDITIONAL LOGIC STEP:

If you know the basic applications of the inverse square law, you know that as distance doubles, intensity decreases by 4. Thus, you could have divided 50 by 4 to determine the second intensity.

*Sample problem 2:*

If the intensity is 100 mR at 2 meters, what is intensity at 1 meter?

PRESOLVING STEP:

Distance is decreasing; intensity must increase (by the inverse of the square).

FORMULA USED:

$$\frac{100}{x} = \left(\frac{1}{2}\right)^2$$

$$x = 400$$

At 1 meter, intensity is 400 mR.

ADDITIONAL LOGIC STEP:

If you know the basic applications of the inverse square law, you know that as distance halves, intensity increases by 4. Thus, you could have multiplied 100 by 4 to determine the second intensity.

*Sample problem 3:*

A technologist stands at one meter, where intensity is 10 mR/hr. How far back must she step to reduce her intensity to 5 mR/hr?

PRESOLVING STEP:

This is slightly different than other problems. The two intensities are known and distance is calculated. Distance must obviously increase. It also will be less than a doubling of the distance, since 2x distance would cut the intensity to one fourth the original value, or 2.5 mR/hr.

FORMULA USED:

$$\frac{10}{5} = \left(\frac{x}{1}\right)^2$$

$$5x^2 = 10$$

$$x^2 = 2$$

$$x = 1.44$$

The new distance needed is 1.44 meters.

## SCREEN SPEED AND RADIATION DOSE

As screen speed decreases, the amount of radiation needed to expose the film increases. The trade-off is image quality—slower speed screens give better detail. Screens are assigned relative speed values. Determine the new exposure needed when changing screen speeds through the formula:

$$\frac{mAs_1}{mAs_2} = \frac{speed_2}{speed_1}$$

The assumption can be made, since mAs and intensity are directly related, that increases or decreases made in mAs to compensate for screen speed will have the same effect on patient exposure (entrance skin exposure). See the section on mAs and exposure if this is unclear. This can be expressed in a formula as follows:

$$\frac{I_1}{I_2} = \frac{speed_2}{speed_1} \text{ (assumes compensated mAs)}$$

*Sample problem 1:*

Original screen speed used is 100. To minimize motion through a faster exposure, a screen speed of 400 is used. If original intensity was 100 mR (entrance skin exposure), what will it be with the new screen?

PRESOLVING STEP:

A screen that is four times as fast is being used. If mAs is decreased to compensate, intensity should decrease by a factor of 4.

FORMULA USED:

$$\frac{100}{x} = \frac{400}{100}$$

$$400x = 10,000$$

$$x = 25$$

New intensity will be 25 mR.

*Sample problem 2:* To improve film quality, a radiologist wants to switch from 400 speed screens to 200. The chief technologist should remind the radiologist that this will cause what change in radiation dose?

PRESOLVING STEP: Halving screen speed will require two times the mAs, and thus twice the intensity will be produced.

FORMULA USED:

$$\frac{I_1}{I_2} = \frac{200}{400}$$

Since we are comparing $I_2$ to $I_1$, we should invert the equation:

$$\frac{I_2}{I_1} = \frac{400}{200}$$

$$= \frac{2}{1}$$

$I_2$ is 2 times $I_1$.

*Sample problem 3:* Which of the following technical factors, with everything else held equal, would result in the lowest patient exposure dose?

   a. 10 mAs, 100 kVp, 200 speed system
   b. 5 mAs, 100 kVp, 400 speed system
   c. 2.5 mAs, 100 kVp, 100 speed system
   d. 1.25 mAs, 100 kVp, 50 speed system

In this case, note that the film/screen system used does not have to be known. It is extra information. Since the kVp levels are the same, the technique with the lowest mAs will provide the lowest exposure (d).

## GRIDS AND RADIATION DOSE

Using a grid increases patient dose as technical factors must be increased. Either mAs or kVp can be used to compensate for the addition of a grid or changing grid ratio. From a radiation protection standpoint, kVp is preferred. From an imaging standpoint, mAs may be a preferred change.

*Sample problem 1:* A no-grid technique is originally used with a technique of 5 mAs and 70 kVp for a knee, providing an entrance skin exposure of 80 mR. If a 6:1 grid is then used with mAs compensated (mAs conversion factor of 3), what would the increase in intensity be?

PRESOLVING STEP: Intensity must increase; it will increase proportionally to the mAs change.

FORMULA USED: Calculate the new mAs needed first:

$$10 \times 3 = 30$$

Then calculate the new intensity using the formula for mAs and intensity:

$$\frac{mAs_1}{mAs_2} = \frac{I_1}{I_2}$$

$$\frac{10}{30} = \frac{80}{240}$$

The second intensity is 240 mR.

*Sample problem 2:* A technique of 40 mAs and 80 kVp and an 8:1 grid is used for an anteroposterior abdomen film, producing an entrance skin exposure of 400 mR. What will happen to intensity if a 12:1 grid is used with mAs to compensate?

8:1 conversion factor = 4x mAs

12:1 conversion factor = 5x mAs

FORMULA USED:

This problem can be solved as follows in two steps:

$$\frac{mAs_1}{mAs_2} = \frac{grid\ factor_1}{grid\ factor_2}$$

$$\frac{40}{x} = \frac{4}{5}$$

$$4x = 200$$

$$x = 50$$

The new mAs needed is 50.

Now use the formula for mAs and intensity:

$$\frac{40}{50} = \frac{400}{x}$$

$$40x = 20,000$$

$$x = 500$$

Intensity increases to 500 mR.

*Sample problem 3:*

If all factors remain the same, which of the following would result in the lowest patient exposure?

a. 10 mAs, 8:1 grid
b. 14 mAs, 8:1 grid
c. 10 mAs, 10:1 grid
d. 14 mAs, 10:1 grid

This type of problem is sometimes seen on certification examinations. We can use the formula above or use logic: look for the lowest mAs (10; answer a). Grid ratio is unimportant; it is *after* the patient. Remember that the goal of the certification examination is to determine your skill as a practitioner; thus, the same logical problem-solving you use in the clinic will often work here too.

## HALF-VALUE LAYER

A half-value layer (HVL) is that thickness of material that will reduce radiation intensity by half.

*Sample problem 1:*

After three HVLs, what intensity of radiation remains with a beginning intensity of 100 mR?

PRESOLVING STEP:

Intensity must decrease.

FORMULA USED:

Divide each intensity by half as follows.

$$I_0 = 100\ mR$$

$$I_1 = 50\ mR$$

$$I_2 = 25\ mR$$

$$I_3 = 12.5\ mR$$

$I_0$ is the intensity before any HVLs are applied (the original intensity); each subscript number indicates the number of HVLs applied.

*Sample problem 2:*

After five HVLs, what percentage of radiation remains?

PRESOLVING STEP:

There must be a decrease in intensity. Also, you must know that we always start with 100% intensity; thus $I_0$ is 100. This type of problem is sometimes confusing since no initial intensity is given.

FORMULA USED:

$$I_0 = 100$$

$$I_1 = 50$$

$$I_2 = 25$$

$$I_3 = 12.5$$

$$I_4 = 6.25$$

$$I_5 = 3.125$$

After five HVLs, 3.125% of radiation remains.

*Sample problem 3:*

How many HVLs would it take to reduce radiation intensity to less than 10% of original value?

PRESOLVING STEP:

The same logic as above applies. In this case, intensity must be divided until less than 10% remains. That HVL is the solution.

FORMULA USED:

$I_0 = 100$

$I_1 = 50$

$I_2 = 25$

$I_3 = 12.5$

$I_4 = 6.25$

After four HVLs, less than 10% (6.25%) of radiation remains.

## COLLIMATION (X-RAY)

Collimation affects radiation dose by increasing the amount of scatter produced. A larger field produces more scatter. This is a fairly simple problem.

*Sample problem:* Which of the following field sizes will produce the greatest amount of scatter —a 10 by 10-inch field or a 10 by 12-inch field?

PRESOLVING STEP: The largest field will produce the greatest amount of scatter.

FORMULA USED:

$10 \times 10 = 100$

$10 \times 12 = 120$

The 10 by 12-inch field will produce the greatest amount of scatter.

## X-RAY DOSE

The formula for output intensity is:

$$\text{output intensity} = \frac{k \ (mAs) \ (kVp)^2}{d^2}$$

Once the constant of k is known by measuring it at 70 kVp and 100 cm (40 inches), new intensity can be calculated as follows:

output intensity = k (mR/mAs)

$$(mAs_2) \left(\frac{kVp}{70}\right)^2 \left(\frac{100cm}{d_2}\right)^2$$

k = measured value at 70 kVp and 100 cm

$mAs_2$ = new technique

$kVp_2$ = new technique

$d_2$ = new FFD (SID)

*Sample problem 1:* The value of k is 4 mR/mAs. If 50 mAs and 90 kVp are used, what is intensity?

FORMULA USED:

(4 mR/mAs) (50 mAs)

$$\left(\frac{90}{70}\right)^2 \left(\frac{100}{100}\right)^2$$

Since distance is the same, it can be eliminated from the calculation.

$$200 \times \left(\frac{8100}{4900}\right)$$

$8100 \div 4900 = 1.653$

$200 \times 1.653 = 330.6$

The intensity is 331 mR.

*Sample problem 2:* The calculated value of k is 5 mR/mAs. For a postero-anterior chest radiograph, 2 mAs, 120 kVp, and 72 inches are used. What is the intensity?

FORMULA USED:

(5 mR/mAs) (2 mAs)

$$\left(\frac{120}{70}\right)^2 \left(\frac{40}{72}\right)^2$$

$$10 \times \left(\frac{14,400}{4900}\right)^2 \times \left(\frac{1600}{5184}\right)^2$$

$14,400 \div 4900 = 2.94$

$1600 \div 5184 = 0.309$

$10 \times 2.94 \times .309 = 9.08$

Intensity would be 9 mR.

Hiss (1993) recommends using the following formula to *approximate* exposure in mR:

$$15 \times \frac{kVp_2 \times mAs}{D^2} = \text{exposure in mR}$$

$D^2$ = distance squared in centimeters

This formula is most useful when k is not known. In our two sample problems using this formula, intensity would have been 337.5 mR (sample problem 1) and 12.9 mR (sample problem 2).

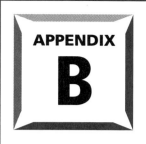

# APPENDIX B

# A Guide to Radiation Protection Resources on the Internet

## Richard Terrass

## THE DEVELOPMENT OF ONLINE RADIATION PROTECTION RESOURCES

The historical development of online radiation protection resources (1, 2) can be traced to the RADSAFE mailing list, which was started by Hector Mandel at the University of Illinois at Urbana–Champaign in 1993. Before that RAD-SAFE was a Fidonet echo running off of The Check Source BBS in Urbana. Responsibility for running the list has since passed to Melissa Woo at UIUC. The development of World Wide Web resources for the radiation protection and health physics community can be traced to Bruce Busby, who started the Radiation Protection and Health Physics Home Page at the University of Michigan in the spring of 1995. Busby writes a monthly column on Net resources in the *Health Physics Journal* and lectures on the subject with Woo at meetings and symposiums. I recently asked Woo and Busby how they would characterize the online resources currently available in this field and what changes they saw coming.

Busby sees online resources as having just begun. "They are a start, but no way would the(y) be considered to be done or complete," according to Busby. He likes the chance that this gives different places to share their experience, their manuals and procedures, and having good information available to the public. Woo sees the online resources in the field as mirroring the state of the entire Internet. The online resources are, in her words, "getting there." According to Woo, "I believe that we've finally bypassed the temporary infatuation with the technology itself, and people are clamoring for 'real' content and utility from the Internet."

"The areas in which the field are lacking," Woo says, "are in access to scientific journal articles, full text of standards (e.g. ANSI), and full text of pertinent guidelines (e.g. NCRP Reports). However, as the limitation on these resources is based on financial considerations, these issues will be resolved only when the Internet as a whole can be engineered into a communications vehicle through which private concerns can still make a profit off of the information they possess."

As far as coming changes goes, Busby sees

[O]n-line training, questions and answers from professionals (already happening), standardization among hospitals, universities, states (regs, manuals, procedures . . .), better dose record keeping, better sharing of dose (and other) information, more public training, on-line courses/tests, video conferencing, more notice of incidents/lessons learned, more helping of each other through communication, NCRP reports on line, NUREGs on line, laws and regulations on line, much better communication with the public, more on-line job resources, . . . and more on-line shopping . . . course announcements, conferences, registration, abstract submittal, on line publishing . . . faster speed, better communication and notification, more on-line computing, virtual offices . . . .

Woo believes that "ways will be found to provide 'for fee' access to the full text of journal articles, standards, and other documents important to our field." She also sees online "distance" training becoming more popular because of time and location constraints inherent in having on-site training seminars.

## AN IMPORTANT NOTE ON ONLINE RESOURCES

The Internet in general, and the World Wide Web in particular, is in a constant state of flux. New resources are constantly coming online and old resources disappear. The resources included in this guide were chosen for their authority and for their relative permanence. Every effort has been made to ensure that the links included in this appendix are accurate but, in time, it is likely that some of these URLs will change. The most current version of this guide can be found online at:

*http://www.radscice.com/dowd.html.*

## ADVISORY BODIES

### International

International Commission on Radiological Protection

*http://www.who.ch/programmes/ina/ngo/ngo-44.htm*
The mission of the ICRP is to ensure progress in the whole field of radiation protection by publishing recommendations on radiation safety standards, mainly dealing with basic principles of radiation protection (3). This page, maintained by the World Health Organization, provides information on the organization and mission of the ICRP.

### United States

National Council on Radiation Protection and Measurement

*http://www.ncrp.com/*
The NCRP seeks to formulate and widely disseminate information, guidance, and recommendations on radiation protection and measurements that represent the consensus of leading scientific thinking. The Council's

mission also encompasses the responsibility to facilitate and stimulate cooperation among organizations concerned with the scientific and related aspects of radiation protection and measurements (4). The site also contains information on ordering NCRP reports.

## COMPREHENSIVE SITES

RadEFX Radiation Health Effects Research Resource

*http://radefx.bcm.tmc.edu/default.htm*
This comprehensive site, maintained by the Baylor College of Medicine, is home to several valuable resources. RadEFX also maintains a substantial links section. Other key sections include:
Ionizing Radiation Health Effects Forum
*http://radefx.med.bcm.tmc.edu/ionizing/ionizing.htm*
USA–Canada Chernobyl Immigrant Registry
*http://radefx.bcm.tmc.edu/usacir/bcm-cr.htm*
Research Software Forum
*http://radefx.bcm.tmc.edu/statsoft/statsoft.htm*

Radiation and Health Physics Home Page
*http://www.sph.umich.edu/group/eih/UMSCHPS/*
This site, maintained by the University of Michigan Student Chapter of the Health Physics Society, is far and away the most comprehensive radiation protection resource on the World Wide Web. Key sections include:
Downloadable Files for Training
*http://www.sph.umich.edu/group/eih/UMSCHPS/Files/download.htm*
History of Radiation Protection
*http://www.sph.umich.edu/group/eih/UMSCHPS/hist.htm*
Natural Radioactivity
*http://www.sph.umich.edu/group/eih/UMSCHPS/natural.htm*
Radiation and Radioactive Material Specific Information
*http://www.sph.umich.edu/group/eih/UMSCHPS/Source.htm*
Radiation and Radioactivity
*http://www.sph.umich.edu/group/eih/UMSCHPS/cover.htm*
Radiation and Risk
*http://www.sph.umich.edu/group/eih/UMSCHPS/risk.htm*

Radiation and Us
  *http://www.sph.umich.edu/group/eih/ UMSCHPS/radrus.htm*
U.S. State Radiation Programs
  *http://www.sph.umich.edu/group/eih/ UMSCHPS/states.htm*
What You Need to Know about Radiation
  *http://www.sph.umich.edu/group/eih/ UMSCHPS/lst.htm*

Radiation Effects Research Foundation
  *http://www.rerf.or.jp/eigo/experhp/rerfhome.htm*
  RERF conducts research and studies—for peaceful purposes—on the effects of radiation exposure on humans with a view toward contributing to the maintenance of the health and welfare of atomic-bomb survivors and to the enhancement of the health of all people (5). This is an excellent comprehensive site and the best source for information and data on atomic bomb survivors but very slow connections from the United States.

## DOSIMETRY

Mucal on the Web
  *http://www.csrri.iit.edu/mucal.html*
  This is a WWW interface to a program used to calculate x-ray absorption coefficients.

Radiation Internal Dose Information Center
  *http://www.orau.gov/ehsd/ridic.htm*
  The RIDIC provides physicians, as well as other nuclear medicine professionals, regulators, manufacturers, and nuclear pharmacy workers with the most up-to-date information on internal dose estimates and internal dosimetry techniques applied to the practice of nuclear medicine. RIDIC, a program at the Oak Ridge Institute for Science and Education (ORISE), also provides information on internal dosimetry in other applications, such as the nuclear fuel cycle (6).

X-Ray Absorption Coefficients of the Elements
  *http://www1.usa1.com/~aic/2121.html*
  Maintained by AIC Software, Inc.

## GENERAL INFORMATION

Ask Your Medical Physicist
  *http://www.medphysics.wisc.edu/~empw/ask1.html*

University of Wisconsin's Electronic Medical Physics World's Q&A on medical physics issues organized by category.

Natural Radioactivity
  *http://www.sph.umich.edu/group/eih/ UMSCHPS/natural.htm*
  This paper on natural radioactivity was developed by the University of Michigan's Student Chapter of the Health Physics Society.

Radiation and Radioactivity
  *http://www.sph.umich.edu/group/eih/ UMSCHPS/cover.htm*
  This self-paced lesson on the basics of radiation and radioactivity was developed by the University of Michigan's Student Chapter of the Health Physics Society.

Radiation and Risk
  *http://www.sph.umich.edu/group/eih/ UMSCHPS/risk.htm*
  Short essays, information, and links from the University of Michigan's Student Chapter of the Health Physics Society.

Radiation and Us
  *http://www.sph.umich.edu/group/eih/ UMSCHPS/radrus.htm*
  Short essays, information, and links from the University of Michigan's Student Chapter of the Health Physics Society.

Radiation and Life
  *http://www.uic.com.au/ral.htm*
  Eric J Hall, Professor of Radiology, College of Physicians and Surgeons, Columbia University, New York. This page is maintained by the Uranium Information Center in Australia.

What You Need to Know about Radiation
  *http://www.sph.umich.edu/group/eih/ UMSCHPS/lst.htm*
  Written by Lauriston S. Taylor for the University of Michigan's Student Chapter of the Health Physics Society.

## HEALTH EFFECTS

### Acute Radiation Syndromes

Health Effects of Acute Radiation Exposure
  *http://radefx.bcm.tmc.edu/ionizing/subject/risk/ acute.htm*
  Some useful data on health effects of acute

radiation exposure from RadEFX at Baylor College of Medicine.

Patient Treatment and Management for Acute Radiation Syndromes
*http://radefx.bcm.tmc.edu/ionizing/subject/risk/ patient.htm*
Minimal, supportive and intensive treatment regimens from RadEFX at Baylor College of Medicine.

Radiation Effects Overview
*http://www.rerf.or.jp/eigo/radefx/toc.htm*
Radiation Effects Research Foundation. Excellent site but very slow connections from the United States.

Ten Years after Chernobyl: What Do We Really Know?
*http://www.iaea.or.at/worldatom/inforesource/ other/chernoten/index.html*
Comprehensive overview of impact and health effects of the Chernobyl accident maintained by the International Atomic Energy Agency.

## Fluoroscopy

Radiation Injuries
*http://www.fda.gov/cdrh/radinj.html*
Advisories on radiation injuries from the Center for Devices and Radiological Health of the U.S. Food and Drug Administration.

Avoidance of Serious X-Ray-Induced Skin Injuries to Patients during Fluoroscopically Guided Procedures
*http://www.fda.gov/cdrh/fluor.html*
Text of a September 30, 1994, FDA Public Health Advisory.

Radiation-Induced Skin Injuries from Fluoroscopy
*http://www.fda.gov/cdrh/rsnaii.html*
Thomas B. Shope, Ph.D., Office of Science and Technology, Center for Devices and Radiological Health, Food and Drug Administration. Presented at the 81st Scientific Assembly and Annual Meeting of the Radiological Society of North America in 1995.

## Low-Level Exposure

Radiation Effects Overview
*http://www.rerf.or.jp/eigo/radefx/toc.htm*

Radiation Effects Research Foundation. Excellent site but very slow connections from the United States.

Ten Years after Chernobyl: What Do We Really Know?
*http://www.iaea.or.at/worldatom/inforesource/ other/chernoten/index.html*
Comprehensive overview of impact and health effects of the Chernobyl accident maintained by the International Atomic Energy Agency.

## Other Health Effects Information

Estimating Radiogenic Cancer Risks
*http://www.epa.gov/radiation/docs/rad_risk.pdf*
U.S. Environmental Protection Agency. (PDF Format)

RadEFX Ionizing Radiation Health Effects Forum
*http://radefx.med.bcm.tmc.edu/ionizing/ ionizing.htm*

Radiation and Health Physics Home Page
*http://www.sph.umich.edu/group/eih/ UMSCHPS/*
Maintained by the University of Michigan Student Chapter of the Health Physics Society.

Radiation and Risk
*http://www.sph.umich.edu/group/eih/ UMSCHPS/risk.htm*
Short essays, information, and links from the University of Michigan Student Chapter of the Health Physics Society.

Ask Your Medical Physicist
*http://www.medphysics.wisc.edu/~empw/ ask1.html*
University of Wisconsin's Electronic Medical Physics World's Q&A on medical physics issues by category.

## History

History of Radiation Protection
*http://www.sph.umich.edu/group/eih/ UMSCHPS/hist.htm*
The University of Michigan Student Chapter of the Health Physics Society's links to articles and sites on the history of radiation protection.

## Human Radiation Experiments

DOE Openness: Human Radiation Experiments
*http://www.ohre.doe.gov/*
The U.S. Department of Energy's Office of Human Radiation Experiments.

## POPULATION REGISTRIES AND DATABASES

### Chernobyl

Project Polyn
*http://polyn.net.kiae.su/polyn/manifest.html*
Kurchatov Institute's Project Polyn.

USA–Canada Chernobyl Immigrant Registry
*http://radefx.bcm.tmc.edu/usacir/bcm-cr.htm*
The USA–Canada Chernobyl Immigrant Registry maintained by the Baylor College of Medicine.

### Hiroshima/Nagasaki

Radiation Effects Research Foundation
*http://www.rerf.or.jp/eigo/experhp/rerfhome.htm*
Excellent site but very slow connections from the United States.

### United States

Comprehensive Epidemiologic Data Resource WWW Home Page
*http://cedr.lbl.gov/CEDRhomepage.html*
Most of the data are from epidemiologic studies conducted as part of the DOE Worker Health and Mortality Study.

## PROFESSIONAL ORGANIZATIONS

American Academy of Health Physics
*http://phantom.ehs.uiuc.edu/~aahp/*

American Association of Physicists in Medicine
*http://www.aapm.org/*

American Society of Radiologic Technologists
*http://www.asrt.org/*

Canadian Radiation Protection Association
*http://www.safety.ubc.ca/crpa*

European Nuclear Society
*http://www.aey.ch/ens/*

Health Physics Society
*http://www2.hps.org/hps/*

International Radiation Protection Association
*http://www.tue.nl/sbd/irpa/irpahome.htm*

International Society of Radiographers and Radiological Technologists
*http://users.aol.com/isrrt/isrrt.html*

National Registry of Radiation Protection Technologists
*http://www.nrrpt.org/*

Society of Nuclear Medicine
*http://www.snm.org/*

The American Nuclear Society
*http://www.ans.org/*

The Radiological Society of North America
*http://www.rsna.org/*

## PUBLICATIONS

### Journals

Radiation Research
*http://www.cjp.com/radres*
The official journal of the Radiation Research Society.

### Papers, Articles, and Reports

Ionizing Radiation: Defining a Research Agenda
*http://radefx.med.bcm.tmc.edu/ionizing/publications/niehsrpt.txt*
Workshop on Priorities in Health Effects Research—Ionizing Radiation: Defining a Research Agenda, NIEHS (Arthur Upton, Chair).

Natural Radioactivity
*http://www.sph.umich.edu/group/eih/UMSCHPS/natural.htm*
This paper on natural radioactivity was developed by the University of Michigan's Student Chapter of the Health Physics Society.

Radiation and the Environment: Assessing Effects on Plants and Animals
*http://www.iaea.or.at/worldatom/inforesource/bulletin/bull391/linsley.html*

IAEA Bulletin 39/1: Radiation and the Environment: Assessing Effects on Plants and Animals.

Radiation-Induced Skin Injuries from Fluoroscopy
*http://www.fda.gov/cdrh/rsnaii.html*
Thomas B. Shope, Ph.D., Office of Science and Technology, Center for Devices and Radiological Health, Food and Drug Administration. Presented at the 81st Scientific Assembly and Annual Meeting of the Radiological Society of North America in 1995.

Radiation Protection Today and Tomorrow
*http://www.nea.fr/html/rp/rp.html*
An assessment of the present status and future perspectives of radiation protection from the NEA.

Radiation risk evaluation
*http://minf.vub.ac.be/~ifmbe/mpbe/no7/radrisk.html*
Fred A. Mettler, Jr., M.D., University of New Mexico, Department of Radiology. Read at the Symposium: "Health Effects of Ionising Radiation" of the Polish Nuclear Medicine Society and the IAEA, October 22–24, 1992.

What You Need to Know about Radiation
*http://www.sph.umich.edu/group/eih/UMSCHPS/lst.htm*
Written by Lauriston S. Taylor for the University of Michigan's Student Chapter of the Health Physics Society.

## Radiation Safety Training Guides

Caltech Radiation Safety Training and Reference Manual
*http://www.cco.caltech.edu/~safety/trm.html*

Downloadable Files for Training from the University of Michigan's Student Chapter of the Health Physics Society
*http://www.sph.umich.edu/group/eih/UMSCHPS/Files/download.htm*

Radiation and Radioactivity
*http://www.sph.umich.edu/group/eih/UMSCHPS/cover.htm*
A self-paced lesson on the basics of radiation and radioactivity developed by the University of Michigan's Student Chapter of the Health Physics Society.

University of Chicago Radiation Safety Training Tutorial
*http://radiant.uchicago.edu/uofcinfo/traini~1/ttutor~1.htm*

Radiological Control Technician (RCT) Academic Lessons from the U.S. Department of Energy
*http://cted.inel.gov/cted/eh_mat.html*

University of Pennsylvania RSO Training Document
*http://www.rso.upenn.edu/htmls/train0(A).html*

## REGULATIONS AND GUIDELINES: UNITED STATES

10 CFR 20
*http://www.saic.com/home/nrc_rad/cfr20.htm*
The copy of 10 CFR 20 that is referenced on this site represents a copy that was obtained on January 1, 1995. This document may not reflect revisions and addenda that have been made since that time.

Public Health Advisory: Avoidance of Serious X-Ray-Induced Skin Injuries to Patients During Fluoroscopically Guided Procedures
*http://www.fda.gov/cdrh/fluor.html*

Department of Energy (DOE) Radiological Control Manual
*http://nattie.eh.doe.gov/docs/rcm/rcm.html*

NRC Regulatory Guides
*http://www.saic.com/home/nrc_rad/reg_gds.htm*

Radiation Internal Dose Information Center
*http://www.orau.gov/ehsd/ridic.htm*

Recording Information in the Patient's Medical Record that Identifies the Potential for Serious X-Ray-Induced Skin Injuries Following Fluoroscopically Guided Procedures
*http://www.fda.gov/cdrh/xrayinj.html*
CDRH Information Paper.

## REGULATORY BODIES

### Canada

Atomic Energy Control Board
*http://www.gc.ca/aecb/index.htm*
Canada's nuclear regulatory authority.

## International

International Atomic Energy Agency
*http://www.iaea.or.at/*

World Health Organization
*http://www.who.ch/*

## United Kingdom

U.K. National Radiation Protection Board
*http://www.nrpb.org.uk/*

## United States

### U.S. Government Agencies

Department of Energy Home Page
*http://www.doe.gov/*
The DOE provides regulations for DOE National Labs and test facilities. Their portion of the CFRs is 10 CFR parts 100–1000.

Environmental Protection Agency
*http://www.epa.gov*
EPA's portion of the CFRs for radiation protection can be found under 40 CFR parts 61, 141, 190, 192, 220–229, 440.

Food and Drug Administration Home Page
*http://www.fda.gov/*
The FDA's portion of the CFRs for radiation protection can be found under 21 CFR 1000.

FDA Center for Devices and Radiological Health
*http://www.fda.gov/cdrh/cdrhhome.html*

Occupational Safety and Health Administration Home Page
*http://www.osha.gov/*
OSHA's portion of the CFRs for radiation protection can be found under 29 CFR parts 1910, 1926.

U.S. Nuclear Regulatory Commission
*http://www.nrc.gov/*
The NRC provides regulations for NRC license holders, including power generation facilities, hospitals and universities. Their portion of the CFRs is 10 CFR parts 1–99.

NRC-Office of State Programs
*http://www.hsrd.ornl.gov/nrc/home.html*

### U.S. States

Colorado Laboratory and Radiation Services Division
*http://www.cdphe.state.co.us/lr/lrhom.htm*

Georgia Department of Natural Resources Environmental Protection Division, Radiation Control in Georgia
*http://www.ganet.org/dnr/environ/branches/progcoord/rad_prog.html*

Idaho
*http://www.idwr.state.id.us/apa/idapa16/0109.htm*

Illinois Department of Nuclear Safety (IDNS)
*http://www.state.il.us/idns/*

Indiana Code Title 16, Article 41, Chapter 35. Radiation: Radiation Control
*http://www.law.indiana.edu/codes/in/16/ch-16-41-35.html*

Louisiana DEQ—Office of Air Quality and Radiation Protection
*http://www.deq.state.la.us/oarp/oarp.htm*

Maine Radiation Control Program
*http://www.state.me.us/dhs/eng/rad/rad.htm*

Nevada—Health Division—BHPS: Radiological Health
*http://www.state.nv.us/health/bhps/rad.htm*

New Jersey Radiation Protection Home Page
*http://www.state.nj.us/dep/rpp/rppindex.htm*

NRC—Office of State Programs
*http://www.hsrd.ornl.gov/nrc/home.html*

Oregon Office of Energy Nuclear Safety
*http://www.cbs.state.or.us/external/ooe/nucsafe/nucsafe.htm*

Pennsylvania Bureau of Radiation Protection
*http://www.dep.state.pa.us/dep/deputate/airwaste/rp/rp.htm*

South Carolina Department of Health and Environmental Control—Radiological Health
*http://www.state.sc.us/dhec/hrrh.htm*

Texas Department of Health, Bureau of Radiation Control
*http://www.tdh.state.tx.us/ech/rad/pages/brc.htm*

Utah Division of Radiation Control
*http://www.eq.state.ut.us/eqrad/drc_hmpg.htm*

Washington Division of Radiation Protection
*http://198.187.0.42:80/ehp/rp/*

## RESEARCH

### Chernobyl Related

International Consortium for Research on the Health Effects of Radiation
*http://radefx.bcm.tmc.edu/icrher/icrher.htm*

Project Polyn
*http://polyn.net.kiae.su/polyn/manifest.html*
Kurchatov Institute's Project Polyn.

Ten Years after Chernobyl: What Do We Really Know?
*http://www.iaea.or.at/worldatom/inforesource/other/chernoten/index.html*
Comprehensive overview of impact and health effects of the Chernobyl accident maintained by the International Atomic Energy Agency.

Ukrainian American Chernobyl Ocular Study at Columbia University
*http://cpmcnet.columbia.edu/dept/eye/rad/uacos.html*

### Hiroshima/Nagasaki

Radiation Effects Research Foundation
*http://www.rerf.or.jp/eigo/experhp/rerfhome.htm*
Far and away the best source for research and information related to atomic bomb survivors. Very slow connection with the United States.

### Other Sites with Research Information

Comprehensive Epidemiologic Data Resource WWW Home Page
*http://cedr.lbl.gov/CEDRhomepage.html*
Most of the data are from epidemiologic studies conducted as part of the DOE Worker Health and Mortality Study.

RadEFX Radiation Health Effects Research Resource
*http://radefx.bcm.tmc.edu/default.htm*
This comprehensive site maintained by the Baylor College of Medicine is home to several valuable research resources.

Radiation and Health Physics Home Page
*http://www.sph.umich.edu/group/eih/UMSCHPS/*
This site maintained by the University of Michigan Student Chapter of the Health Physics Society is far and away the most comprehensive radiation protection resource on the World Wide Web.

## E-MAIL DISCUSSION GROUPS

The following e-mail discussion groups frequently host discussions related to radiation protection of interest to radiologic sciences professionals. To subscribe to one of these lists, send an e-mail to the subscription address with the message: SUBSCRIBE "listname" "your name." "Listname" is the list you want to subscribe to and "your name" is your name. When your request is received you will be added to the list and you will be sent instructions on how to use the list. In general, it is considered good etiquette to spend the first week or so "lurking," which simply means silently following the discussion to pick up the unwritten rules and customs of the group.

### Mail Server Description and Subscription E-Mail Address

Airnews: Australian Institute of Radiography listserver.
*LISTSERV@giant.bnc.com.au*

BNCT Discussion list: Forum to exchange ideas on Boron Neutron Capture Therapy.
*LISTSERV@mitvma.mit.edu*

DOSE-NET: Provides services related to internal dosimetry.
*mailserv@orau.gov*

MEDPHYS: Forum for professionals interested in matters related to radiation therapy.
*LISTSERV@cwis-20.wayne.edu*

NUCMED: Nuclear medicine forum to exchange ideas, reports of meetings, reviews of books, etc.
*LISTSERV@largnet.uwo.ca*

PET mail: Provides information of interest to the PET imaging community.
*pet_mail-request@pet.bgsm.edu*

Radiobiology: Forum for discussion on animal, cellular, or molecular radiobiology or clinical radiotherapy.
*mailbase@mailbase.ac.uk*

RADAHRA: American Healthcare Radiology Administrators listserver.
*majordomo@majordomo.microserve.net*

RADSAFE: Forum for professionals interested in matters related to Radiation Protection.
*LISTSERV@romulus.ehs.uiuc.edu*

RADSCI-L mailing list: Forum to explore topics of all concerns related to all radiological sciences.
*majordomo@listmail.western.tec.wi.us*

## REFERENCES

1. Busy, Bruce. July 20, 1997. Personal e-mail.
2. Woo, Melissa. July 22, 1997. Personal e-mail.
3. International Commission on Radiological Protection. January 12, 1996. Available online. *http://www.who.ch/programmes/ina/ngo/ngo-44.htm*
4. National Council on Radiation Protection and Measurement. May 19, 1997. Available online. *http://www.ncrp.com/goals.html*
5. Radiation Effects Research Foundation. June 24, 1997. Available online. *http://wwwo.who.ch/programmes/ina/ngo/ngo-44.htm*
6. Radiation Internal Dose Information Center. May 2, 1996. Available online. *http://\www.orau.gov/ehsd/ridicint.htm*

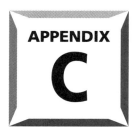

# APPENDIX C

# Greek Alphabet

| | | |
|---|---|---|
| A | α | alpha |
| B | β | beta |
| Γ | γ | gamma |
| Δ | δ | delta |
| E | ε | epsilon |
| Z | ζ | zeta |
| H | η | eta |
| Θ | θ | theta |
| I | ι | iota |
| K | κ | kappa |
| Λ | λ | lambda |
| M | μ | mu |
| N | ν | nu |
| Ξ | ξ | xi |
| O | ο | omicron |
| Π | π | pi |
| P | ρ | rho |
| Σ | σ | sigma |
| T | τ | tau |
| Y | υ | upsilon |
| Φ | φ | phi |
| X | χ | chi |
| Ψ | ψ | psi |
| Ω | ω | omega |

# Bibliography

AAPM Monograph No. 23. Frey GD, Sprawls PS (eds): *The Expanding Role of Medical Physics in Diagnostic Imaging.* Proceedings of the 1997 Summer School. Advanced Medical Publishing Inc., 1997.

AAPM Report No. 38: *The Role of a Physicist in Radiation Oncology.* 1993.

AAPM Report No. 42: *The Role of the Clinical Medical Physicist in Diagnostic Radiology.* 1994.

AAPM Report No. 53: *Radiation Information for Hospital Personnel.* 1995.

Abramson N: Radiation therapy: What is it? *South Med J* 67:1333–1336, 1974.

Adler AM, Carlton RR, Wold B. An analysis of radiographic repeat rate data. *Radiol Technol* 63(5): 308–314, 1992.

Albert RW, et al: Follow-up study of patients treated by x-ray epilation for tinea capitis. *Arch Environ Health* 17:899, 1968.

American Society of Radiologic Technologists Code of Ethics. ASRT, 15,000 Central Avenue SE, Albuquerque, NM 87123.

Ancel P, Vitemberger P: Sur la radiosensibilité cellulaire. *C R Soc Biol* 92:517, 1925.

Arena V: *Ionizing Radiations and Life.* St Louis, CV Mosby, 1971.

Bacq AM, Alexander P: *Fundamentals of Radiobiology,* 2nd ed. New York, Pergamon Press, 1961.

Baker M, Dalrymple GV: Radiation and the fetus. *In* Hendee WR (ed): *Health Effects of Low-Level Radiation.* Norwalk, CT, Appleton-Century-Crofts, 1984.

Barcham N, Egan I, Dowd SB: Gonadal protection methods in neonatal chest radiography. *Radiol Technol* 69(2):157–161, 1997.

Barnett M, Eccleston R: *Radiation Protection During Medical X-Ray Examinations.* Rockville, MD, U.S. Department of Health, Education, and Welfare, 1976.

Beck TJ, Gayler B: Image quality and radiation levels in videofluoroscopy for swallowing studies: A review. *Dysphagia* 5:118–128, 1990.

*BEIR III: The Effects on Populations of Exposure to Low Levels of Ionizing Radiation.* Washington, DC, National Academy Press, 1980.

*BEIR IV: Health Risks of Radon and Other Internally Deposited Alpha Emitters.* Washington, DC, National Academy Press, 1988.

*BEIR V: Health Effects of Exposure to Low Levels of Ionizing Radiation: Report of Advisory Committee on the Biological Effects of Ionizing Radiation.* National Academy of Sciences, National Research Council, Washington, DC, 1990.

Berdjis CC: *Pathology of Irradiation.* Baltimore, Williams & Wilkins, 1971.

Bergonie J, Tribondeau L: De quelques résultats de la radiothérapie et essai de fixation d'une technique rationelle. *C R Acad Sci* (Paris) 143:983, 1906.

Black WC, Nease RF, Tosteson AN: Perceptions of breast cancer risk and screening effectiveness in women younger than 50 years of age. *J Nat Cancer Inst* 87:720–731, 1995.

Boice JD, Mandel JS, Doody MM, et al: A health study of radiologic technologists. *Cancer* 69: 586–597, 1992.

Boice JD Jr, Land CE, Shore RE, et al: Risk of breast cancer following low dose exposure. *Radiology* 131:589–597, 1979.

Boice JD, Monson RR: X-ray exposure and breast cancer. *Am J Epidemiol* 104:349–350, 1976.

Bonte RJ: Chernobyl retrospective. *Semin Nucl Med* 18:16–24, 1988.

Boone JM, Levin DC: Radiation exposure to angiographers under different fluoroscopic imaging conditions. *Radiology* 180:861–865, 1991.

Brown MR, Greenberg LH: Fluoroscopic measurement in Saskatchewan. *J Can Assoc Radiol* 32:118, 1981.

Burks J, Griffith P, McCormick K, et al: Radiation exposure to nursing personnel from patients receiving diagnostic radionuclides. *Heart Lung* 11:217–220, 1982.

Burns C. Using computed digital radiography effectively. *Semin Radiol Technol* 1(1):24–36, 1993.

Burns CB, Turner GW: The effect of decreased developer activity on patient exposure. *Radiol Technol* 54:391–392, 1983.

Bushong, S. *Radiologic Science for Technologists. Physics, Biology, and Protection*, 6th ed. St. Louis: Mosby Yearbook, 1997.

Bushong SC: Radiation protection. *In* Ballinger, PW (ed): *Merrill's Atlas of Radiographic Positions and Radiologic Procedures*, 5th ed. St Louis, CV Mosby, 1982.

Bushong SC: Policies for managing the pregnant employee. *Radiol Manage* 6(3):2–7, 1984.

Bushong SC: Quality assurance in mammography. Presented at the 1992 Annual Meeting of the Alabama State Society of Radiologic Technologists, Gulf Shores, AL.

Butler PF, Thomas AW, Thompson WE, et al: Simple methods to reduce patient exposure during scoliosis radiography. *Radiol Technol* 57:411–417, 1986.

Cameron J: Are we exaggerating fear? *Radiol Technol* 62:336, 1991.

Cancer induction and dose response models. *In* Mettler FA, Mosely RD (eds): *Medical Effects of Ionizing Radiation*. Orlando, Grune & Stratton, 1985, pp 74–92.

Caprio ML: The pregnant x-ray tech: Providing adequate radiation protection for the fetus. *Radiol Technol* 52:161, 1980.

Carey JE, Swanson DP: Thyroid contamination from airborne I-131. *J Nucl Med* 20:362, 1979.

Carlton RR, Adler AM: *Principles of Radiographic Imaging: An Art and a Science*, 2nd ed. Albany, Delmar, 1996.

Carroll QB: *Fuchs's Principles of Radiographic Exposure, Processing, and Quality Control*, 3rd ed. Springfield, IL, Charles C Thomas, 1985.

Carson V, Arnold E: *Mental Health Nursing*. Philadelphia, WB Saunders, 1996.

Casarett AP: *Radiation Biology*. Englewood Cliffs, NJ, Prentice-Hall, 1968.

Chu RYL, Parry C, Eaton BG. Entrance skin exposure in PA chest radiography. *Radiol Technol* 69(3):251–254, 1998.

Clarke MT, Galie E. Radionuclide therapy of osseous metastatic disease. *J Nucl Med Technol* 21:3–6, 1993.

Code of Ethics: *Can J Med Rad Technol* 22:6, 1991.

Cohen B: The cancer risk from low-level radiation, *Health Phys* 39:659–678, 1980.

Cohen N: Quality assurance as an optimizing procedure in diagnostic radiology. *Br J Radiol* 18, 134, 1985.

Coia LR, Moylan DJ: *Introduction to Clinical Radiation Oncology*. 2nd ed. Madison, WI, Medical Physics Publishing, 493–511, 1994.

Conard RA, et al: Thyroid nodules as a late sequela of radioactive fallout in a Marshall Island population exposed in 1954. *N Engl J Med* 274:1391, 1966.

Conard RA, et al: Thyroid neoplasia as late effect of exposure to radioactive iodine in fallout. *JAMA* 214:316, 1970.

Conard RA, Hicking A: Medical findings in Marshallese people exposed to fallout radiation: Results from a ten-year study. *JAMA* 192:457, 1965.

Connett R: A Survey into Radiation Dose Received by Staff Working in Angiography Suites. London, HDCR, Module F Thesis, 1987.

Conway BJ, McCrohan JL, Antosen RG, Rueter FG, Slayton RJ, Suleiman OH: Average radiation dose in standard CT examinations of the head: Results of the 1990 NEXT survey. *Radiology* 184(1):135–40, 1992.

Costanza ME: Clinical breast examination, breast self-examination: What is the evidence for utility in screening for breast cancer? *Women's Health Issues* 2(4):220–235, 1992.

Costanza ME, Stoddard A, Gaw VP, et al: The risk factors of age and family history and their relationship to screening mammography utilization. *J Am Geriatr Soc* 40:774–778, 1992.

Court-Brown WM, Doll R: Expectation of life and mortality from cancer among British radiologists. *Br Med J* 2:181, 1958.

Court-Brown WM, Doll R: Mortality from cancer and other causes after radiotherapy for ankylosing spondylitis. *Br Med J* 2:1327, 1965.

Court-Brown WM, et al: The incidence of leukaemia after the exposure to diagnostic radiation in utero. *Br Med J* 2:1599, 1960.

Cousin AJ, Lawdahl RB, Charaborty DP, et al: The case for radioprotective eyewear/facewear: Practical implications and suggestions. *Invest Radiol* 22:688–692, 1987.

Crawford ES, Quain BC, Zaken AM: Air and surface contamination resulting from lung ventilation aerosol procedures. *J Nucl Med Technol* 20:151–154, 1992.

Cullinan AM: *Producing Quality Radiographs*. Philadelphia, JB Lippincott, 1987.

Curry TS, Dowdey JE, Murry RC: *Christensen's Physics of Diagnostic Radiology*, 3rd ed. Philadelphia, Lea & Febiger, 1990.

Cusworth RJ: *Quality Assurance in Diagnostic Radiology: An Eight-Step Methodology*. Denver, Multi-Media Publishing, 1983.

Davidhizar RE, Dowd SB: Fear in the patient with undiagnosed symptoms. *J Nucl Med Technol* 24(4):325–328, 1996.

Davidhizar RE, Dowd SB: Should technologists tell everything they know? *Radiol Manage* 19:3, 1997.

Dekaban AS: Abnormalities in children exposed to x-radiation during various stages of gestation: Tentative timetable of radiation injury to the human fetus. *J Nucl Med* 9:471, 1968.

Dendy PP, Heaton B: *Physics for Radiologists*. Chicago, Year Book Medical Publishers, 1987.

DeVos D: *Basic Principles of Radiographic Exposure*. Philadelphia, Lea & Febiger, 1990.

Dickinson CZ, Hendrix NS. Strontium-89 therapy in painful bony metastases. *J Nucl Med Technol* 21:133–137, 1993.

Donohue DP: *An Analysis of Radiographic Quality*. Baltimore, University Park Press, 1980.

Dowd SB: A continuum for evaluating risks and benefits of ionizing radiation. *Appl Radiol* 13:81–82, 1984.

Dowd SB: The basics of radiation protection for hospital workers. *Hosp Topics* 69(4):31, 1991.

Dowd SB: *Informed Consent*. Albuquerque, NM: American Society of Radiologic Technologists, 1994a. (Homestudy).

Dowd SB: The practice of radiobiology in the radiologic sciences. *Radiol Technol* 66(1):25–33, 1994b.

Dowd SB: *Teaching in the Health-Related Professions*. Chapel Hill, NC, Carolina Academic Press, 1996.

Dowd SB, Steves AM: *Patient Education*. Albuquerque, NM, American Society of Radiologic Technologists, 1997. (Homestudy).

Dowd SB, Wilson B: Informed patient consent: A historical perspective. *Radiol Technol* 67(2):119–124, 1995.

Drafke M: *Trauma and Mobile Radiography*. Philadelphia, FA Davis, 1990.

Dreyer NA, Loughlin JE, Friedlander ER, et al: Choosing populations to study the health effects of low-dose ionizing radiation. *Am J Public Health* 71:1247–1252, 1981.

Early PJ, Sodee DB: *Principles and Practice of Nuclear Medicine*. St Louis, Mosby, 1985, pp 88–112, 471–538.

*Essentials and Guidelines of an Accredited Program for the Radiographer*. Chicago, Joint Review Committee on Education in Radiologic Technology, 1990.

Fabrikant JI: Radiation and health. *West J Med* 138:387–390, 1983.

Fischoff B, et al: How safe is safe enough? A psychometric study of attitudes towards technological risks and benefits. *Pol Sci* 9:127, 1978.

Foley JJ: Radiation and its genetic sequelae. *Radiol Technol* 54:198–205, 1983.

Food and Drug Administration: *Code of Federal Regulations, 21 CFR 1020.32*. Washington, DC, U.S. Government Printing Office, 1997.

Ford DD, et al: Fetal exposure to diagnostic x-rays and leukemia and other malignant disease in childhood. *J Natl Cancer Inst* 22:1093, 1959.

Frank E, Stears J, Gray J, et al: Use of the PA projection: A method of reducing x-ray exposure to specific radiosensitive organs. *Radiol Technol* 54:343–347, 1983.

Frankel R: *Radiation Protection for Radiologic Technologists*. New York, McGraw-Hill, 1975.

Franz KH: Radiation protection in radiologic technology: Apathy versus active involvement. *Radiol Technol* 54:119–122, 1982.

Friedell HI. Radiation protection—Concepts and trade-offs. *In Perception of risk*. Proceedings of the National Council on Radiation Protection and Measurements (NCRP). Washington, DC, 1980.

Frigerioi NA, Stowe RS: Carcinogenic and genetic hazard from background radiation. *In Biological and Environmental Effects of Low-Level Radiation*, vol 2. Vienna, IAEA, 1976, pp 385–393.

Gaulden ME, Murry RC: Medical radiation and possible adverse effects on the human embryo. *In* Meyn RE, Withers R (eds): *Radiation Biology in Cancer Research*. New York, Raven Press, 1980.

Geise RA, Hunter DW: Personnel exposure during fluoroscopy. *Postgrad Radiol* 8:557, 1988.

Giomuso CA, Early PJ: Radiation health safety. *In* Early PJ, Sodee DB: *Principles and Practice of Nuclear Medicine*. St Louis, Mosby, 1985, pp 471–517.

Glaze S, LeBlanc AD, Bushong SC: Defects in new protective aprons. *Radiology* 152:217, 1984.

Goldsmith JR: Incorporation of epidemiological findings into radiation protection standards. *Public Health Rev* 19:19–34, 1991.

Gray JE, Swee RG: The elimination of grids during intensified fluoroscopy and photofluoro spot imaging. *Radiology* 144:426–429, 1982.

Griem ML, et al: Analysis of the morbidity and mortality of children irradiated in fetal life. *Radiology* 88:347, 1967.

Hackett MT, Perdikaris N, Ruffin TT. Additional radiation safety concerns involving sodium iodide-131 capsules. *J Nucl Med Technol* 23:289–290, 1995.

Hale J, Thomas JW: Radiation risks for patients having x-rays. *Nurse Pract* 10:16–27, 1985.

Hall EJ: *Radiobiology for the Radiologist*, 4th ed. Philadelphia, JB Lippincott, 1993.

Hammer-Jacobsen E: Therapeutic abortion on account of x-ray examination during pregnancy. *Dan Med Bull* 6:113, 1959.

Hassey K: Care of patients with radioactive implants. *In* Professional Education Publication. Atlanta, American Cancer Society, 1988.

Hatfield S: Act encourages RTs to report faulty equipment. *Advance* 6(28):7, 1993.

Hendee WR: Real and perceived risks of medical radiation exposure. *West J Med* 138:380–386, 1983.

Hendee WR: Estimation of radiation risks: BEIR V and its significance for medicine. *JAMA* 268:620–624, 1992.

Hendee WR, Ritenour R: *Medical Imaging Physics,* 3rd ed. St Louis, Mosby Yearbook, 1993.

High Background Radiation Research Group, China: Health survey in high background radiation areas in China. *Science* 209:877–880, 1980.

Hiss S: *Understanding Radiography,* 3rd ed. Springfield, IL, Charles C Thomas, 1993.

Holleb AI, Fink DJ, Murphy GP (eds): *American Cancer Society Textbook of Clinical Oncology.* Atlanta, American Cancer Society, 1991.

Holmes P: Off beam. *Nurs Times* 87(4):20, 1991.

Horiot JC: What has radiation biology contributed to the evolution of radiotherapy? *Eur J Cancer* 27:399–402, 1991.

Howard BY: Safe handling of radioiodinated solutions. *J Nucl Med Technol* 4:28–30, 1976.

Huda W, Gordon K, Greenberg ID: Diagnostic thyroid and corresponding radiation doses in Manitoba: 1981–1985. *Health Phys* 59:287–293, 1990.

Indiana State Board of Health. *Low Dosage Medical Roentgenography,* Indianapolis, IN, 1964.

International Commission on Radiological Protection (ICRP). (1982). *Protection of the Patient in Diagnostic Radiology.* Elmsford, NY: Pergamon Press.

ICRP Publication No. 26: *Recommendations of the International Commission on Radiological Protection.* New York, Pergamon Press, 1977.

ICRP Publication No. 34. *Protection of the Patient in Diagnostic Radiology.* New York, Pergamon Press, 1982.

ICRP Publication No. 43: *Principles of Monitoring for the Radiation Protection of Population,* vol. 15, no. 1. New York, Pergamon Press, 1985.

Implications of Prenatal Radiation Exposure (videotape and educational packet). Birmingham, University of Alabama at Birmingham, 1988.

Ionising Radiation Regulations, 1985. London, HMSO.

Jacobson AP, Plato PA, Toeroek D: Contamination of the home environment by patients treated with iodine-131: Initial results. *Am J Public Health* 68:225–230, 1978.

Jankowski CB: Radiation exposure of nurses in a coronary care unit. *Heart Lung* 13:55–58, 1984.

Janssen JHA, Wellen HJJ: What do medical students know about in-hospital radiation hazards? *Angiology* 40:36, 1989.

Katsuda T, Okazaki M, Kuroda C: Using compensating filters to reduce patient dose. *Radiol Technol* 68(1):18–22, 1996.

Kebart RC, James CD: Benefits of increasing focal film distance. *Radiol Technol* 62:434–442, 1991.

Kelsey CA: *Radiation Safety Manual for Laboratory Technicians.* St. Louis, Warren H. Green, Inc., 1983.

Khan FM. *The Physics of Radiation Therapy,* 2nd ed. Baltimore, Williams & Wilkins, 1994.

Kimme-Smith C, Bassett L, Gold R: Radiation dose. *Admin Radiol* 11:34–43, 1992.

Kohn HI, Fry RJ: Radiation carcinogenesis. *N Engl J Med* 310:504–511, 1984.

Kondo S: *Health Effects of Low Level Radiation.* Oska, Japan, Kinki University Press, and Madison, WI, Medical Physics Publishing, 1993.

Krestel E: *Imaging Systems for Medical Diagnostics.* Munich, Siemens Aktiengesellschaft, 1990.

Kumagai E, et al: Effects of long-term radiation exposure on chromosomal aberrations in radiological technologists. *J Radiat Res* 31:270–279, 1990.

Land CE: Estimating cancer risks from low doses of ionizing radiation. *Science* 209:1197–1203, 1981.

Lea DE: *Actions of Radiations on Living Cells,* 2nd ed. Cambridge, UK, Cambridge University Press, 1962.

Lewis F: Patient's response to illness and hospitalisation. *Radiography* 52(602):91–93, 1986.

Linnemann RE: Soviet medical response to the Chernobyl nuclear accident. *JAMA* 258:637–643, 1987.

*Low Level Radiation Effects: A Fact Book.* New York, Society of Nuclear Medicine, 1985.

Lushbaugh CC: Reflections on some recent progress in human radiobiology. *In* Augestein LG (ed): *Advances in Radiation Biology.* New York, Academic Press, 1969, pp 277–314.

Lyon JL: Radiation exposure and cancer. *Hosp Pract* 19:159–169, 1984.

Maguire WJ: A precaution for minimizing radiation exposure from iodine vaporization. *J Nucl Med Technol* 8:90–93, 1980.

Mallie HD, et al: Effect of patient size on doses received by patients in diagnostic radiology. *Health Phys* 42:665–670, 1982.

March HC: Leukemia in radiologists in a 20-year period. *Am J Med Sci* 220:282, 1950.

Martigoni K, Nitschke J: A new radiation protection dose limit for occupationally exposed personnel in the Federal Republic of Germany. *Radiology* 31:235–239, 1991.

Martin JE: Latitude in mobile chest radiography: How much is too much? *RT Image,* June 17:23, 1991.

McGraw RS, Culver CM, Juni JE, et al: Lung ventilation studies: Surface contamination associated with technetium-99m DTPA aerosol. *J Nucl Med Technol* 20:228–230, 1992.

McLemore J: *Quality Assurance in Diagnostic Radiology.* Chicago, Year Book Medical Publishers, 1981.

Merriam GR, Focht EF: Clinical study of radiation cataracts and the relation to dose. *AJR* 77:759, 1957.

Miller GA: The magical number seven. *Psychol Rev* 63:81, 1956.

Miller KL, Bott SM, Velkley DE, et al: Review of contamination and exposure hazards associated with therapeutic uses of radioiodine. *J Nucl Med Technol* 7:163–166, 1979.

Miller PE: Biological effects of diagnostic irradiation. *Radiol Technol* 48:11–17, 1976.

Miller RW: Effects of prenatal exposure to ionizing radiation. *Health Phys* 59:57–61, 1990.

MIRD dose estimate report no. 5: Summary and current radiation dose estimates to humans from I-123, I-124, I-125, I-126, I-130, I-131, and I-132 as sodium iodide. *J Nucl Med* 16:857–860, 1975.

Mole RH: The ten-day rule: A misnomer. *Radiography* 50:229–230, 1984.

Moore R: Ionizing radiations in chromosomes. *J Coll Radiol* 9:272, 1965.

Muller HJ: Artificial transmutation of the gene. *Science* 66:84, 1927.

National Council on Radiation Protection and Measurements (NCRP): Report No. 37: *Precautions in the Management of Patients Who Have Received Therapeutic Amounts of Radionuclides.* Bethesda, MD, 1970.

NCRP Report No. 39: *Basic Radiation Criteria.* Washington, DC, 1971.

NCRP Report No. 49: *Structural Shielding Design and Evaluation for Medical Use of X-Rays and Gamma Rays of Energies up to 10 MeV.* Bethesda, MD, 1976.

NCRP Report No. 51: *Quantities and Units in Radiation Protection Dosimetry.* Bethesda, MD, 1987.

NRCP Report No. 54: *Medical Radiation Exposure of Pregnant and Potentially Pregnant Women.* Washington, DC, U.S. Government Printing Office, 1977.

NCRP Report No. 57: *Instrumentation and Monitoring Methods for Radiation Protection.* Bethesda, MD, 1978.

NRCP Report No. 91: *Recommendations on Limits for Exposure to Ionizing Radiation.* Washington, DC, U.S. Government Printing Office, 1987.

NRCP Report No. 93: *Ionizing Radiation Exposure of the Population of the United States.* Bethesda, MD, 1987.

NCRP Report No. 94: *Exposure of the Population in the United States and Canada from Natural Background Radiation.* Bethesda, MD, 1987.

NCRP Report No. 105: *Radiation Protection for Medical and Allied Health Personnel.* Bethesda, MD, 1989.

NRCP Report No. 107: *Implementation of the Principle of ALARA for Medical and Dental Personnel.* Bethesda, MD, 1990.

NCRP Report No. 115: *Risk Estimates for Radiation Protection.* Bethesda, MD, 1987.

NCRP Report No. 116: *Limitation for Exposure to Ionizing Radiation.* Bethesda, MD, 1993.

Neel JV, Satoh C, Goriki K, et al: Search for mutations altering protein charge or function in children of atomic bomb survivors: Final report. *Am J Hum Genet* 42:663–676, 1988.

Nicklason, LT, Marx MV, Chan HP: Interventional radiologists: Occupational radiation doses and risks. *Radiology* 187:729, 1993.

Noz ME, Maguire GQ: *Radiation Protection in the Radiologic and Health Sciences,* 2nd ed. Philadelphia, Lea & Febiger, 1985.

Palmer L: Exposed (synopsis of a presentation by Dr. SC Bushong). *RT Image,* June 22:32, 1992.

Payne JT, Loken MK: A survey of the risks and benefits of ionizing radiation. *In CRC Critical Reviews of Clinical Radiology and Nuclear Medicine.* Cleveland, CRC Press, 1975.

Pizzarello D, Witcofski RL: *Basic Radiation Biology,* 2nd ed. Philadelphia, Lea & Febiger, 1975.

Plaut S: *Radiation Protection in the X-Ray Department.* London, Butterworth-Heinemann, 1993.

Preston DL, Kato H, Kopecky K, Fujita S: Studies of the mortality of A-bomb survivors: Cancer mortality 1950–1982. *Radiat Res* 111:151–178, 1987.

Preston-Martin S, et al: Diagnostic radiograph as a risk factor for chronic myeloid and monocytic leukemia. *Br J Cancer* 59:639–644, 1989.

Proposed rules, specific area gonad shielding, guidelines for use on patients during medical diagnostic x-ray procedures. *Fed Register* 40:42749, 1975.

Puck TT, Marcus TI: Action of x-rays on mammalian cells. *J Exp Med* 103:653, 1956.

Raven PH, Johnson GB: *Biology.* Boston, William C. Brown Publishers, 1996.

Renaud L: A five-year follow-up of the radiation exposure to in-room personnel during cardiac catheterization. *Health Phys* 62:10–15, 1992.

Riley SA: Radiation exposure from fluoroscopy during orthopedic surgical procedures. *Clin Orthop Rel Res* 248:257–260, 1989.

Rimer BK: Putting the "informed" in informed consent about mammography. *J Nat Cancer Inst* 87:703–704, 1995.

Rossi RP: Radiation protection. *In* Carlton RR, Adler A (eds): *Principles of Radiographic Imaging: An Art and a Science.* Albany, Delmar Publishers, 1992.

Royal HD: Cancer and genetic radiation effects. Unpublished.

Rubin P, Casarett GW: *Clinical Radiation Pathology.* Philadelphia, WB Saunders, 1968.

Rubin P, Siemann D: Principles of radiation oncology and cancer radiotherapy. *In* Rubin P (ed): *Clinical Oncology for Medical Students and Physicians: A Multidisciplinary Approach,* 7th ed. Atlanta, American Cancer Society, 1991.

Rudin S, Bednarek DR: Dose reduction during fluoroscopic placement of feeding tubes. *Radiology* 178:647–651, 1991.

Ruegesegger DR: Radiation exposure levels in an intensive care nursery. *Pediatr Nurs* 8:244–247, 1982.

Rugh R: Ionizing radiations: Their possible relation to the etiology of some congenital anomalies in human disorders. *Milit Med* 124:401, 1959.

Seeram E: *Radiation Protection.* Philadelphia, JB Lippincott, 1997.

Selman J: *Elements of Radiobiology.* Springfield, IL, Charles C Thomas, 1983.

Seltser R, Sartwell PE: Influence of occupational exposure to radiation on mortality of American radiologists and other medical specialists. *Am J Epidemiol* 81:2, 1965.

Silverman C: Thyroid tumors associated with radiation exposure. *Public Health Rep* 99:369–373, 1984.

Sloboda RS, Schmid MG, Willis CP: Technologist radiation exposures from nuclear medicine imaging procedures. *J Nucl Med Technol* 15:16–24, 1987.

Smith S, Spencer NM, Faulkener K, et al: Effect of automatic exposure control on patient dose. *In* Moore BM, Wall BF, Erikstat H, et al (eds): *Optimisation of Image Quality and Patient Exposure in Diagnostic Radiology*. London, British Institute of Radiology Report 20, 1989, pp 198–200.

Sprawls P: *Principles of Radiography for Technologists*. Rockville, MD, Aspen, 1990.

Society of Nuclear Medicine Technologist Section Code of Ethics. Society of Nuclear Medicine, 1150 Samuel Morse Drive, Reston, VA 22090–5316, adopted 1985.

St. Germain J: The radioactive patient. *Semin Nucl Med* 16:179–183, 1986.

Stanton R, Stinson D, Shahabi S: *An Introduction to Radiation Oncology Physics*. Madison, WI, Medical Physics Publishing, 1992.

Statkiewicz-Sherer MA, Visconti P, Ritenour ER: *Radiation Protection in Medical Radiography*. St. Louis: Mosby Yearbook, 1993.

Steves AM: *Review of Nuclear Medicine Technology*. New York, Society of Nuclear Medicine, 1992.

Strandqvist M: Studien ueber die kumulative Wirkung der Roentgenstrahlen bei Fraktionierung. *Acta Radiol* 55:1–300, 1944.

Thomas DC, Preston-Martin S: Risk of leukemia caused by diagnostic x-rays. *Health Phys* 63:576–578, 1992.

Tilson ER: Educational and experiential effects on radiographer's radiation safety behavior. *Radiol Technol* 53:321–325, 1982.

Tortorici M: *Concepts in Medical Radiographic Imaging: Circuitry, Exposure, and Quality Control*. Philadelphia, WB Saunders, 1992.

Travis EL: *Primer of Medical Radiobiology*, 2nd ed. Chicago, Year Book Medical Publishers, 1989.

Trout ED, Kelley JP, Cathey CA: The use of filters to control radiation exposure to the patient in diagnostic roentgenology. *AJR* 67:946–963, 1952.

Upton AC: Radiological effects of low doses: Implications for radiological protection. *Radiat Res* 71:51–71, 1977.

Upton AC: The Biological Effects of Low-Level Ionizing Radiation. *Sci Am* 246:41–49, 1982.

U.S. Nuclear Regulatory Commission: U.S. Nuclear Regulatory Guide 8.13: *Instruction Regarding Prenatal Radiation Exposure*. Washington, DC, U.S. Government Printing Office, 1987.

U.S. Nuclear Regulatory Commission: *Code of Federal Regulations, Title 10, Chapter 1, Energy, Parts 19, 20 and 35*. Washington, DC, U.S. Government Printing Office, 1995.

U.S. Nuclear Regulatory Commission: U.S. Nuclear Regulatory Guide 8.39: *Release of Patients Administered Radioactive Materials*. Washington, DC, U.S. Government Printing Office, 1997.

van Servellen G: *Communications Skills for the Health Care Professional. Concepts and Techniques*. Gaithersburg, MD, Aspen Publishers, Inc., 1997.

Wagner LK, Fabrikant JI, Fry RJM, et al: *Radiation Bioeffects and Management Test and Syllabus*. Reston, VA, American College of Radiology, 1991.

Wagner LK, Hayman LA: Pregnancy and women radiologists. *Radiology* 145:559–562, 1982.

Wagner LK, Lester RG, Saldana LR: *Exposure of the Pregnant Patient to Diagnostic Radiations: A Guide to Medical Management*. Philadelphia, JB Lippincott, 1985.

Walter JB: *An Introduction to the Principles of Disease*, 3rd ed. Philadelphia, WB Saunders, 1992.

Warner, R: Using technique factors to predict patent ESE. *Radiol Technol* 65(1):21–29, 1994.

Warner R. Focus on quality. Grid cutoff as a result of improper FFD. *Radiol Technol* 69(3):265–266, 1998.

Watson DA, Walsh ML: The perception of harm from radiation exposure. *Health Phys* 38:845–846, 1980.

Watson JD: *Molecular Biology of the Gene*. New York, WA Benjamin, 1965.

Weart SR: *Nuclear Fear: A History of Images*. Cambridge, MA, Harvard University Press, 1988.

Whalen JP, Balter S: *Radiation Risks in Medical Imaging*. Chicago: Year Book Medical Publishers, 1984.

Wheldon TE, Abdelaal AS, Nias AHW: Tumor curability, cellular radiosensitivity and clonogenic cell number. *Br J Radiobiol* 50:843–844, 1977.

Wight P: Pregnancy and RTs. *Advance* July 22:7, 1991.

Williamson BDP, Le Heron JC: Radiographic quality and radiation protection in general medical practice and small hospitals. *NZ Med J* 102:104–107, 1989.

Winkler NT: Minimizing radiation exposure of patients and personnel: Screen-film, TFD, filters, shields, and grid ratio. *Radiol Technol* 41:142, 1969.

Wochos JF, Cameron JR: Effect of operator training on patient exposure: An analysis of the NEXT data. *Radiol Technol* 48:19–22, 1976.

Woodruff K: Here's a way to make filters. *Advance* 4:23, 1991.

Yoshizumi TT, et al: Radiation safety and protection of neonates in radiological examinations. *Radiol Technol* 58:405–408, 1987.

# Index

Note: Page numbers in *italics* indicate illustrations; those followed by t refer to tables.

Bone marrow syndrome, 129
Brachytherapy, 43, 296
distance in, 301
high-dose-rate, 297
intracavitary devices in, 296, *298*
intrastitial devices in, 296, *298*
patient care guidelines in, 302
radiation protection in, 301, 302–303
shielding in, 302–303
time in, 301
Breast, radiography of. See *Mammography.*
shielding for, 236
Breast cancer, absolute risk in, 149t
mammography and, 149
radiation exposure in, 114, 148–149
Breast-feeding, discontinuance of, after radiopharmaceutical administration, 274, 275t
Bremsstrahlung radiation, 27
BRH Test Method, 181
Bucky grid, 231, 232

Canada, regulatory bodies in, 330
Cancer. See also *Tumor.*
childhood, 162
from Three Mile Island accident, 141–142
in radiologic technologists, 146
metastasis in, 95
model for, 289, *289*
radiation dose and, 207t, 208
radiation-induced, 145–151, 146t, 149t, 150t
studies on, 150–151, 150t
radiodermatitis and, 131, *131*
risk for, after irradiation, 144
treatment of, 289
Cancer cells, hematogenous spread of, 289
vs. normal cells, 95
Carbohydrates, 88–89
Carbon fiber, in screens, 230
Carcinogen effect, 115–116
Carcinogenesis, radiation, 150, 150t
epidemiology of, 143
Cardiac catheterization, chromosomal defects after, 137t
occupational exposure minimization in, 187
shield design for, 177–178, *179, 180*
Cardiac cineangiography, patient protection in, 253
Cardiovascular system, radioresistance of, 154
C-arm units, 212, *214*
Cartilage, late radiation effects on, 155
Catabolism, 92
Cataractogenesis, radiation, 152, *153*
Catheterization, cardiac, chromosomal defects after, 137t
occupational exposure minimization in, 187

Catheterization *(Continued)*
shield design for, 177–178, *179, 180*
Cathode, of x-ray tube, 26, *26*
Cell, 86–95
cancer in, radiation and, 115–116
chemical components of, 87–89
cytoplasm of, 89, 90t, 92–93
in tissue composition, 120–121, 121t
isomotic, 87
isostonic, 87
nucleoplasm of, 90t
nucleus of, 89, 90–92, *91*
organelles of, 89–90, 90t
osmotic pressure of, 87
properties of, 86–87
protoplasm of, 86–87
radiation absorbed by, 109–111, *109–111*
radiation interactions with, *105,* 105–106
radiosensitivity of, 97, 295
repopulation of, 295
somatic mutation of, 135–136
structure of, *89,* 89–93, 90t, *91*
target theories about, 118
Cell cycle, 94, *95*
radiation effect on, 295
redistribution in, 295
Cell division, 94, *94*
Cell membrane, 90t, 92
Cell survival curves, *118,* 118–119, *119,* 120
Center for Devices and Radiological Health (CDRH), 10, 181
Centigray, 47
Central nervous system, late radiation effects on, 155–156
Central nervous system syndrome, 129–130
Centromere, 94
Certainty effects, 112
Certification, 16–17
in patient protection, 248–249, 249t
Cesium-137, Chernobyl accident and, 142
Characteristic cascade, in photoelectric interactions, 70, *71*
Characteristic radiation, 27
Chernobyl, 142
childhood thyroid cancer incidence after, 143
Internet population registries for, 329
Internet research sites about, 332
Chest radiography, chromosomal defects after, 137t
collimation in, 239
exposure dose in, 237t
gonadal protection in, 236–237
Children, malignancy in, 162
radiation protection in, 249–250, *250*
radiosensitivity of, 114
Chondroblasts, radiosensitivity of, 155

Chromatids, 94
Chromosome(s), 90t, 91
aberrations of, after examination, 136, 137t
radiation and, 134–136, *136, 137,* 137t
acentric fragment formation in, 117, *117*
dicentric fragment formation in, 117, *117*
diploid number of, 92
duplication in, 116, *116*
frameshift mutations in, 114
haploid number of, 92
interstitial deletion in, 116, *116*
inversion in, 116, *116*
one-break effect in, 116, *116*
point mutations in, 114, 118
radiation effect on, 114, *116,* 116–117, *117,* 135
radiation mutation in, 117
ring, 117, *117*
terminal deletion in, 116, *116*
translocation of, 135
two-break effects in, 116–117, *117*
Cineangiography, cardiac, patient protection in, 253
Classic scatter, 73, *74*
Cobalt-60, radiation therapy with, 296
Coherent scatter, 73, *74,* 77t
Collimation, cones in, 231, *232*
cylinders in, 231, *232*
formula for, 324
gonadal dose effect of, 235, *235*
in mobile radiography, 256
in patient protection, 228, *229,* 231, 231–232, *232,* 232t
on chest radiograph, 239
Communication, in patient education, 310–311, 312t
Compounds, inorganic, 87, 88
organic, 87, 88
Compton electron, 70
Compton scatter, 70–73, *72,* 77t
energy level and, 81
formula for, 70
Computed tomography, 24
radiation protection in, 257
Conference of Radiation Control Program Directors (CRCPD), 172
Congenital malformation, radiation exposure and, 161–162
Consumer-Patient Radiation Health and Safety Act (1981), 16–17
Continuous quality improvement, 245–246, 246t
Control booth, shield design for, 186
Conversion factors, 191
formulas for, 316–318
Coulombs, 43, 44–45, 44t
conversion formula for, 316
Cumulative dose, 78
Curative dose, 293, 293t